Principles of Sports Training

Principles of Sports Training

Edited by Patrick Clinton

SYRAWOOD
PUBLISHING HOUSE
New York

Published by Syrawood Publishing House,
750 Third Avenue, 9th Floor,
New York, NY 10017, USA
www.syrawoodpublishinghouse.com

Principles of Sports Training
Edited by Patrick Clinton

International Standard Book Number: 978-1-68286-563-7 (Hardback)

Cataloging-in-Publication Data

Principles of sports training / edited by Patrick Clinton.
p. cm.
Includes bibliographical references and index.
ISBN 978-1-68286-563-7
1. Sports. 2. Physical education and training.
3. Sports medicine. I. Clinton, Patrick.
GV565 .P75 2018
613.7--dc23

Printed in China.

TABLE OF CONTENTS

PREFACE

Sports training refers to the enhancement of skills for physical activities and sports in particular. Different types of sports require different types and levels of training. Athletes spend a major share of their time practicing routines in order to perform their best. Different approaches, evaluations, methodologies and advanced studies on sports training have been included in this book. It will prove immensely beneficial to students and researches in this field.

Various studies have approached the subject by analyzing it with a single perspective, but the present book provides diverse methodologies and techniques to address this field. This book contains theories and applications needed for understanding the subject from different perspectives. The aim is to keep the readers informed about the progresses in the field; therefore, the contributions were carefully examined to compile novel researches by specialists from across the globe.

Indeed, the job of the editor is the most crucial and challenging in compiling all chapters into a single book. In the end, I would extend my sincere thanks to the chapter authors for their profound work. I am also thankful for the support provided by my family and colleagues during the compilation of this book.

Editor

1

Impact of Nintendo Wii Games on Physical Literacy in Children: Motor Skills, Physical Fitness, Activity Behaviors, and Knowledge

Amanda M. George, Linda E. Rohr *,† and Jeannette Byrne †

Academic Editor: Eling de Bruin

School of Human Kinetics and Recreation, Memorial University, St. John's, NL A1C 5S7, Canada; amg205@mun.ca (A.M.G.); jmbyrne@mun.ca (J.B.)
* Correspondence: lerohr@mun.ca
† These authors contributed equally to this work.

Abstract: Physical literacy is the degree of fitness, behaviors, knowledge, and fundamental movement skills (agility, balance, and coordination) a child has to confidently participate in physical activity. Active video games (AVG), like the Nintendo Wii, have emerged as alternatives to traditional physical activity by providing a non-threatening environment to develop physical literacy. This study examined the impact of AVGs on children's (age 6–12, $N = 15$) physical literacy. For six weeks children played one of four pre-selected AVGs (minimum 20 min, twice per week). Pre and post measures of motivation, enjoyment, and physical literacy were completed. Results indicated a near significant improvement in aiming and catching ($p = 0.06$). Manual dexterity significantly improved in males ($p = 0.001$), and females felt significantly less pressured to engage in PA ($p = 0.008$). Overall, there appears to be some positive impact of an AVG intervention on components of physical literacy.

Keywords: physical literacy; children; active video games; motivation

---

1. Introduction

Physical literacy is an important factor in child development. Developing basic skills to move around confidently at an early age is critical, enabling lifelong participation in various physical activities, including rhythmic (dance) and sports [1,2]. Physical literacy includes four main domains; physical activity behaviors, physical fitness, awareness/knowledge and understanding, and motor skills [2]. Physical activity behaviors include directly measurable daily activities, such as wearing a pedometer to track daily steps. Physical fitness encompasses factors such as cardio-respiratory fitness, flexibility, and muscular strength [2]. Awareness, knowledge, and understanding summarize how an individual thinks about physical activity and its importance [2]. The motor skills domain refers directly to an individual's physical competency, and includes mastery of fundamental movement skills, including balance, coordination and agility. It is critical that these skills are developed for future success in physical activities [1,2].

Active video games (AVG) are popular with the general population. These games—sometimes called exergames—can simulate real life activities, sports, and dances [3]. Research exploring the impact of AVG use by children shows positive improvements in physical activity levels [4], and a reduction in sedentary behaviors [5] during leisure time. Dally (2009) has extended the benefits of AVGs for children with motor control difficulties, low self-confidence, or previous negative physical activity experiences [6]. Despite the ability of AVGs to allow individuals to engage in physical activity in the relative safety of their own homes, little is known regarding their effects on the development of physical literacy. As a potential alternative to regular physical activity, understanding the effect of AVG systems in the acquisition of physical literacy skills is important.

Numerous AVG systems are available for public purchase, each with its own set of games, unique features, benefits, and limitation. The popular Nintendo Wii uses handheld controllers fitted with motion sensors to detect players' movements. The Nintendo Wii has a high enjoyment rating compared to other systems such as the Gamercize Power Stepper, sedentary games, and treadmill walking [7]; however, a drawback is the reduced energy expenditure during gameplay as compared to Dance Dance Revolution (DDR), Monster 4 × 4, various Gamercize and Play Station games, and the Xbox Kinect [3,8]. The use of the Nintendo Wii in research is supported by factors such as a variety of available games, low-to-moderate cost, and popularity with children. The popularity of various gaming systems fluctuates over time and is impacted by the release of new systems [9]. From 2008 to 2014, the Nintendo Wii sold 82.18 million units worldwide, compared to 68.04 million for the Xbox, and 75.27 for the PS3 [9].

Previous research indicates that girls tend to play online games for intrinsic reasons, whereas boys are more motivated by external rewards [10]. The research regarding the motivation of children to play AVGs is still new [11], but indicates that there may be several factors that influence how children play. The motivation of children is greater when playing with others, as opposed to alone [11], ultimately increasing intrinsic motivation [12]. Additionally, boys traditionally reduce extraneous movements to increase the efficiency of their game play [13]. The difference in motivation for playing AVGs may also impact boys' style of gameplay; minimalist movements are typically more efficient and may produce higher scores, whereas larger movements more closely resemble real-world play but may not be as efficient. Overall, boys may therefore not achieve similar physical activity levels as girls due to their focus on efficiency, and ultimately high scores in the AVG.

The present study investigated the effect of AVGs (Nintendo Wii) on the physical literacy, enjoyment, motivation, and competency in children. Based on earlier research [3,4,6,14,15] it is expected that children who play AVGs will experience benefits in each of the four areas of physical literacy; physical activity behaviours (measured with pedometers), physical fitness (measured with a walk test), knowledge and awareness (measured by questionnaires) and motor skills (measured with a movement assessment). Additionally, AVG play is expected to increase children's physical literacy, enjoyment and motivation for physical activity. Differences based on gender are expected, where boys will show greater improvements in manual dexterity [13], and girls will show greater improvements in enjoyment of physical activity [10].

2. Methods

2.1. Participants

Participants were recruited from the After School Activity Center at the Memorial University Campus Childcare Center. All boys and girls aged 6–12 who attended the Activity Center two or more days per week were invited to participate. Of the 28 children in the Center, 17 agreed to participate. In total 14 children ranged in age from 6–8 and three were between 11 and 12 years. Two of the children in the 6–8 group were excluded from the analysis (one due to not completing the intervention while the other was not available for the post-test). Ethics for this project was approved by the Interdisciplinary Committee on Ethics in Human Research, 20131719-HK.

2.2. Apparatus

The physical activity intervention utilized several active video games from the Nintendo Wii system; Wii Sport, Wii Sport Resort, Wii Play and Just Dance 2. Games were chosen based on how much physical activity they promote and their ability to produce increases in heart rate [4]. Children played on one of two identical Wii systems, each attached to 40 in. TV screens. Both Wii Motion Plus controllers and the associated nunchucks were available.

To directly measure exercise intensity during each AVG play sessions, participants wore a wrist-worn Garmin Vivofit Activity Trackers and associated chest-strap heart rate sensor. The Vivofit device recorded the heart rate and the data was subsequently uploaded to the online Garmin Connect Website. In addition, participants completed the OMNI Scales of Perceived Exertion [16] after each activity session. This data provided indirect feedback on the perceived intensity of the movement experience for the participants.

In attempt to better understand the overall physical activity behaviours, participants wore a Yamax Digi-Walker Electronic Pedometer. Each child was asked to attach the pedometer to the waistband of their pants upon waking, and wore the pedometer until bed, except during water activities (such as swimming or showering). Each participant was provided with a recording chart and was asked to complete this chart each night. Steps were recorded daily for six weeks.

To assess the knowledge and awareness component of physical literacy a variety of questionnaires were used. These questionnaires included were the Physical Activity Enjoyment Scale (PACES) [17], the Intrinsic Motivation Inventory (IMI) [18], and the Rosenberg Self-Esteem Scale (RSE) [19]. The PACES is a 16-question assessment of enjoyment levels of physical activity, with responses ranging from 1 (disagree a lot) to 5 (agree a lot). The IMI consists of 21 questions divided into four subscales; perceived competence, pressure/tension, perceived choice, and enjoyment. The RSE contains ten 5-point Likert-scale questions to assess children's self-esteem. Overall these questionnaires provided feedback on enjoyment, perceived competency, and movement knowledge.

The Movement Assessment Battery for Children (ABC) [20] assessed manual dexterity, aiming and catching, and balance; all scales are components of the motor skill domain for physical literacy. Fitness was evaluated using the six-minute walk test (6 MWT), where the distance (meters) walked in six minutes was recorded.

2.3. Procedures

A pre/post-test design was followed; all domains of physical literacy were measured prior to and at the end of a 6-week intervention period. Younger children (ages 6 to 8) had the PACES, IMI and RSE questionnaires explained and read to them, and then dictated their responses; older children (ages 11 to 12) were given the option of having the questionnaires read to them or completing them independently. The two physical assessments (Movement ABC and the 6MWT) were completed in the gymnasium with the researcher demonstrating what actions were required. For the Movement ABC participants were given a practice trial before the actual assessment, and results were scored as per the official guidelines [20].

The intervention consisted of, at minimum, two weekly Nintendo Wii game sessions for 20 min or more. Children played each game in pairs. Four games were provided at each of two Wii stations—Wii Sports Resort, Wii Sports, Wii Play, and Just Dance 2—and participants self-selected in order to increase ecological validity. Participants were encouraged to do their best and have fun. Games could be changed part way through play to ensure that each participant had an opportunity to select a game. During each session, participants' heart rates were recorded with Vivofit activity trackers and heart sensors to determine level of exertion. At the end of each session, participants completed an OMNI scale of Perceived Exertion [16] to assess how tired they felt. The length of play and games played was recorded for each play session over the 6-week period. As noted earlier pedometers were worn daily for the duration of the study.

Upon completion of the intervention, the pre-tests were repeated; each scale was administered by the same research to ensure consistency. The older children that chose to complete questionnaires on their own during the pre-test also did so during the post-test. Younger children again had the questionnaires read to them and dictated their responses.

2.4. Data Analysis

Heart rate data was automatically calculated on the online Garmin Connect website. The peak and average heart rate values were then extracted and analyzed in SPSS. During each session the duration and type of games played were manually recorded. Total time play for each week, as well as overall time was calculated along with number of times each game was selected by each participant.

A paired samples t-test compared change over time for the 6 MWT to assess physical fitness. Comparisons were made for all participants as well as separately for boys and girls. A regression analysis used total playtime as a predictor for changes in physical fitness. Participant's change in exertion were examined though linear trends in heart rate data and OMNI scores. A repeated measures ANOVA analyzed pedometer data changes over time. Changes in steps taken per week were also analyzed using linear trends for each participant.

Paired samples *t*-tests evaluated questionnaire data. Correlations to test the reliability between each of the scales (IMI, RSE and PACES) at pre-test and post-test were completed. A regression, using total amount of game play as a predictor, determined the influence of amount of game play. The Movement ABC, where scales include manual dexterity, aiming and catching, and balance assessed motor skills. Paired samples t-tests looked at changes over time for all participants, as well as separately for boys and girls. Total game playtime was used to predict changes in motor skills using a linear regression analysis.

3. Results

3.1. Participants

The final sample contained 15 children (7 boys, 8 girls) aged 6 to 12 ($M = 7.9$, $SD = 2.12$). Fitness was assessed at baseline with the 6MWT. On average, the sample was below average [21], but was not significantly different than the normal range for boys, $t(6) = -4.857$, $p = 0.869$, Cohen's $d = 0.06$, or for girls, $t(7) = -10.825$, $p = 0.662$, Cohen's $d = 0.15$. For mean 6MWT values see Table 1. Due to differences in attendance at the Childcare Center, amount of play varied between participants. Children played an average of 13.54 times ($SD = 2.23$), for an average of 25.71 min ($SD = 4.06$) per session (see Table 2).

Table 1. Six minute walk test (meters) means and standard deviations.

Participants	Pre-Test	Post-Test
All ($n = 15$)	549.93 (68.82)	542.30 (75.53)
Boys ($n = 7$)	559.14 (74.94)	562.29 (90.05)
Girls ($n = 8$)	541.88 (67.08)	524.81 (60.91)

Table 2. Frequency and average play duration.

Variable	Total	Boys	Girls
# Times Played	13.54 (2.23)	13.57 (1.62)	13.25 (2.25)
Wii Sports Resort	12.07 (2.52)	13.28 (2.06)	11.00 (2.51)
Wii Sports	0.33 (0.49)	0.28 (0.49)	0.38 (0.52)
Wii Play	1.27 (1.94)	0.86 (0.90)	1.62 (2.56)
Just Dance 2	2.73 (2.71)	0.86 (1.07)	4.38 (2.67)
Average Minutes	25.71 (4.06)	28.07 (3.53)	23.65 (3.45)
Wii Sports Resort	27.32 (3.99)	29.36 (4.10)	25.34 (2.72)
Wii Sports	20.8 (13.16)	10.00 (7.07)	28.00 (11.27)
Wii Play	14.1(1.47)	15.31 (1.55)	13.95 (1.16)
Just Dance 2	21.98 (9.30)	25.46 (14.92)	19.45 (5.17)

Notes: Frequency of each game played, mean and standard deviation. Average play duration (min), mean and standard deviation.

3.2. *Physical Fitness*

Physical fitness was assessed with the 6MWT, and exertion was measured both directly (heart rate) and indirectly (10 point OMNI scale of perceived exertion). There was no significant differences in the distance walked by participants from pre-test to post-test, indicating that children's fitness did not change over the study duration.

A 2 × 6 (gender by week) repeated measures ANOVA was conducted for both average and peak heart rate; neither test revealed a significant difference in heart rate over time for boys or girls. The average (M = 113.50 bpm; SD = 10.34 bpm) and peak (M = 150.12 bpm; SD = 16.72 bpm) heart rates at the beginning of the intervention were not significantly different than the average (M = 114.92 bpm; SD = 9.41 bpm) and peak (M = 156.49 bpm; SD = 14.71 bpm) heart rates at the end of the intervention. A paired samples t-test comparing exertion from the first and last weeks of the intervention found a decrease on the OMNI scale ($M_{difference} = 1.35$, $SD_{difference} = 1.67$), $t(13) = 3.029$, $p = 0.010$, Cohen's $d = 0.81$. A post-hoc power analysis indicated an 83% chance of detecting a significant effect at the 5% level (two-tailed). Linear trends were computed for each participant to examine the changes in heart rate and perceived exertion. There was no significant change in heart rate (average or peak) over time, but there was a significant decrease in OMNI scores, $t(14) = -3.961$, $p = 0.001$, Cohen's $d = 1.02$. A post-hoc power analysis indicated a 96% chance of detecting a significant effect at the 5% level (two-tailed). Overall, these data suggest that although no changes were noted for actual exertion, physical fitness or heart rate, participant's level of exertion decreased.

3.3. *Physical Activity Behaviors*

To assess daily physical activity behaviors, participants were asked to wear pedometers for the duration of the study. Nine children (5 girls, 4 boys) complied with this requirement for at least five weeks. Data is presented in Table 3. A 2 × 5 (gender by week) repeated measures ANOVA revealed no significant differences over time for either gender. An independent samples t-test compared average steps taken by boys and girls, and found a trend towards boys being more active than girls, $t(7) = -2.313$, $p = 0.054$, Cohen's $d = 1.54$. A post-hoc power analysis indicated a 46% chance of detecting a significant effect at the 5% level (two-tailed). Linear trends for each participant showed no significant overall changes in average daily steps.

Table 3. Average daily steps.

Week	All Participants	Boys (n = 4)	Girls (n = 5)
Total	10,389 (2,157)	11,887 (2526)	9192 (700)
Week 1	11,603 (3,151)	13,310 (3124)	9327 (1242)
Week 2	10,763 (2,017)	10,852 (2547)	10,645 (1560)
Week 3	10,222 (2,646)	11,068 (3391)	9094 (646)
Week 4	11,655 (2,696)	13,333 (2229)	9417 (1098)
Week 5	10,406 (2,766)	10,869 (3445)	9787 (2037)

3.4. *Knowledge and Awareness*

Motivation was assessed using the four scales of the Intrinsic Motivation Inventory (Table 4). The pressure/tension scale of the IMI indicated a positive trend for all children, suggesting that they felt less pressured after the intervention. The pressure/tension subscale of the IMI is theorized to be a negative predictor of intrinsic motivation [18]. A significant improvement was evident for girls ($t(7) = 3.65$, $p = 0.008$, Cohen's $d = 1.29$), but not for boys. A post-hoc power analysis indicated an 88% chance of detecting a significant effect at the 5% level (two-tailed). The other scales of the IMI (choice, competence, and enjoyment) were not impacted by the intervention. There were no significant changes in self-esteem (assessed with the RSE) or in enjoyment (assessed with the PACES) over the course of the intervention (see Table 4).

Table 4. Pre-test and post-test enjoyment, motivation, and self-esteem scores.

Test/Group		All (n = 15)		Boys (n = 7)		Girls (n = 8)	
		Pre	Post	Pre	Post	Pre	Post
PACES		71.20 (5.57)	68.20 (7.21)	70.86 (6.67)	66.86 (7.60)	71.50 (4.87)	69.38 (7.15)
Rosenberg Self-Esteem		22.47 (3.54)	22.60 (3.09)	23.29 (4.07)	22.71 (3.64)	21.75 (3.10)	22.50 (2.78)
IMI	Enjoyment	44.40 (4.98)	43.07 (5.35)	42.86 (5.15)	42.00 (7.21)	45.75 (4.74)	44.00 (3.25)
	Choice	29.47 (4.41)	30.53 (4.72)	32.14 (2.34)	31.29 (3.90)	27.13 (4.55)	29.88 (5.52)
	Competence	28.80 (4.77)	28.40 (4.31)	28.00 (5.89)	27.14 (5.82)	29.50 (3.82)	29.50 (2.27)
	Pressure	14.33 (4.48)	12.73 (5.28)	13.43 (3.50)	13.86 (5.21)	15.13 (5.30)	11.75 (5.50) **

Notes: Maximum scores for each scale are as follows: Physical Activity Enjoyment Scale (PACES) = 80; Rosenberg Self-Esteem Scale (RSE) = 30; Enjoyment = 49; Choice = 35; Competence = 35; Pressure = 35; ** = $p < 0.01$. Intrinsic Motivation Inventory = IMI).

To assess the degree to which the scales are related, Pearson's correlations were conducted (Table 5). All assessments showed a high correlation between their pre and post-test scores. This is important as it demonstrates the relationship between the three scales; although the scales measure separate concepts they are related to each other. Additionally, many of the scales were correlated with each other at both pre and post-test.

Table 5. Test correlations.

Time Point	Variable	Post-test					
		IMI Enjoyment	IMI Competence	IMI Choice	IMI Pressure	RSE	PACES
Pre-test	IMI Enjoyment	0.583 *	0.674 **	−0.358	0.223	0.563 *	0.514 *
	IMI Competence	0.758 **	0.651 **	0.182	0.134	0.512	0.535 *
	IMI Choice	0.014	0.253	0.592 *	0.129	−0.126	−0.127
	IMI Pressure	−0.099	0.023	−0.410	0.767 **	−0.016	−0.034
	RSE	0.474	0.737 **	0.571 *	−0.136	0.684 **	0.639 *
	PACES	0.553*	0.798 **	0.319	−0.114	0.610 *	0.648 **

Notes: Left half of the diagonal is correlations between assessments at pre-test, right half of the diagonal is correlation between assessments at post-test. Highlighted boxes along the diagonal represent the correlation between the test at pre-test and post-test.* $p < 0.05$; ** $p < 0.01$.

Regression analyses used total game play as a predictor. For the choice subscale of the IMI, there was a trend towards a significant prediction for all participants (R^2 = 0.223, p = 0.076), and a significant improvement for girls (R^2 = 0.727, p = 0.007). Amount of game play was not a significant predictor for any other the other scales.

3.5. *Motor Skills*

Data from the manual dexterity, aiming and catching, and balance scales of the Movement ABC were compared using a paired samples t-test (Table 6). Aiming and catching approached significance ($t(14) = -2.044$, $p = 0.06$, Cohen's $d = 1.09$) for all participants. A post-hoc power analysis indicated a 48% chance of detecting a significant effect at the 5% level (two-tailed). Manual dexterity improved for boys ($t(6) = -6.00$, $p = 0.001$, Cohen's $d = 2.26$), with younger boys ($p = 0.016$, Cohen's $d = 2.45$) showing greater improvement than older boys ($p = 0.057$, Cohen's $d = 2.30$). The post-hoc power analysis indicated a 99% chance of detecting a significant effect for all boys, 88% for younger boys and

56% for older boys, significant at the 5% level (two-tailed). There were no significant differences in balance for any participant.

Table 6. Movement Assessment Battery for Children standard scores.

Variable	All (n = 15)		Boys (n = 7)		Girls (n = 8)	
	Pre	Post	Pre	Post	Pre	Post
Total	9.33 (2.92)	10.00 (2.93)	7.86 (2.12)	8.86 (2.34)	10.63 (3.02)	11.00 (3.16)
Aiming and Catching	8.40 (2.13)	9.73 (2.40) *	8.71 (2.50)	9.86 (2.12)	8.13 (1.88)	9.63 (2.77)
Balance	10.80 (2.73)	9.93 (2.76)	9.29 (1.98)	9.43 (2.99)	12.13 (2.70)	10.38 (2.67)
Manual Dexterity	9.40 (3.94)	10.60 (3.60)	7.00 (2.45)	8.71 (2.63) **	11.50 (3.89)	12.25 (3.66)

Notes: Mean scores for the motor skills assessments at pre-test and post-test. Maximum score for each scale is 19. * = $p < 0.06$ ** = $p < 0.01$.

To further investigate the impact of AVGs on motor skills, regression analyses were conducted using playtime as a predictor. Analyses used total playtime over six weeks, as well as time spent playing each game. Overall, playtime significantly predicted total motor skills ($R^2 = 0.310$, $p = 0.031$) for all participants. Follow up analyses found that total playtime was not significant for boys ($R^2 = 0.024$), but was significant for girls ($R^2 = 0.506$, $p = 0.048$). There was a trend towards a significant prediction of manual dexterity ($R^2 = 0.236$, $p = 0.067$) for all participants. For individual games, the model to predict total motor skills was not significant; however, several games had trends towards significance. For all participants both Wii Play ($p = 0.071$) and Wii Sports Resort ($p = 0.059$) had a positive trend. This was also seen in girls, with positive trends found for Wii Play ($p = 0.051$) and Wii Sports Resort ($p = 0.077$), as well as for Just Dance 2 ($p = 0.089$). The model predicting manual dexterity for all participants (R2 = 0.636, $p = 0.027$) was significant. Both Wii Play ($p = 0.005$) and Wii Sports Resort ($p = 0.051$) significantly predicted manual dexterity scores. When analyzed singly, there were no significant results for boys. Although girls did not have a significant model predicting manual dexterity, Wii Play ($p = 0.023$) was still a significant predictor; additionally, Wii Sport Resort ($p = 0.088$) and Just Dance 2 ($p = 0.072$) had a trend towards a significant impact.

4. Discussion

Each of the four domains of physical literacy (physical activity behaviours, physical fitness, motor skills, and knowledge and understanding) were assessed in this study. Significant improvements however, were only found in two domains—motor skills, and knowledge and understanding. Improvements in motor skills were mixed; girl's manual dexterity improved as their gameplay time increased, whereas boys significantly improved their manual dexterity regardless of gameplay. Additionally, manual dexterity (as opposed to balance or aiming and catching) was most closely related to overall motor skills. Knowledge and awareness in terms of motivation and enjoyment significantly improved for participants. Girls reported feeling less pressure, indicating the Wii had a positive impact on their attitude towards physical activity.

Physical activity behaviors, specifically average daily step count, did not change over the six-week intervention. Previous research with school based activity interventions have impacted school-time behaviours, but do not change activity behaviours outside of school [22]. This intervention took place at a childcare center—a structured environment outside of the home—and did not require children to change their daily routines. It is possible that their activity levels at the center may have been altered by the intervention, but similar to school-based interventions the effect did not carry over to their daily lives.

Physical fitness levels did not change over the duration of the study. Although participants reported lower levels of exertion at the post-test there was no change in their heart rate or distance walked in the 6MWT. Potentially participants gained a better understanding of how to rate their exertion throughout the study. Many adults have difficulty accurately rating their level of exertion [23], it is likely that children would experience similar difficulties. Conceivably, as participants engaged in more physical activity sessions their understanding of rating exertion improved, ultimately changing their responses. An alternative explanation for the lack of change in heart rate may be that the breaks in between playing games (loading times) allowed for children's heart rates to lower before new games.

Boys and girls may take different approaches to the Wii games. Previous studies indicate boys are more likely to reduce unnecessary movements, thus being more efficient [13]. This may have impacted their manual dexterity, as smaller movements can sometimes be more effective for game success [13]. For example, in a basketball game, rather than completing a jumping and throwing motion, players can achieve the same results using a simple wrist flick. Regardless of game type or play duration, boys experienced improvements in manual dexterity, whereas girl's improvements were related to the games that they played. It is probable that for all games boys were more apt use minimalist movements, thus all game play impacted their manual dexterity. Girls are less likely to reduce to minimalist movements for all games [13], and thus games that naturally use smaller movements (e.g., table tennis, cycling) as opposed to full body movements (e.g., dance based games) may have had a greater impact on their manual dexterity. However, these smaller movements do require less energy, which may also account for some of the decrease in exertion reported during the intervention [6].

Girls, as opposed to boys, are more likely to participate in games for fun or enjoyment and social interactions [24]. Rather than competition to win, girls generally engage in games for intrinsic reasons. The IMI subscale pressure is a negative predictor of intrinsic motivation, with greater scores indicating lower levels of motivation [18]. The present study found significant changes in the pressure scale for females, with a trend towards significance for all participants. When the goal is not to win the game, but rather to have fun, AVG gameplay reflects real-world game situations [13]. Unlike boys who use minimalist, efficient movements to increase performance, girls play more closely reflects standard gameplay movements.

Limitations and Future Directions

Based on attendance at the Activity Centre some children had a greater opportunity for Wii play. Although all played a minimum of twice per week, the children who attended the Center more frequently received extra time when other children were unavailable to play in pairs [11]. Additionally, children were allowed to both self-select and change games during the play sessions. This flexibility was time consuming, resulting in children with less game playtime. The rationale for playing in pairs and allowing children to select their own games was to maximize ecological validity. Studies in a laboratory are often not "natural," and participants may behave differently than in the real world [25]. By attempting to maximize ecological validity the responses of the participants typically mirrors real-world responses. As a trade-off the methodology is not as rigorous. Future research should aim to balance ecological validity and solid methodologies to accurately determine the effects of playing AVGs and their benefits in real world situations.

A limitation of many AVG systems, including the Nintendo Wii, is that motion is recorded through a handheld controller. While full body movements are encouraged they are not compulsory for game success. More experienced Wii players are able to utilize smaller wrist and arm movements while maintaining high levels of performance [13]. As children gained experience with the Wii they may have adopted this minimalist approach. Regardless, the data suggest that heart rate values and rates of perceived exertion remained consistent across the study, suggesting that our participants maintained similar movement levels.

5. Conclusions

Overall, playing Wii games produces some benefits to specific domains of physical literacy. Although authentic game play is still the best activity for children, AVGs are a good alternative for many individuals, providing a safe environment for children to develop basic physical literacy skills. Ultimately physical literate children are enabled to participate in a variety of activities throughout life. Though no change in daily activity or fitness levels after the Wii intervention were evident, there was an improvement in both motor skills and attitudes towards physical activity. Based on the differential impact of the games on various physical literacy skills, further investigation into the specific benefits of gameplay is warranted.

Author Contributions: All authors designed and conceived the study. Amanda M. George analyzed the data. Amanda M. George and Linda E. Rohr wrote the original article. All authors reviewed and approved the manuscript.

Conflicts of Interest: The authors declare no conflict of interest.

References

1. Fisher, A.; Reilly, J.J.; Kelly, L.A.; Montgomery, C.; Williamson, A.; Paton, J.Y.; Grant, S. Fundamental movement skills and habitual physical activity in young children. *Med. Sci. Sports Exerc.* **2005**, *37*, 684–688. [CrossRef] [PubMed]
2. Tremblay, M.; Lloyd, M. Physical literacy measurement–The missing piece. *Phys. Health Educ. J.* **2010**, *76*, 26–30.
3. Shayne, R.K.; Fogel, V.A.; Miltenberger, R.G.; SKochler, S. The effects of exergaming on physical activity in the third grade physical education class. *J. Appl. Behav. Anal.* **2012**, *45*, 211–215. [CrossRef] [PubMed]
4. Graf, D.L.; Pratt, L.V.; Hester, C.N.; Short, K.R. Playing active videogames increases energy expenditure in children. *Pediatrics* **2009**, *124*, 534–540. [CrossRef] [PubMed]
5. Marshall, S.J.; Biddle, S.J.H.; Sallis, J.F.; McKenzie, T.L.; Conway, T.L. Clustering of sedentary behaviors and physical activity among youth: A cross-national study. *Phys. Exerc. Sci.* **2002**, *14*, 401–417.
6. Daley, A.J. Can exergaming contribute to improving physical activity levels and health outcomes in children? *Pediatrics* **2009**, *124*, 763–771. [CrossRef] [PubMed]
7. Duncan, M.J.; Dick, S. Energy expenditure and enjoyment of exergaming: A comparison of the Nintendo Wii and the gamercize power stepper in young adults. *Med. Sportiva* **2012**, *16*, 92–98. [CrossRef]
8. O'Donovan, C.; Hirsch, E.; Holohan, E.; McBride, I.; McManus, R.; Hussey, J. Energy expended playing Xbox Kinect™ and Wii™ games: A preliminary study comparing single and multiplayer modes. *Physiotherapy* **2012**, *98*, 224–229. [CrossRef] [PubMed]
9. Statista (2015). Global unit sales of current video game consoles from 2008 to 2014 (in million units). Available online: http://www.statista.com/statistics/276768/global-unit-sales-of-video-game-consoles/ (accessed on 15 December 2015).
10. Yee, N. Motivations for play in online games. *Cyber. Psych. Behav.* **2006**, *9*, 772–775. [CrossRef] [PubMed]
11. Paw, M.; Jacobs, M.W.; Vaessen, E.P.; Titze, S.; van Mechelen, S.W. The motivation of children to play an active video game. *J. Sci. Med. Sport* **2008**, *11*, 163–166. [CrossRef] [PubMed]
12. Staiano, A.E.; Abraham, A.A.; Calvert, S.L. The Wii Club: Gaming for weight loss in overweight and obese youth. *Games Health J.* **2012**, *1*, 377–380. [CrossRef] [PubMed]
13. Pasch, M.; Bianchi-Berthouze, N.; van Dijk, B.; Nijholt, A. Movement-based sports video games: Investigating motivation and gaming experience. *Lect. Notes Comput. SC* **2009**, *1*, 49–61. [CrossRef]
14. Sheehan, D.; Katz, L. Using interactive fitness and exergames to develop physical literacy. *Phys. Health Educ. J.* **2010**, *76*, 12–19.
15. Smallwood, S.R.; Morris, M.M.; Fallows, S.J.; Buckley, J.P. Physiologic responses and energy expenditure of Kinect active video game play in schoolchildren. *Arch. Pediat. Adol. Med.* **2012**, *166*, 1005–1009. [CrossRef] [PubMed]
16. Robertson, R.J.; Goss, F.L.; Boer, N.F.; Peoples, J.A.; Foreman, A.J.; Dabayebeh, I.M. Children's OMNI scale of perceived exertion: Mixed gender and race validation. *Med. Sci. Sports Exerc.* **2000**, *32*, 452–458. [CrossRef] [PubMed]
17. Kendzierski, D.; de Carlo, K.J. Physical Activity Enjoyment Scale: Two validation studies. *J. Sport Exerc. Psych.* **1991**, *13*, 50–64.

18. McAuley, E.; Duncan, T.; Tammen, V.V. Psychometric properties of the Intrinsic Motivation Inventory in a competitive sport setting: A confirmatory factor analysis. *Res. Q. Exerc. Sport* **1989**, *60*, 48–58. [CrossRef] [PubMed]
19. Robins, R.W.; Hendin, H.M.; Trzesniewski, K.H. Measuring global self-esteem: Construct validation of a single-item measure and the Rosenberg Self-Esteem Scale. *Pers. Soc. Psych. B* **2001**, *27*, 151–161. [CrossRef]
20. Henderson, S.E.; Sugden, D.A.; Barnett, A.L. *Movement Assessment Battery for Children-2: Movement Abc02;* Examiner'S Manual; Pearson: London, UK, 2007.
21. Geiger, R.; Strasak, A.; Treml, B.; Gasser, K.; Kleinsasser, A.; Fischer, V.; Stein, J.I. Six-minute walk test in children and adolescents. *J. Pediatr.* **2007**, *150*, 395–399. [CrossRef] [PubMed]
22. Dobbins, M.; DeCorby, K.; Robeson, P.; Husson, H.; Tirilis, D. School-based physical activity programs for promoting physical activity and fitness in children and adolescents aged 6–18. *The Cochrane Library* [online]. 2009. Available online: http://www.thehealthwell.info/node/3674 (accessed on 29 September 215).
23. Testa, M.; Noakes, T.D.; Desgorces, F.D. Training state improves the relationship between rating of perceived exertion and relative exercise volume during resistance exercises. *J. Strength Cond. Res.* **2012**, *26*, 2990–2996. [CrossRef] [PubMed]
24. O'Loughlin, E.K.; Dugas, E.M.; Sabiston, C.M.; O'Loughlin, J.L. Prevalence and correlates of exergaming in youth. *Pediatrics* **2012**, *30*, 806–814. [CrossRef] [PubMed]
25. Schmuckler, M.A. What is ecological validity? A dimensional analysis. *Infancy* **2001**, *2*, 419–436. [CrossRef]

2

America's Cup Sailing: Effect of Standing Arm-Cranking ("Grinding") Direction on Muscle Activity, Kinematics, and Torque Application

Simon N. Pearson [1,2,*], Patria A. Hume [1], John Cronin [1] and David Slyfield [1,3]

[1] Sports Performance Research Institute New Zealand (SPRINZ), School of Sport and Recreation, Faculty of Health and Environmental Science, Auckland University of Technology, Private Bag 92006, Auckland 1020, New Zealand; patria.hume@aut.ac.nz (P.A.H.); john.cronin@aut.ac.nz (J.C.); david.slyfield@hpsnz.org.nz (D.S.)

[2] Queensland Academy of Sport, QLD Sport & Athletics Centre, Kessels Rd, Nathan QLD 4111, Australia

[3] High Performance Sport New Zealand, PO Box 302 563, North Shore 0751, New Zealand

* Correspondence: simon.pearson@npsr.qld.gov.au

Academic Editor: Eling Douwe de Bruin

Abstract: Grinding is a key physical element in America's Cup sailing. This study aimed to describe kinematics and muscle activation patterns in relation to torque applied in forward and backward grinding. Ten male America's Cup sailors (33.6 ± 5.7 years, 97.9 ± 13.4 kg, 186.6 ± 7.4 cm) completed forward and backward grinding on a customised grinding ergometer. In forward grinding peak torque (77 Nm) occurred at 95° (0° = crank vertically up) on the downward section of the rotation at the end of shoulder flexion and elbow extension. Backward grinding torque peaked at 35° (69 Nm) following the pull action (shoulder extension, elbow flexion) across the top of the rotation. During forward grinding, relatively high levels of torque (>50 Nm) were maintained through the majority (72%) of the cycle, compared to 47% for backward grinding, with sections of low torque corresponding with low numbers of active muscles. Variation in torque was negatively associated with forward grinding performance ($r = -0.60$; 90% CI −0.88 to −0.02), but positively associated with backward performance ($r = 0.48$; CI = −0.15 to 0.83). Magnitude and distribution of torque generation differed according to grinding direction and presents an argument for divergent training methods to improve forward and backward grinding performance.

Keywords: yachting; biomechanics; movement analysis; performance

---

1. Introduction

The America's Cup is generally regarded as the most prestigious competition in sailing and is the oldest active trophy in international sport, dating back to 1851 [1]. On-water performance in America's Cup competition is determined by numerous factors including tactics, crew work and yacht design, however, in terms of physical human performance during racing, grinding is considered to be the primary physical activity [2].

Grinding is a cyclic upper body task requiring the manual arm cranking of winches which control the movement of the mast and sails, making it a crucial component of manoeuvres such as tacking (turning on an upwind leg) and gybing (turning on a downwind) [3]. Grinding is performed in a standing position and the set-up of the winch system means that sailors are required to perform grinding in both a forward direction—pushing away from their body at the top of the rotation; and backward—pulling towards their body at the top of the rotation [2]. In race analysis of the 32nd America's Cup and associated Louis Vuitton Challenger series, Neville, Calefato et al. [4] reported that an average of 20 tacks (5.5 ± 0.5 s in duration) and 8 gybes (11.2 ± 1.4 s) were performed during a race. These values were lower than previously reported figures of 30 tacks and 15 gybes per race [5]. However, it was calculated that when combined with mark roundings and the more frequent but less demanding grinding activity of sail trimming, a sailor whose principle role was grinding could expect a work to rest ratio of ~1:6 over an average 82 min race, and up to 1:3 in close racing. More accomplished crews (top four of the 11 challengers) completed manoeuvres in significantly shorter time than less accomplished crews [4], a finding that highlights the important relationship between grinding capability and overall race performance.

In addition to the performance aspects, grinders have been identified in a number of epidemiological studies as having the highest rate of injury amongst America's Cup crew members [6–10]. Although these studies reported sometimes conflicting findings (possibly due to different methodologies), soft tissue injuries to the upper limb made up a large proportion of the preventable (non-accident/impact) injuries suffered by grinders, with the grinding activity itself directly attributed to 30% of injuries in this group [11]. A review of sailing injuries by Neville and Folland [10] suggested that poor technique and strength deficiencies may be risk factors when looking at the grinding task, and as such a better understanding of the muscles, movements, and loading patterns utilised may provide useful information for the preventative conditioning of sailors who perform grinding as part of their on-board role.

In recent years there has been an increasing body of research focussed on America's Cup sailing from sport science and medicine perspective. With regards to the grinding activity in particular, studies examining the physiological [2,5] and strength and power [12] factors associated with performance, along with descriptions of the physical characteristics [4,13], nutritional requirements [14], and competition demands [4,15] have all been published. From a biomechanical perspective, an examination of grinding pedestal (crank-axle) height and crank length reported ground reaction force and kinematic data for forward grinding [16]. Results of this study indicated that while the standard crank length of America's Cup yachts (250 mm) was near optimal for peak power generation, peak power was significantly greater for forward grinding at higher crank-axle heights (950–1150 mm) than was typically in use (850 mm). While this appears somewhat contradictory to results from seated arm-cranking which concluded that shoulder height relative to the crank axis has no influence on performance [17], Neville et al. identified substantial contribution of the legs to the standing arm cranking movement whereby restricting movement at the knees and ankles (achieved by joint splinting) reduced peak unilateral vertical ground reaction forces (indicating reduced lateral body mass transfer) and significantly increased the physiological strain [18]. Additional factors associated with improved power output through increased pedestal height were a more extended hip position (reduced forward trunk lean), and increased resultant ground reaction force, while it was noted that further examination of upper body function is required [16].

Away from the specific grinding or standing arm-cranking movement there have been a number of other papers on the kinematically similar seated arm cranking exercise, which is often used in rehabilitation and for wheelchair users [19]. Arm cranking papers have reported that hand-grip/forearm orientation affects muscle activation patterns [20], and that backward arm cranking is less proficient than forward, based on reduced kinematic variability at the elbow [21]. Possibly of most relevance, Bressel [19], in a comparison of forward and reverse (backward) seated arm cranking, observed little difference in either upper limb kinematics or oxygen consumption, but found that backward arm cranking required significantly greater activity of the biceps brachii, deltoid, and infraspinatus muscles.

While there may be some cross-over from the findings of this body of research, the differences in body position and posture due to the standing position adopted during America's Cup grinding mean that there is justification in examining the mechanics of this activity in its own right. Concomitantly, of the current research examining the standing arm-cranking movement, so far none have examined both the forward and backward movements. The purpose of this study was therefore to describe the kinetic, kinematic, and muscular activation characteristics of the forward and backward grinding movements in America's Cup sailing. It was hypothesised that the biomechanical requirements of the two movements would be substantially different, therefore necessitating different approaches to training.

2. Materials and Methods

2.1. Participants

Ten male America's Cup sailors (33.6 ± 5.7 years, 97.9 ± 13.4 kg, 186.6 ± 7.4 cm) participated in this study by completing the grinding protocol. While the sailors varied in their primary role within the team, all performed grinding regularly as part of their on-board role. As maximal strength has previously been shown to be a key predictor of grinding performance, one-repetition maximum (1 RM) scores for the concentric only bench press (121.7 ± 26.1 kg) and bench pull (99.6 ± 17.1 kg) resistance strength training exercises was measured as an additional classification variable.

All procedures used in this study complied with the guidelines of the Auckland University of Technology Ethics Committee and had been granted ethical approval (reference 04/221).

2.2. Procedures: Performance Testing

Grinding performance testing was conducted on a custom-built grinding ergometer (Dynapack, Wellington, New Zealand) for which the technical specifics and reliability have previously been reported [22]. The ergometer was set up with standard pedestal (870 mm vertical) and crank arm (250 mm) dimensions for a main sheet grinding pedestal on an America's Cup class yacht (see Figure 1).

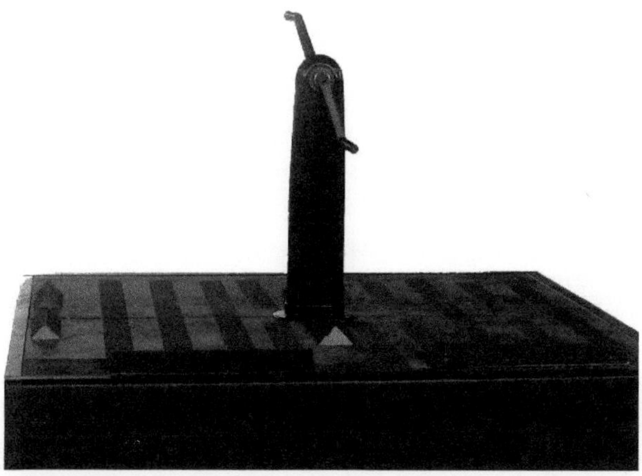

Figure 1. Ergometer for grinding performance testing.

Prior to testing, the sailors completed a self-determined warm-up on the grinding ergometer, typically consisting of 4–5 short bursts (5–10 s) of grinding, moving from low to high intensity, along with individually selected stretches. Performance testing consisted of two eight-second maximal-effort grinds for four conditions: Forward and backward directions, each performed against a moderate (48 Nm) and heavy (68 Nm) resistance. All trials were separated by a rest period of at least two minutes (representing a minimum 1:15 work:rest ratio). Testing loads were selected to correspond with moderate and heavy load conditions during on-water grinding manoeuvres, based on grinding speed ranges for a primary grinder. Testing conditions were presented in the following order: moderate-forward, moderate-backward, heavy-forward, heavy-backward; moving from what was generally perceived to be the easiest to hardest conditions in order to minimize the potential influence of any residual fatigue not removed by the two minute rest period. This was consistent with the protocol used regularly as part of the sailors general fitness monitoring and assessment, therefore meaning no specific familiarization was required for this testing.

Torque and velocity from both arms were recorded instantaneously by the ergometer. For the grinding performance measure raw power values were calculated by the Dynapack ergometer software using the formula: Power (W) = Torque $\times$ 2π $\times$ (rpm)/60. Raw power curves were smoothed using a second order recursive Butterworth low pass filter with a cut-off frequency of 6 Hz. Peak power and external work were calculated using a customised Labview (National Instruments, Austin, TX, USA) analysis program. Total work (J) performed during the five-second period following the attainment of peak power was determined for each trial, and the two-trial mean calculated. External work was used as the performance measure as this variable has been shown to be more reliable than peak power [22].

2.3. Procedures: Motion Analysis

Grinding for the motion analysis section of this study was conducted independently (within four weeks) of the grinding performance testing, although the protocol used was very similar. The primary point of difference was that the ergometer resistance was not set at an absolute level; rather, tests were performed against relative set loads customised to the individual sailor so that all participants were grinding within a similar speed range when grinding maximally (120–90 rpm), which incorporated the typically observed drop-off of 20–30 rpm during an eight-second trial. Individual loads were selected based on data from the medium and heavy load conditions in the performance testing. Those who typically met the speed range criteria at either of the standard testing loads (68 Nm, Heavy; 48 Nm, Moderate) were tested at those resistances, while those who didn't meet those criteria were given an intermediate resistance of either 55 or 62 Nm, as judged most appropriate based on typical performance at the two standard loads. No participants were tested against a resistance higher or lower than this Moderate-Heavy range.

The decision to use relative loads was made due to the reasonably wide range of grinding abilities represented in the sample of interest to this study. As this section of study was focused on the mechanics of the movement rather than direct performance comparisons the desire was to examine grinding performance at high load (which has the biggest influence on boat performance) without inducing the degradation in basic technique that can be observed when an individual is performing at an excessively high load relative to their capability. If a set load was used for all participants, individuals either performing at loads much too easy or much too hard for their ability would likely have confounded the description of the grinding movement. As such, all individuals performed two maximal effort grinds in each of the forward and backward direction (four in total), against a moderate-heavy resistance, scaled relative to capability.

Biomechanical data, consisting of muscle activation patterns using surface electromyography (EMG), torque applied to the grinding handles, and sagittal plane kinematics; were averaged over five complete grinding revolutions during the middle of the eight-second trial, avoiding the initial start/acceleration phase. All data were referenced based on handle motion relative to a 0° position where the handle vertically was above the hub (Figure 2) and angle moving positively in the direction of motion (Figure 3), which is consistent with conventions used in other arm cranking research [19].

EMG signals were collected using a Bortec AMT-8 system (Bortec, Calgary, Alberta, Canada) with pre-gelled Ag/AgCl surface electrodes, sampling at 1000 Hz. EMG activity data was collected on six upper body muscles: posterior deltoid, latissimus dorsi, triceps brachii (lateral head), anterior deltoid, pectoralis major (sternocostal head), and biceps brachii. Standard skin preparation was completed for electrodes placed according to the guidelines of Basmajian and Blumenstein [23]. Wires connected to electrodes were secured with tape to avoid movement artefacts. EMG data were full-wave rectified and low-pass filtered (15 Hz cut-off frequency). The signal from each muscle was normalised to a 100% scale of its own activation throughout the five-revolution analysis period, with 0% as the lowest recorded signal and 100% as the highest recorded signal. Muscle activation data was presented by dividing the grinding cycle into quartiles: upper (315°–44°), descending (45°–134°), lower (135°–224°), and ascending (225°–314°). Data are presented as the average relative activation during each quartile.

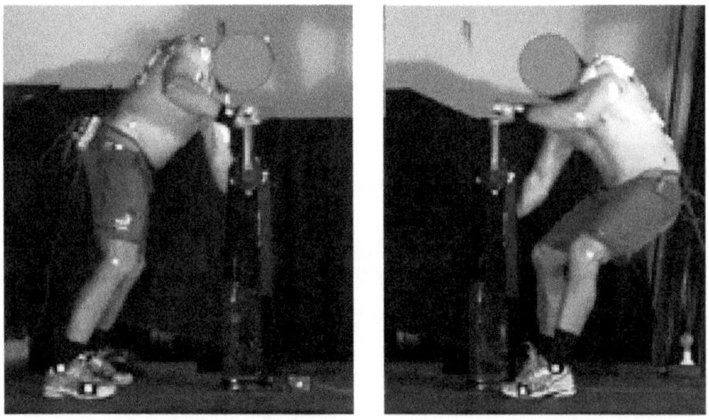

(a) (b)

Figure 2. Examples of forward (**a**) and backward (**b**) body position at 0° crank angle.

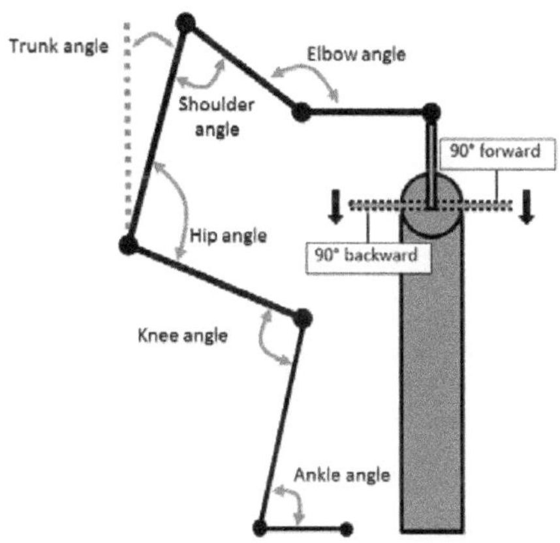

Figure 3. Analysis convention for joint angles and crank arm position, relative to sailor position.

Torque application and angular position data were collected using an SRM Powermeter Science Road system (Schoberer Rad Messtechnik, Jülich, Germany) with torque analysis module sampling at 200 Hz. Characteristics of the captured torque-angle data output from the SRM system were such that averaging of the five cycles of interest was conducted without any additional smoothing. The SRM Powermeter was attached to the hub of the grinding pedestal using a custom-made mounting plate which enabled collection of data independently from a single crank arm, eliminating the issue of standard SRM mounting in bicycles, which captures combined torque from both cranks. Data was therefore captured from one crank arm and one side of the body only for any particular trial. As the grinding ergometer was optimized for hub rotation in a single direction, the single side analysis corresponded to the sailor's right hand side for forward grinding and left hand side for backward grinding (see Figure 2).

Full body sagittal plane motion was recorded using a video camcorder (Sony DCR-TRV120E, Sony Corporation, Tokyo, Japan) recording at 50 fields/s with a 1/500 shutter speed. To aid digitisation, markers were placed on the distal head of the fifth metatarsal bone, lateral malleolus of the ankle, lateral condyle of the tibia, greater trochanter, lateral aspect of the acromion process, lateral epicondyle of the humerus, and the styloid process of the ulna. Two-dimensional sagittal plane relative joint angles in degrees (°) were obtained through digitisation using APAS (Ariel Dynamics, Trabuco Canyon, CA,

USA) for the ankle, knee, hip, shoulder, and elbow (Figure 3). Shoulder angle was measured using the trunk as a relative 0° position, with a positive value moving anteriorly into flexion. Trunk angle was measured relative to vertical, with a positive value indicating the shoulder was anterior to the hip. Kinematic data were summarised using four reference points during the grinding cycle based on handle position: 0° = handle vertically above the point of rotation (hub); 90° = horizontal to the hub, moving from 0° in the direction of rotation (on the sailor's side of the pedestal for forward grinding, away from the sailor for backward); 180° = vertically below the hub; 270° = horizontal to the hub, on the way back up towards the 0° position.

Data were synchronised using the onset of a five-volt pulse to the computer-based data acquisition system, generated simultaneously with the activation of an LED light in the line of view of the video camera. Due to the collection of torque-angle (SRM) data being limited to a single crank, all data were analysed for only the right side during forward grinding and the left side for backward grinding.

2.4. *Statistical Analyses*

Descriptive statistics for all variables are represented as mean and standard deviation (SD). The presence of significant systematic discrepancies between forward and backward grinding for given variables during the cycle were determined using a two-tailed paired *t*-test with alpha set at $p < 0.05$. In addition to descriptive data the relationship between variability in torque application throughout a revolution and grinding performance was also examined using Pearson correlation analysis. Grinding performance (J) for an individual was log transformed (ln) and corrected for maximal strength (1RM—also log transformed), with the residuals from this correction plotted against the sailor's variation in torque application, as represented by the standard deviation of the log-transformed SRM data. To make inferences about true (population) values of the relationship, the uncertainty in the effect was expressed as likelihoods that the true value of the effect represents substantial change (harm or benefit) using the methods of Hopkins [24], with the smallest worthwhile change set as 0.10 standardised Cohen units [25] and confidence limits set at 90%.

3. Results

3.1. *Torque Application and Grinding Performance*

Forward grinding produced significantly more work and higher mean torque throughout the cycle than backward grinding (Table 1). Greatest torque application occurred through 60°–200° for forward grinding and 300°–40° for backward grinding (see Figure 4). Peak torque for the group average torque-angle data was 77.5 ± 4.1 Nm at 95° for forward grinding and 68.8 ± 2.9 Nm at 35° for backward grinding. Variation in torque application throughout the grinding cycle was negatively associated with strength corrected forward grinding performance ($r = -0.60$; $p = 0.09$; 90% CI = −0.88 to −0.02) but positively associated with backward performance ($r = 0.48$; $p = 0.19$; 90% CI = −0.15 to −0.83). While these relationships were non-significant, inference-based statistics, which take into account the population size and confidence limits, indicate that it was likely or probable that these correlations represented clinically meaningful relationships.

Table 1. Summary data (Mean ± SD) for grinding performance, mean torque application and variability in torque application.

Direction	Grinding Performance (J)	Torque Application	
		Mean (Nm)	Variability (SD of ln (J))
Fwd	2938 ± 317	56.0 ± 10.9	38.3 ± 5.7
Back	2738 ± 316	49.9 ± 10.2	35.6 ± 13.4
Diff in Mean (%)	*7.3% **	*12.2% **	*7.5%*

* Significant difference between forward and backward grinding ($p < 0.05$).

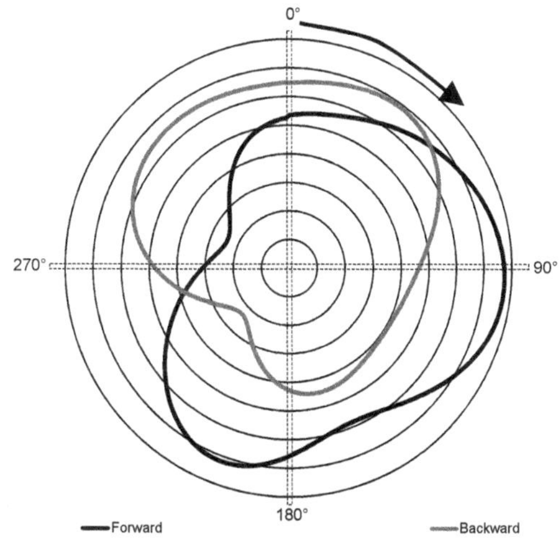

Figure 4. Average torque-angle curves for forward (black) and backward (grey) grinding. Torque increases as the traces move away from the centre (lines = 10 Nm increments). Arrow indicates the direction of handle rotation. 0° = crank handle vertically upwards from the centre.

3.2. *Joint Kinematics*

When grinding forward the sailors typically stood more upright and leaned over the grinding pedestal when compared to backward grinding (see Figure 2), as indicated by significantly less hip flexion and more forward trunk lean throughout the cycle (see Table 2). Sailors also tended to have a more plantar flexed ankle and greater knee flexion during backward grinding. Elbow and shoulder angles differed significantly at 90° and 270° but tended to be more similar at 0° and 180°.

Table 2. Average (±SD) joint angles for forward (Fwd) and backward (Back) grinding presented at four positions (in degrees) during the cycle. Position (°) increases in the direction of motion.

Position	Direction	Ankle	Knee	Hip	Shoulder	Elbow	Trunk
0°	Fwd	103 ± 11 *	136 ± 12	133 ± 5 *	15 ± 15 *	93 ± 19	39 ± 4 *
	Back	136 ± 8 *	134 ± 9	101 ± 6 *	39 ± 5 *	100 ± 14	26 ± 5 *
90°	Fwd	98 ± 9 *	134 ± 15	128 ± 8 *	72 ± 10 *	166 ± 7 *	46 ± 6 *
	Back	130 ± 10 *	131 ± 4	106 ± 5 *	−1 ± 9 *	92 ± 7 *	20 ± 5 *
180°	Fwd	102 ± 9 *	139 ± 12 *	122 ± 6 *	51 ± 9	154 ± 8	50 ± 4 *
	Back	124 ± 9 *	122 ± 4 *	94 ± 11 *	47 ± 9	162 ± 7	33 ± 7 *
270°	Fwd	114 ± 13	150 ± 14 *	133 ± 7 *	2 ± 7 *	105 ± 9 *	44 ± 3 *
	Back	127 ± 8	123 ± 5 *	97 ± 8 *	73 ± 10 *	162 ± 15 *	30 ± 6 *

* Significant difference between forward and backward grinding ($p < 0.05$).

3.3. *Muscle Activation*

EMG activity patterns for forward and backward grinding are presented numerically in Table 3 and graphically in Figure 5, with muscles paired according to approximate agonist-antagonist relationships based on typical involvement in joint actions. In backward grinding there was a high level of activation (>50%) from five of the six muscles monitored during the ascending (pectoralis major, latissimus dorsi, and biceps brachii) and upper (latissimus dorsi, posterior deltoid, and triceps brachii) quartiles of the rotation where torque increased rapidly and peaked before declining again as the crank arm came in close to the sailors body at ~90°. Through the descending and lower quartiles of the cycle, as the crank arm passed down to its lowest point (180°) and then started moving away from the sailor the only notable activity was from smaller muscles—anterior deltoid and the triceps and biceps brachii. At the point of minimum backward grinding torque (227°, 23 Nm), biceps brachii was the only muscle showing any meaningful level of activation, with pectoralis major and latissimus dorsi just beginning to fire.

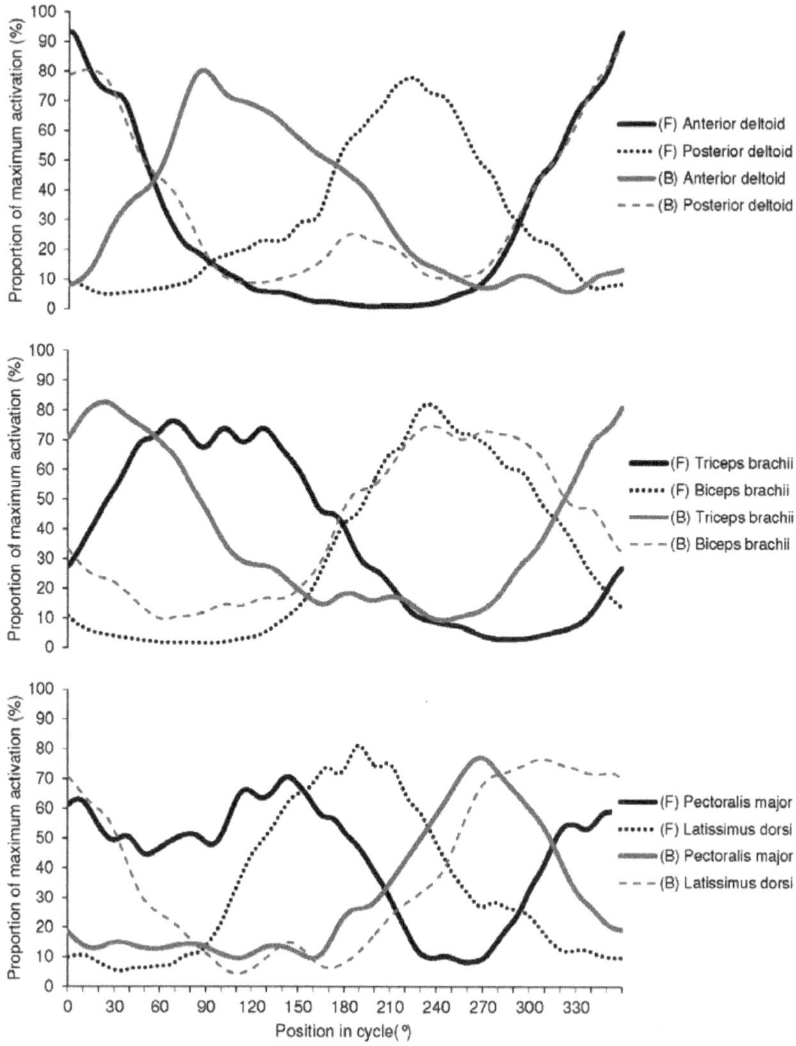

Figure 5. Average EMG activity patterns during forward (F) and backward (B) grinding for 10 grinders. Crank angle defined as 0° when positioned vertical and above the pedestal. Crank angles are positive in the direction of motion.

Table 3. Mean (±SD) relative muscle activation (% of maximum) per quartile of the grinding cycle for forward (Fwd) and backward (Back) grinding. Dark grey shading indicates mean activation over 60%, light grey shading indicates 40%–60%.

Quartile		PD	LD	TB	AD	PM	BB
Upper	Fwd	19 ± 7	15 ± 2	20 ± 9	72 ± 10	44 ± 12	35 ± 16 *
(315°–44°)	Back	72 ± 11	64 ± 11	71 ± 11	16 ± 10	22 ± 10	34 ± 12 *
Descending	Fwd	12 ± 2	21 ± 12	63 ± 14	38 ± 17	56 ± 4	7 ± 2
(45°–134°)	Back	24 ± 15	14 ± 9	48 ± 17	65 ± 13	13 ± 2	13 ± 2
Lower	Fwd	31 ± 15	67 ± 10	43 ± 15	6 ± 3	58 ± 5	33 ± 18
(135°–224°)	Back	18 ± 5	15 ± 7	18 ± 3	44 ± 13	23 ± 11	42 ± 18
Ascending	Fwd	52 ± 5	45 ± 17	14 ± 5	19 ± 13	20 ± 9	76 ± 5
(225°–314°)	Back	21 ± 13	59 ± 17	19 ± 10	11 ± 3	64 ± 9	71 ± 4

Muscles presented are: Posterior deltoid (PD), latissimus dorsi (LD), triceps brachii (TB), anterior deltoid (AD), pectoralis major PM), and biceps brachii (BB); Comparisons between grinding direction were significant for all muscles in all quartiles other than biceps brachii in the upper quartile (shaded grey).

In contrast, forward grinding showed a much more even spread of muscle activity throughout the rotation, with anterior deltoid, pectoralis major and triceps brachii dominant through the upper and descending quartiles (315°–134°) and latissimus dorsi, biceps brachii, pectoralis major and posterior deltoid highly active through the majority of the lower and ascending phases. As with backward grinding, the point of minimum torque application for forward grinding (294°, 24 Nm) was on the ascending section and corresponded with a period during which only biceps brachii was notably active.

4. Discussion

This study provided torque-angle curves for upper limb arm grinding for America's Cup sailors, along with kinematic and muscle activation data characterizing the movement. Cycling literature [26–28] has consistently reported that torque or applied force for a single limb occurs almost entirely in the down stroke (0°–180°, with 0° crank position again vertically upward) with virtually no positive force, and in many cases a negative force applied during the following up stroke [27–29]. In contrast torque during grinding was never negative, with the mean curve remaining above 20 Nm throughout the entire 360° cycle. The torque application differed between forward and backward grinding. While backward grinding followed a similar pattern to cycling in which the majority of torque was applied through half of the rotation (270°–80°) with a considerable drop-off through the remaining half-circle, in forward grinding a high level of force at the handles was maintained through a much greater proportion of the rotation (340°–240°), leaving only a relatively small "dead spot" of ~100° in which torque was reduced. This was in contrast to cycling literature, with Neptune, Kautz and Zajac [29] observing very little difference in tangential pedal force between forward and backward pedalling. A potential reason for the difference in torque throughout the cycle may relate to foot position adopted, which in the case of forward grinding is away from the pedestal, characterised by a relatively dorsiflexed ankle and forward trunk lean, enabling notable contribution from the lower limb and body mass [16,18]. In contrast, the position adopted in backward grinding is much less balanced with the feet close to the grinding pedestal, greater flexion at the hips and more upright trunk, which results in effectively "hanging" off the handles, which is likely to limit the ability to apply force to the handles consistently.

Relative levels of torque throughout the rotation were also reflected in muscle activation patterns. On an individual basis muscle activation patterns were consistent with the bi-phasic nature of grinding with distinct periods of activation and in-activation, which has also been seen previously in seated arm cranking [19]. However, the spread of muscles active at any one time differed with grinding direction, with more consistent contributions from the muscles examined (most notably latissimus dorsi and pectoralis major) throughout the forward grinding cycle compared to backward.

In addition to the importance of identifying causes of low torque zones or "dead spots" which can impact on performance, it is also of interest to examine where grinding biomechanics are optimum. In terms of maximum force application, both peak and mean torque were ~12% higher for forward grinding than for backward grinding, which was consistent with previous findings where work performed over five seconds of maximal grinding was 12%–15% greater in the forward direction [22]. Fujii and Nagasaki [21] concluded that reverse arm cranking was less proficient than forward arm cranking. In the average torque-angle curve for the cohort, peak torque occurred at 95° and 35° crank angles for forward and backward grinding respectively, aligning with the end of shoulder horizontal flexion and elbow extension (push movement) in forward grinding, and at the completion of shoulder extension and elbow flexion (pull movement) in backward grinding. Although forward grinding has a more even distribution of torque throughout the cycle, the location of the peaks does support the view that the primary "work generating" movements are upper body push and pull for forward and backward grinding respectively.

The importance of the areas of maximum torque application to the respective grinding directions also appears to differ. Analysis of the relationship between torque application and strength-corrected grinding performance (removing strength as a covariate to focus on technical performance) showed that greater variation in torque throughout the grinding cycle was positively associated with backward performance ($r = 0.48$). Although not conclusive, this does indicate some justification in focusing on the primary pull movement (maximising the peak) to improve backward grinding performance. In contrast, the negative association between torque variability and forward grinding performance ($r = -0.60$) suggest that improvements in forward grinding are likely to be achieved through the ability to maintain torque throughout the entire cycle. These findings also align with previous research where maximum muscular force was related to forward grinding performance, while power and rate of force development were important for backward grinding [12,30]. While maximal strength and force were important in both directions, the additional importance of the speed of force generation for backward grinding was consistent with the torque profile observed in this study with cyclic loading, unloading, and re-loading having to be repeated during a short period of time.

Limitations of the study include whether the two minutes for rest period was long enough for recovery given metabolic disturbance from the maximal 8-s effort, and whether there is the effect of limb dominance may have influences the findings. However, given the magnitude of the differences observed, it seems unlikely that the observed patterns would be fundamentally different, although the strength of the relationships may well be altered. It should also be noted from a kinematic perspective, that although the majority of the grinding movement occurs in the sagittal plane, three dimensional analysis would improve accuracy of some of the measures taken in the upper body (elbow, shoulder and trunk). The use of absolute loads rather than relative loads could also be considered given competition involves high load maximal effort grinding and inevitably some breakdown of technique. Further investigations could consider the use of force plates to better understand lower limb contribution to backward grinding, while from an injury perspective a prospective investigation could provide valuable insight into whether movement or torque application patterns predispose sailors to certain types of injuries.

5. Conclusions

Overall, the disparities observed between the biomechanical characteristics of forward and backward grinding are somewhat at odds with previous literature from cycling [29] and seated arm-cranking [19] which observed relatively little directional difference. While the discrepancy with cycling can be explained by the substantial differences in lower limb structure and function, the same does not apply for seated arm cranking. It would seem that the additional degrees of positional freedom along with the potentially greater contribution of body weight allowed by the standing position used in grinding makes a difference to the variation in biomechanics between cranking direction. This is observable at the most basic level by the different postural positions selected by the sailors when grinding backward *versus* forward, as compared to the relatively fixed position in seated arm cranking.

In terms of specific information that could potentially be used to improve performance, we have identified the movements and muscles involved in the grinding activity and the factors involved in periods of high and low torque. In many sporting movements it is the reduction in inefficiencies as much as maximum capability that determines overall proficiency and so it may be that working to improve the areas of weakness in the grinding cycle, whether through conditioning or technical changes, can improve grinding performance. However, further investigation would be required to determine whether this is in fact a practical solution or if it is the result of an unchangeable factor such as structurally limited function of the upper limb in that position. Even within the findings of this study, there is evidence that the influence of biomechanical factors on performance differ according to direction, and as such any intervention should be customised for forward and backward grinding.

Acknowledgments: This research was funded by the Tertiary Education Commission (New Zealand) and Emirates Team New Zealand. The authors have no professional relationships with any companies or manufacturers identified in this study.

Author Contributions: Simon Pearson had the idea for the study, reviewed literature and conducted the collection and analysis of data, and drafted the first version of the paper. Patria Hume provided advice on the methods, reviewed the data analysis and edited the paper. David Slyfield and John Cronin provided advice on the methods and edited the paper.

Conflicts of Interest: The authors declare no conflict of interest.

References

1. Rayner, R.; Thompson, T. *The Story of the America's Cup 1851–1995*; Warwick Publishing: Toronto, ON, Canada, 1996; p. 94.
2. Neville, V.; Pain, M.T.; Folland, J.P. Aerobic power and peak power of elite America's Cup sailors. *Eur. J. Appl. Physiol.* **2009**, *106*, 149–157. [CrossRef] [PubMed]
3. Whiting, P. *The 32nd America's Cup: A Simple Guide*; John Wiley & Sons: Chichester, UK, 2007; p. 71.
4. Neville, V.; Calefato, J.; Perez-Encinas, C.; Rodilla-Sala, E.; Rada-Ruiz, S.; Dorochenko, P.; Folland, J.P. America's Cup yacht racing: Race analysis and physical characteristics of the athletes. *J. Sports Sci.* **2009**, *27*, 915–923. [CrossRef] [PubMed]
5. Bernardi, M.; Quattrini, F.M.; Rodio, A.; Fontana, G.; Madaffari, A.; Brugnoli, M.; Marchetti, M. Physiological characteristics of America's Cup sailors. *J. Sports Sci.* **2007**, *25*, 1141–1152. [CrossRef] [PubMed]
6. Allen, J.B. Sports medicine injuries in the America's Cup 2000. *N. Z. J. Sports Med.* **2005**, *33*, 43–47.
7. Hadala, M.; Barrios, C. Different strategies for sports injury prevention in an America's Cup yachting crew. *Med. Sci. Sports Exerc.* **2009**, *41*, 1587–1596. [CrossRef] [PubMed]
8. Hadala, M.; Barrios, C. Sports injuries in an America's Cup yachting crew: A 4-year epidemiological study covering the 2007 challenge. *J. Sports Sci.* **2009**, *27*, 711–717. [CrossRef] [PubMed]
9. Neville, V.; Molloy, J.; Brooks, J.H.; Speedy, D.B.; Atkinson, G. Epidemiology of injuries and illnesses in America's Cup yacht racing. *Br. J. Sports Med.* **2006**, *40*, 304–311. [CrossRef] [PubMed]
10. Neville, V.; Folland, J.P. The epidemiology and aetiology of injuries in sailing. *Sports Med.* **2009**, *39*, 129–145. [CrossRef] [PubMed]
11. Allen, J.B.; De Jong, M.R. Sailing and sports medicine: A literature review. *Br. J. Sports Med.* **2006**, *40*, 587–593. [CrossRef] [PubMed]
12. Pearson, S.N.; Cronin, J.B.; Hume, P.A.; Slyfield, D. Strength and power determinants of grinding performance in America's Cup sailors. *J. Strength Cond. Res.* **2009**, *23*, 1883–1889. [CrossRef] [PubMed]
13. Pearson, S.N.; Hume, P.A.; Mellow, P.; Slyfield, D. Anthropometric dimensions of Team New Zealand America's Cup sailors. *N. Z. J. Sports Med.* **2005**, *33*, 52–57.
14. Bernardi, E.; Delussu, S.A.; Quattrini, F.M.; Rodio, A.; Bernardi, M. Energy balance and dietary habits of America's Cup sailors. *J. Sports Sci.* **2007**, *25*, 1153–1160. [CrossRef] [PubMed]
15. Neville, V.; Gant, N.; Folland, J.P. Thermoregulatory demands of Elite Professional America's Cup Yacht Racing. *Scand. J. Med. Sci. Sports* **2009**. [CrossRef] [PubMed]

16. Neville, V.; Pain, M.T.; Kantor, J.; Folland, J.P. Influence of crank length and crank-axle height on standing arm-crank (grinding) power. *Med. Sci. Sports Exerc.* **2010**, *42*, 381–387. [CrossRef] [PubMed]
17. Cummins, T.D.; Gladden, L.B. Responses to submaximal and maximal arm cycling above, at, and below heart level. *Med. Sci. Sports Exerc.* **1983**, *15*, 295–298. [CrossRef] [PubMed]
18. Neville, V.; Zaher, N.; Pain, M.T.; Folland, J.P. Lower limb influence on standing arm-cranking ("grinding"). *Int. J. Sports Med.* **2009**, *30*, 713–718. [CrossRef] [PubMed]
19. Bressel, E.; Heise, G.D. Effect of arm cranking direction on EMG, kinematic, and oxygen consumption responses. *J. Appl. Biomech.* **2004**, *20*, 129–143.
20. Bressel, E.; Bressel, M.; Marquez, M.; Heise, G.D. The effect of handgrip position on upper extremity neuromuscular responses to arm cranking exercise. *J. Electromyogr. Kinesiol.* **2001**, *11*, 291–298. [CrossRef]
21. Fujii, N.; Nagasaki, H. Efficiency and proficiency of bimanual cranking: Differences between two cranking patterns. *Percept. Mot. Skills* **1995**, *80*, 275–283. [CrossRef] [PubMed]
22. Pearson, S.N.; Hume, P.A.; Slyfield, D.; Cronin, J.B. External work and peak power are reliable measures of ergometer grinding performance when tested under load, deck heel and grinding direction conditions. *Sports Biomech.* **2007**, *6*, 71–80. [CrossRef] [PubMed]
23. Basmajian, J.V.; Blumenstein, R. *Electrode Placement in EMG Biofeedback*; Williams & Wilkins: Baltimore, MD, USA, 1980.
24. Hopkins, W.G. Calculating likely (confidence) limits and likelihoods for true values (Excel spreadsheet). Available online: http://sportsci.org/resource/stats/xcl.xls (accessed on 27 June 2016).
25. Cohen, J. *Statistical Power Analysis for the Behavioral Sciences*, 2nd ed.; Lawrence Erlbaum: Hillsdale, NJ, USA, 1988.
26. Bertucci, W.; Grappe, F.; Girard, A.; Betik, A.; Rouillon, J.D. Effects on the crank torque profile when changing pedalling cadence in level ground and uphill road cycling. *J. Biomech.* **2005**, *38*, 1003–1010. [CrossRef] [PubMed]
27. Neptune, R.R.; Hull, M.L. Evaluation of performance criteria for simulation of submaximal steady-state cycling using a forward dynamic model. *J. Biomech. Eng.* **1998**, *120*, 334–341. [CrossRef] [PubMed]
28. Reiser, R.F.; Peterson, M.L.; Broker, J.P. Instrumented bicycle pedals for dynamic measurement of propulsive cycling loads. *Sports Eng.* **2003**, *6*, 41–48. [CrossRef]
29. Neptune, R.R.; Kautz, S.A.; Zajac, F.E. Muscle contributions to specific biomechanical functions do not change in forward *versus* backward pedaling. *J. Biomech.* **2000**, *33*, 155–164. [CrossRef]
30. Pearson, S.N.; Cronin, J.B.; Hume, P.A.; Slyfield, D. Effects of a power-focussed resistance training intervention on backward grinding performance in America's Cup sailing. *Sports Biomech.* **2009**, *8*, 334–344. [CrossRef] [PubMed]

3

The Effects of Exercise on Natriuretic Peptides in Individuals without Heart Failure

Hidetaka Hamasaki [1,2]

[1] Department of Internal Medicine, National Center for Global Health and Medicine Kohnodai Hospital, 1-7-1 Kohnodai, Chiba 272-8516, Japan; hhamasaki78@gmail.com

[2] Hamasaki Clinic, 2-21-4 Nishida, Kagoshima 890-0046, Japan

Academic Editor: Eling Douwe de Bruin

Abstract: Cardiac natriuretic peptides (NPs) play an important role in the regulation of energy expenditure in skeletal muscle and adipose tissue. A systematic review on the effects of exercise on NPs in patients with heart failure reported that aerobic and resistance training reduced NPs; however, the effects of exercise on NPs and the underlying mechanism of exercise-induced NP secretion in subjects without heart failure remain unknown. In athletes and young, healthy subjects, the NP concentration at rest is not elevated, but strenuous endurance exercise significantly increases NPs. The exercise-induced increase in NPs may be caused by transient myocardial wall stress, cardiomyocyte metabolic changes, or neuroendocrinological response, which may have cytoprotective and growth-regulating effects on the heart. On the other hand, in elderly, overweight/obese subjects, and patients with hypertension, NP concentrations also increase during exercise; however, NP secretion may be more susceptible to cardiac stress compared to young, healthy individuals. Recent studies have shown that NPs are associated with thermogenesis in fat tissue and oxidative capacity in skeletal muscles. NPs may also have a protective role for skeletal muscle in humans, although further studies are warranted to elucidate the physiological mechanism of exercise-induced NP secretion.

Keywords: exercise; natriuretic peptide; atrial natriuretic peptide; B-type natriuretic peptide; metabolic disease

1. Introduction

Cardiac natriuretic peptides (NPs) including atrial natriuretic peptide (ANP), B-type natriuretic peptide (BNP), and C-type natriuretic peptide (CNP) play an important role in the regulation of cardiac function [1]. NPs have vasodilator and diuretic effects, leading to decreased circulating blood volume, arterial pressure, central venous pressure, and cardiac output [2]. Plasma BNP and N-terminal proBNP (NT-proBNP) have become useful biomarkers for the diagnosis and prognosis of heart failure in clinical practice [3–7]. In addition, their levels are inversely associated with visceral fat [8], body mass index, waist circumference, and serum insulin levels [9–12], suggesting that obesity may be ameliorated by the lipolytic effects of BNP and NT-proBNP [13]. Previous studies have shown that ANP is also a lipolytic hormone that increases free fatty acids and enhances oxidation in skeletal muscle, liver, and adipose tissue [14–16]. Recently, a number of studies have suggested the CNP and its specific receptor, natriuretic peptide receptor B play an important role in regulating cardiovascular system and endothelial functions, but its physiological role has not been fully investigated [17]. For example, a randomized study suggested that the change in CNP concentrations after aerobic physical training represent an improvement of endothelial function in patients with heart failure [18]. NPs play a key role in regulating energy expenditure and fat metabolism as well as cardiovascular homeostasis (Figure 1) [19].

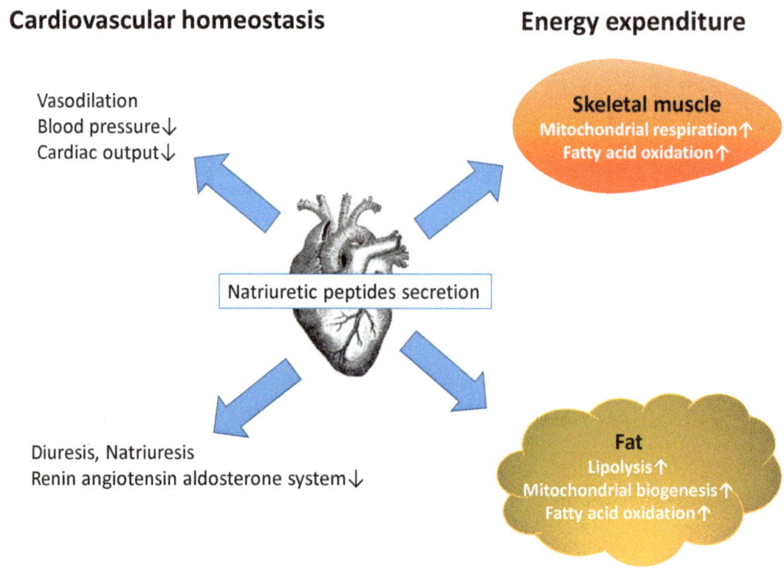

Figure 1. Natriuretic peptides (NPs) released by the heart have various physiological functions. NPs reduce blood pressure, cardiac burden, and renin-angiotensin-aldosterone system activity and increase renal sodium and water excretion. Moreover, NPs enhance lipolysis in human adipose tissue and increase fatty acid oxidation in both adipose tissue and skeletal muscle. NPs also enhance mitochondrial respiration in skeletal muscle and mitochondrial biogenesis in white adipose tissue, leading to increased energy expenditure in humans.

A systematic review of randomized controlled trials (RCTs) investigating the effects of exercise on BNP and NT-proBNP in patients with heart failure showed that aerobic and resistance training had a favorable effect on NPs and decreased BNP levels (mean difference −79 pg/mL; 95% confidence intervals (CI), −141 to −17 pg/mL) and NT-proBNP levels (mean difference −621 pg/mL; 95% CI, −844 to −398 pg/mL) [20]. However, this analysis was among patients with heart failure; the effects of exercise on NPs in subjects without heart failure, especially in older individuals and/or patients with metabolic diseases, have not been fully elucidated. Exercise such as long distance running [21], cycling [22,23], and hand grip exercises [24] have been reported to increase levels of NPs in healthy subjects. Recently, low-intensity daily physical activity was also suggested to be associated with increased plasma BNP levels in patients with type 2 diabetes [25,26]. A cross-sectional study showed that plasma BNP levels were inversely associated with both visceral fat area and thigh muscle mass [27], suggesting that BNP levels increase in response to muscle loss (e.g., sarcopenia) to protect against muscle damage [27]. Larsen *et al.* reported that muscle fiber roundness, an indicator of histological skeletal muscle damage because of intramuscular edema, is positively correlated with NT-proBNP levels [28]. The crosstalk between NPs, fat tissue, and skeletal muscle in humans should be studied to reveal the various physiological actions of NPs.

This review is aimed at summarizing clinical studies investigating the effects of exercise on NPs, specifically ANP and BNP, concentrations in subjects without heart disease and at providing clinicians with current knowledge on the roles of NPs in humans.

2. Methods

The author searched the literature on NPs and exercise using Pubmed from its inception to March 2016. The search terms were "natriuretic peptide" and "exercise." The search returned 1402 published articles; however, 1261 articles were related to heart diseases, and they were excluded from this review. The titles and abstracts of the identified articles were reviewed to determine their relevance. If the study participants had heart diseases such as heart failure, coronary artery disease, and myocardial infarction, the studies were excluded from this review. Not only controlled trials but also before-after studies, as well as cross-sectional studies, were reviewed. A total of 18 articles were eligible.

3. The Effects of Exercise on NPs in Athletes and Healthy Subjects

To the best of the author's knowledge, no RCTs have investigated the effects of aerobic and/or resistance exercise on NPs in subjects without heart diseases. However, some non-randomized and non-controlled clinical studies have found changes in the levels of NPs due to exercise. Ohba *et al.* recruited 10 amateur male athletes (mean age = 46.2 $\pm$ 10.7 years) who participated in a 100-km ultramarathon. Their levels of plasma ANP and BNP increased two- and five-fold, respectively, immediately after running [29]. Interestingly, plasma ANP levels decreased in two athletes (23 and 36 years, respectively), but not in any older subjects. The release of ANP after exercise was greater in older subjects than in young individuals [30], and this study also suggested that the pattern of ANP secretion after prolonged strenuous exercise is related to age. Similarly, Siegel *et al.* measured changes in BNP in 82 runners without smoking habits or coronary heart disease (mean age = 47 $\pm$ 8 years) after the Boston Marathon [31]. The results showed that BNP levels did not increase 4 h after running, but significantly increased within normal limits 24 h after the race. However, other cardiac markers such as creatinine kinase-MB and cardiac troponin I were significantly increased at both 4 and 24 h after running. These results suggest that BNP secretion due to endurance exercise cannot be attributed only to exercise-related myocardial damage. Neumayr *et al.* measured NT-proBNP as a marker of cardiac injury in 29 recreational cyclists to investigate whether strenuous exercise induced cardiac dysfunction [22]. The NT-proBNP levels of study subjects without cardiovascular risk factors (mean age = 34 $\pm$ 8 years) were measured after they finished the cycling race (total distance = 230 km, altitude difference = 5500 m). The plasma levels of NT-proBNP significantly increased immediately after the race, decreased on the following day, and returned to baseline values after one week. The increase of NT-proBNP may be related to the physiologic endocrine response against the myocardial stress induced by exercise, which is not so much cardiac injury as cardiac fatigue. A study with a larger number of subjects was conducted to examine the increase of NT-proBNP and its relationship to the increases in cardiac troponin I and T after prolonged strenuous exercise [32]. A total of 105 healthy endurance athletes (mean age = 40 $\pm$ 8 years) were investigated at three endurance exercise events (a marathon, a 100-km ultramarathon, and a mountain bike marathon). The NT-proBNP levels increased in the participants after all three exercise events and exceeded the upper reference limit in 81 athletes 3 h after endurance exercise. The increases in NT-proBNP were not associated with increases in cardiac troponin I and T; however, they were related to exercise time, suggesting that BNP secretion during and after exercise is not caused by myocardial damage, but instead by cytoprotective and growth-regulating effects, as previously reported in experimental studies [33,34]. NPs have a role as anti-inflammatory and antioxidant regulators inhibiting the induction of inflammatory mediators such as tumor necrosis factor-α, interleukin-1, monocyte chemoattractant protein-1, nitric oxide, cyclooxygenase-2, and reducing oxidative stress [35,36]. Exercise may trigger such cytoprotective effects of NPs.

Scherr *et al.* investigated the 72-h kinetics of cardiac biomarkers such as high-sensitive cardiac troponin T, heart-type fatty acid-binding protein, and NT-proBNP, inflammation markers, and renal function in marathon participants [37]. A total of 102 healthy men (mean age = 42 $\pm$ 9.5 years) were recruited, and cardiac biomarkers were measured before the race and 0, 24, and 72 h after the marathon. The NT-pro BNP levels increased significantly at 0, 24, and 72 h after the race compared to one week before the race. The NT-proBNP and heart-type fatty acid-binding protein kinetics showed similar patterns after the race. Other cardiac biomarkers increased immediately after the race but returned to normal levels within 72 h. These results suggest that the increase in cardiac markers due to endurance exercise may not be explained by myocardial damage but by transient stress or altered cardiomyocyte metabolism. To confirm the evidence of exercise-induced myocardial damage, Scharhag *et al.* conducted two endurance exercise trials in healthy athletes [38]. Twenty male athletes (mean age = 36 ± 7 years) performed both 1 h of exercise at an intensity of 100% of the individual's anaerobic threshold and 3 h of exercise at 75% intensity (running or mountain biking). Myocardial damage was evaluated by echocardiography and magnetic resonance imaging. The levels of cardiac troponin I- and NT-proBNP significantly increased after both exercise sessions, whereas the cardiac troponin T levels did not change. No significant correlations were observed between the exercise-induced increase in NT-proBNP and cardiac troponins. Moreover, no evidence for myocardial damage was detected in echocardiography or magnetic resonance imaging. Considering the absence of relationships among NT-proBNP, cardiac troponins, and cardiac function, the exercise-induced increase in cardiac markers including NT-proBNP may represent a physiological reaction in cardiomyocytes without pathological damage. However, the cardiac effects of such physiological elevation of NT-proBNP remain unknown. Faviou *et al.* investigated whether the release of NT-proBNP after exercise had cytoprotective effects or was caused by myocardial damage during exercise [39]. A total of 99 subjects were assigned to three groups: 43 male soccer and basketball players (mean age = 24 ± 4 years); 21 age-matched patients with left ventricular hypertrophy or impaired left ventricular function; and 35 age-matched healthy controls. The athlete group performed regular training for 11–18 h per week, and the control group engaged in exercise occasionally (2–3 times a week) for 3–6 h per week. The cardiac troponin T and NT-proBNP levels at rest were measured in all three groups. After intense exercise, the changes in cardiac troponin T and NT-proBNP in the athlete group were examined. Cardiac function was evaluated by electrocardiography and echocardiography in all participants. The NT-proBNP levels in patients were significantly higher than those in the healthy controls and athletes. After intense exercise, the NT-proBNP levels were elevated compared to the levels at rest, although they were lower than those in patients at rest. In athletes, cardiac troponin T did not change after exercise. The elevation of NT-proBNP within the normal limit may not represent cardiac dysfunction; instead, it likely indicates the activation of a counter-regulatory system (e.g., the adrenergic system). NPs may be considered as an indicator of the neuroendocrine system rather than a marker of cardiac dysfunction [40]. To date, human and experimental animal studies have shown that various neuroendocrine alterations occur as a result of exercise stress and negative energy balance caused by strenuous and repetitive exercise (Table 1) [41,42]. Hypothalamic-pituitary-adrenocortical axis, antidiuretic hormone and NPs responses to exercise may contribute to integrative regulation of cardiovascular homeostasis.

Table 1. Effects of exercise on neuroendocrine system.

Hormone Concentrations	Dynamics
Adrenocorticotrophic hormone	↑
Cortisol	↑
Antidiuretic hormone	↑
Growth hormone	↑
Gonadotropins	↓
Testosterone	↓
Estradiol	↓
Natriuretic peptides	↑
Sympathetic nerve system	↑

An interesting open-labeled, randomized, crossover study investigating the ANP response to exercise in water was conducted in Germany [43]. Seventeen healthy men (mean age = 31 ± 3.6 years) were studied. The subjects performed two exercise tests on a bicycle ergometer on land and in water. Exercise in water attenuated norepinephrine and epinephrine concentrations during peak exercise in comparison to exercise on land. On the other hand, the increases in ANP levels were significantly augmented when subjects exercised in water, particularly at the anaerobic threshold. Water immersion causes physiological changes such as intracellular-intravascular fluid shifts and increased cardiac output, resulting in an increase in circulating blood volume [44]. Exercise in water may stimulate ANP secretion not by the activation of sympathetic nervous system but by such physiological changes in water. When discussing the effects of exercise on NPs, we should also note the conditions under which exercise is performed (e.g., on land, in water, outside, inside, a high place, or underground). Table 2 shows a list of published articles investigating the effects of exercise on NPs in athletes and healthy subjects. These studies in athletes have focused on whether NPs reflect myocardial damage because several cases of sudden death due to cardiovascular causes have been reported in athletes. However, recent studies suggest that NPs also play a role in mediating the metabolic and endocrine systems in individuals with low levels of physical fitness [2]. This review focuses on the associations between NPs and metabolism in non-athletes, older people, and patients with metabolic disturbance.

Table 2. Clinical studies investigating the effects of exercise on NP levels in athletes and healthy subjects.

Authors, Year	Subjects	Exercise	Results
Ohba *et al.*, 2001 [29]	10 amateur male athletes, 46.2 ± 10.7 years	100 km ultramarathon	ANP↑, BNP↑ in older athletes ANP↓, BNP↑ in younger athletes
Siegel *et al.*, 2008 [31]	82 healthy runners, 47 ± 8 years	Marathon	BNP→ 4 h after running BNP↑ 24 h after running Creatinine kinase-MB↑, cardiac troponin I↑ both 4 and 24 h after running
Neumayr *et al.*, 2005 [22]	29 healthy recreational cyclists, 34 ± 8 years	Cycle race	NT-proBNP↑ after the race NT-proBNP decreased to baseline values after a week
Scharhag *et al.*, 2005 [32]	105 healthy endurance athletes, 40 ± 8 years	Marathon, 100-km ultramarathon and mountain bike marathon	NT-proBNP↑ Increased NT-proBNP was not associated with increases in cardiac troponin I and T
Scherr *et al.*, 2011 [37]	102 healthy men, 42± 9.5 years	Marathon	NT-pro BNP↑ 0, 24 and 72 h after the race Other cardiac biomarkers returned to normal levels within 72 h
Scharhag *et al.*, 2006 [38]	20 male athletes, 36 ± 7 years	Running or mountain biking 1-h and 3-h exercise with an intensity of 100% and 75% of the individual anaerobic threshold, respectively	NT-proBNP↑, cardiac troponin I↑, cardiac troponin T→ No evidence for myocardial damage was detected after exercise
Faviou, *et al.*, 2008 [39]	43 male soccer and basketball players, 24 ± 4 years, age-matched 21 patients, and 35 healthy controls	Regular training for 11–18 h/week (athletes) Occasional exercise 3–6 h/week (controls)	NT-proBNP↑, cardiac troponin T→

NPs = natriuretic peptides; ANP = atrial natriuretic peptide; BNP = B-type natriuretic peptide; NT-proBNP = N-terminal pro B-type natriuretic.

4. The Effects of Exercise on NPs in the Elderly and in Patients with Metabolic Diseases Who Do Not Suffer from Heart Failure

Evidence related to the effects of exercise on NPs in non-athletes without heart failure is limited. Engelmann *et al.* investigated the responses of plasma ANP and BNP to exercise (cycle ergometer) in patients with atrial fibrillation and in healthy control subjects [45]. As expected, the plasma ANP and BNP levels at rest, during exercise, and after exercise were significantly higher in patients with atrial fibrillation than in the control subjects. The mean age of the control group was 67.9 ± 4.5 years, which is relatively high compared to the ages of athletes in clinical studies. During exercise, the ANP and BNP levels significantly increased in elderly, healthy subjects. Interestingly, no changes in ANP and BNP levels were observed between the peak exercise levels and the levels 30 min after exercise in the healthy controls. However, the decrease in plasma BNP in patients with atrial fibrillation was significantly higher than that in healthy controls, whereas the decrease in plasma ANP did not differ between the two groups. These results suggest that BNP may respond rapidly to exercise-induced left ventricular overload as an emergency hormone.

Tanaka *et al.* measured the plasma ANP and BNP levels in 19 patients with hypertension (mean age = 44 ± 2.6 years) and 14 normotensive subjects (mean age = 40 ± 2.2 years) during exercise using a bicycle ergometer [46]. The plasma ANP and BNP levels, blood pressure, heart rate, and plasma norepinephrine levels significantly increased during exercise in both hypertensive and normotensive subjects. Norepinephrine was a significant stimulus for ANP secretion in normotensive subjects, while the changes in ANP levels were associated only with heart rate in hypertensive patients. On the other hand, systolic blood pressure and epinephrine levels were strongly associated with BNP secretion in normotensive subjects, while the changes in BNP levels were associated only with heart rate in hypertensive patients. These results suggest that exercise-induced NP secretion is more sensitive to sympathetic activity in normotensive subjects compared to in patients with hypertension. Thus, in patients with hypertension, the increase in NPs during exercise may represent cardiac stress rather than neuroendocrinological response, which is a potential mechanism of exercise-induced NP secretion in healthy athletes.

A prospective, randomized study assessed the proANP concentrations at rest and after incremental exhaustive exercise in overweight and obese patients [47]. A total of 125 overweight and obese but otherwise healthy subjects were recruited. The 75 subjects that lost more than 5% of their weight during the six-month dietary intervention were analyzed. The subjects performed a stepwise incremental exercise test (bicycle ergometer) until exhaustion. After six months of dietary weight reduction with a low-fat or low-carbohydrate diet, the proANP levels did not change; however, exercise-induced acute increase in proANP levels were observed during exercise both before and after dietary intervention. In addition, natriuretic peptide receptor C (NPR-C) expression in abdominal fat tissue significantly decreased after the six-month hypocaloric diet intervention. These results indicate that physical exercise acutely increases proANP levels in overweight and obese patients, and weight reduction by diet therapy chronically decreases ANP clearance by NPR-C. NP deficiency in obese patients may be ameliorated by the combination of diet and exercise. Increased NP levels stimulate lipolysis [48] and increase lipid oxidation [15] and adiponectin secretion [49] in adipose tissue. NPs regulate thermogenesis in skeletal muscle as well as in adipose tissue [16,50]. Exercise is essential for the management of obesity-associated metabolic and cardiovascular disease, both directly (weight loss) and indirectly (lipolysis by NPs). Two studies have investigated the effects of resistance training on NPs; these studies are different from those mentioned above in that they evaluated the chronic effect of exercise on NT-proBNP rather than the acute effect. The results are controversial.

Bordbar *et al.* investigated the effects of an eight-week resistance training program on the release of NT-proBNP [51]. A total of 22 subjects were allocated to four groups: sedentary individuals who performed eight weeks of aerobic exercise; sedentary individuals who performed eight weeks of resistance training; bodybuilders who did not use anabolic androgenic steroids; and bodybuilders who regularly used anabolic androgenic steroids. Aerobic exercise was treadmill running, and resistance training consisted of 15 min of machine training and 20 min of isometric exercise using dumbbells. NT-proBNP levels significantly increased immediately after aerobic exercise, but decreased after eight weeks of aerobic exercise. On the other hand, NT-proBNP levels significantly increased after eight weeks of resistance training, although they did not change immediately after resistance training. The authors mentioned the possibility of myocardial damage induced by strength training.

Beltran Valls *et al.* investigated the effects of 12 weeks of low-frequency, moderate-intensity resistance training on muscle strength and motor function in the elderly [52]. Twenty-eight elderly subjects (mean age = 72 ± 1 years) without cardiovascular, metabolic, pulmonary, or orthopedic diseases were randomly assigned to the training group or control group. Subjects in the training group engaged in resistance training for 12 weeks. They performed the resistance training at an intensity of 40%–50% 1-repetition maximum during the first two weeks, and the resistance was increased approximately every two weeks. Five subjects dropped out of the study. The muscle power of the upper and lower extremities increased by approximately 30% in the training group. Muscle strength also increased by 15%–20% after the 12 weeks of resistance training. However, NT-proBNP concentrations did not change after resistance training. Thus, moderate-intensity resistance training may be a safe and effective strategy for improving muscle fitness in the elderly without inducing cardiac stress. However, a previous cross-sectional study showed that muscle mass is independently and inversely associated with BNP levels [27]; therefore, the change in NPs concentrations due to resistance training may have no relation to NP secretion caused by myocardial stress.

A total of 1431 healthy middle-aged to elderly subjects were investigated. Thigh muscle mass was evaluated by measuring muscle cross-sectional area using computed tomography. Visceral fat area was also measured using computed tomography at the umbilicus level. Plasma BNP levels were found to be negatively associated with thigh muscle mass and visceral fat area. After adjustment for confounding parameters such as age, gender, body weight, blood pressure, and adiponectin levels, BNP levels were still negatively associated with thigh muscle mass [27]. A previous study in rats showed that BNP protects skeletal muscle mass by decreasing oxidative stress and mitochondrial dysfunction after ischemia-reperfusion [53]. BNP is also secreted from satellite cells within the ischemic skeletal muscle, which can improve the regeneration of neighboring endothelial cells after ischemia. Hence, BNP may also have a protective role against muscle damage in humans. Another cross-sectional study analyzed the association between objectively measured daily physical activity and cardiac biomarkers including NT-proBNP and high-sensitive troponin T in elderly subjects [54]. A total of 1253 community-dwelling subjects (mean age = 75.6 ± 6.5 years) were examined, and their daily physical activity was measured using an accelerometer. After adjustment for age, sex, smoking status, and history of cardiovascular disease, an inverse dose-response relationship with daily walking duration was found for troponin T and NT-proBNP levels. Walking is known to have beneficial effects on cardiovascular morbidity and mortality [55,56], and this study also suggests that daily walking is associated with the reduction of cardiac stress. However, 24.7% of the subjects had a history of cardiovascular disease, and cardiac function tests were not performed; thus, the results should be interpreted carefully. Hamasaki *et al.* showed that objectively measured daily physical activity was positively and independently associated with plasma BNP levels in subjects with glucose intolerance and type 2 diabetic patients [25]. Although this was a small-scale cross-sectional study, light-intensity daily physical activity may also increase BNP levels in patients with metabolic diseases. Table 3 shows a list of published articles investigating the effects of exercise on NPs in the elderly and in patients with metabolic diseases without heart failure.

Table 3. Clinical studies investigating the effects of exercise on NP levels in the elderly or in patients with metabolic diseases.

Authors, Year	Study Design	Subjects	Exercise	Results
Engelmann *et al.*, 2005 [45]	Before-after study with control group	38 patients with atrial fibrillation and age-matched 43 older (67.9 ± 4.5 years) healthy controls	Cycle ergometer	ANP↑, BNP↑ during exercise ANP→, BNP→ 30 min after exercise in older healthy controls BNP↓ 30 min after exercise in patients with atrial fibrillation
Tanaka *et al.*, 1995 [46]	Before-after study with control group	19 patients with hypertension (44 ± 2.6 years) and 14 normotensive subjects (40 ± 2.2 years)	Cycle ergometer	ANP↑, BNP↑ during exercise Changes in ANP and BNP levels were associated with only heart rate in hypertensive patients
Haufe *et al.*, 2015 [47]	Randomized, non-controlled trial	125 middle-aged overweight and obese subjects	Cycle ergometer	proANP↑ during exercise proANP→, NPR-C expression↑ after 6-months dietary intervention
Beltran Valls *et al.*, 2014 [52]	Randomized controlled trial	28 elderly subjects, 72 ± 1 years	12-week low-frequency, moderate-intensity resistance training	NT-proBNP→ Muscle strength and power↑

NPs = natriuretic peptides; ANP = atrial natriuretic peptide; BNP = B-type natriuretic peptide; NT-proBNP = N-terminal pro B-type natriuretic; NPR-C = natriuretic peptide receptor C.

5. The Influence of Exercise Duration and Intensity on NPs Secretion

Differential effects of exercise duration and intensity on exercise-induced NPs secretion should be discussed. Several studies investigating the influence of exercise duration and intensity on the release of cardiac biomarkers have shown that exercise intensity was responsible for the release of cardiac troponin; however, exercise-induced increase of NT-proBNP was associated with exercise duration, but not exercise intensity [57–59]. Recently, Benda *et al.* [60] showed that exercise-induced changes in cardiac troponin and BNP is similar between endurance training and a single bout of high-intensity interval training in heart failure patients and healthy controls. Even though exercise is performed at high-intensity, if the duration was short, excessive cardiac stress could be preventive. Although the optimal intensity, frequency, and duration of exercise for health in individuals with and without heart diseases were not fully elucidated, engaging in exercise at above high-intensity and for above a certain duration, which depends on individuals' physical fitness, may not be beneficial for health.

6. Conclusions

In athletes and young healthy subjects, NP concentrations at rest are not elevated, but strenuous endurance exercise significantly increases NP secretion. Even if NP levels exceed the cutoff values, the increase in NPs does not represent myocardial damage, as detected in patients with heart diseases such as myocardial ischemia. Table 4 summarizes the distinct effects of acute exercise, endurance training, and physical deconditioning/disability including older age on NP concentrations. However, further standardized investigations will be required because there are considerable heterogeneities of exercise interventions (intensity, frequency, and duration) between clinical studies.

Table 4. Effects of acute exercise, endurance training, and deconditioning/disability on NP concentrations.

Types of Exercise	at Rest	During or Immediately after Exercise	After (⩾72 h) Exercise
Healthy younger individuals			
Acute exercise	→	↑	↓ (return to normal levels)
Endurance training	→	→ or ↑	→ or ↓ (return to normal levels)
Older individuals or Individuals with disabilities or disturbances			
Older individuals	↗	→ or ↑	↘
Obesity	↘	↑	↓ NPR-C↑
Heart diseases (e.g., heart failure, myocardial infarction and atrial fibrillation)	↑	↑↑	↓ (Appropriate exercise programs may reduce NPs levels less than those at baseline)

NPs = natriuretic peptides; NPR-C = natriuretic peptide receptor C.

The exercise-induced increase in NPs may be caused by transient myocardial wall stress, cardiomyocyte metabolic changes, or neuroendocrinological response, which may have cytoprotective and growth-regulating effects on the heart. On the other hand, in the elderly, obese subjects, and patients with metabolic diseases, the physiological mechanism of NP secretion due to exercise seems to be different from that in young, healthy subjects, although NP concentrations also increase during exercise in young, healthy subjects. NP secretion may be more susceptible to cardiac stress in elderly subjects than in young, healthy individuals. In short, exercise-induced increases in NPs may be dependent on the balance between the intensity of exercise and the physical fitness level of the individual. The elderly and patients with metabolic diseases generally have low physical strength; thus, even light-to moderate-intensity exercise could elevate NP levels. However, a number of studies have demonstrated that NP levels are reduced in patients with metabolic diseases including obesity [61–64], although how exercise contributes to the change in NP levels remains unknown. To elucidate the underlying mechanism of exercise-induced NP secretion in patients with metabolic diseases, further studies are warranted. Recently, the roles of NPs in thermogenesis in fat tissue and oxidative capacity in skeletal muscle have been investigated [14–16]. Specifically, BNP may have a protective role for skeletal muscle along with cardioprotective effects in humans. The role of NPs in skeletal muscle beyond a cardiac biomarker will be an issue of study. The acute effects of exercise on NPs have also been investigated in many clinical studies; however, the long-term effects of exercise on NPs are still unknown. Well-designed, prospective studies with large numbers of subjects, preferably RCTs, are needed to elucidate the long-term effects of exercise on NPs in both healthy subjects and patients with metabolic diseases such as type 2 diabetes, hypertension, dyslipidemia, and cardiovascular disease.

Conflicts of Interest: The authors declare no conflict of interest.

Abbreviations

The following abbreviations are used in this manuscript:

NP	natriuretic peptide
ANP	atrial natriuretic peptide
BNP	B-type natriuretic peptide
NT-proBNP	N-terminal proBNP
RCT	randomized controlled trial
CI	confidence intervals
NPR-C	natriuretic peptide receptor C

References

1. Potter, L.R.; Abbey-Hosch, S.; Dickey, D.M. Natriuretic peptides, their receptors, and cyclic guanosine monophosphate-dependent signaling functions. *Endocr. Rev.* **2006**, *27*, 47–72. [CrossRef] [PubMed]
2. Schlueter, N.; de Sterke, A.; Willmes, D.M.; Spranger, J.; Jordan, J.; Birkenfeld, A.L. Metabolic actions of natriuretic peptides and therapeutic potential in the metabolic syndrome. *Pharmacol. Ther.* **2014**, *144*, 12–27. [CrossRef] [PubMed]
3. Maeda, K.; Tsutamoto, T.; Wada, A.; Mabuchi, N.; Hayashi, M.; Tsutsui, T.; Ohnishi, M.; Sawaki, M.; Fujii, M.; Matsumoto, T.; *et al.* High levels of plasma brain natriuretic peptide and interleukin-6 after optimized treatment for heart failure are independent risk factors for morbidity and mortality in patients with congestive heart failure. *J. Am. Coll. Cardiol.* **2000**, *36*, 1587–1593. [CrossRef]
4. Wang, T.J.; Larson, M.G.; Levy, D.; Benjamin, E.J.; Leip, E.P.; Omland, T.; Wolf, P.A.; Vasan, R.S. Plasma natriuretic peptide levels and the risk of cardiovascular events and death. *N. Engl. J. Med.* **2004**, *350*, 655–663. [CrossRef] [PubMed]
5. Alehagen, U.; Lindstedt, G.; Levin, L.A.; Dahlström, U. Risk of cardiovascular death in elderly patients with possible heart failure. B-type natriuretic peptide (BNP) and the aminoterminal fragment of ProBNP (N-terminal proBNP) as prognostic indicators in a 6-year follow-up of a primary care population. *Int. J. Cardiol.* **2005**, *100*, 125–133. [CrossRef] [PubMed]
6. Kroon, M.H.; van den Hurk, K.; Alssema, M.; Kamp, O.; Stehouwer, C.D.; Henry, R.M.; Diamant, M.; Boomsma, F.; Nijpels, G.; Paulus, W.J.; *et al.* Prospective associations of B-type natriuretic peptide with markers of left ventricular function in individuals with and without type 2 diabetes: An 8-year follow-up of the Hoorn Study. *Diabetes Care* **2012**, *35*, 2510–2514. [CrossRef] [PubMed]
7. Olsen, M.H.; Wachtell, K.; Tuxen, C.; Fossum, E.; Bang, L.E.; Hall, C.; Ibsen, H.; Rokkedal, J.; Devereux, R.B.; Hildebrandt, P. N-terminal pro-brain natriuretic peptide predicts cardiovascular events in patients with hypertension and left ventricular hypertrophy: A LIFE study. *J. Hypertens.* **2004**, *22*, 1597–1604. [CrossRef] [PubMed]
8. Neeland, I.J.; Winders, B.R.; Ayers, C.R.; Das, S.R.; Chang, A.Y.; Berry, J.D.; Khera, A.; McGuire, D.K.; Vega, G.L.; de Lemos, J.A.; *et al.* Higher natriuretic peptide levels associate with a favorable adipose tissue distribution profile. *J. Am. Coll. Cardiol.* **2013**, *62*, 752–760. [CrossRef] [PubMed]
9. McCord, J.; Mundy, B.J.; Hudson, M.P.; Maisel, A.S.; Hollander, J.E.; Abraham, W.T.; Steg, P.G.; Omland, T.; Knudsen, C.W.; Sandberg, K.R.; *et al.* Breathing Not Properly Multinational Study Investigators. Relationship between obesity and B-type natriuretic peptide levels. *Arch. Intern. Med.* **2004**, *164*, 2247–2252. [CrossRef] [PubMed]

10. Mehra, M.R.; Uber, P.A.; Park, M.H.; Scott, R.L.; Ventura, H.O.; Harris, B.C.; Frohlich, E.D. Obesity and suppressed B-type natriuretic peptide levels in heart failure. *J. Am. Coll. Cardiol.* **2004**, *43*, 1590–1595. [CrossRef] [PubMed]
11. Koizumi, M.; Watanabe, H.; Kaneko, Y.; Iino, K.; Ishida, M.; Kosaka, T.; Motohashi, Y.; Ito, H. Impact of obesity on plasma B-type natriuretic peptide levels in Japanese community-based subjects. *Heart Vessels.* **2012**, *27*, 287–294. [CrossRef] [PubMed]
12. Olsen, M.H.; Hansen, T.W.; Christensen, M.K.; Gustafsson, F.; Rasmussen, S.; Wachtell, K.; Borch-Johnsen, K.; Ibsen, H.; Jørgensen, T.; Hildebrandt, P. N-terminal pro brain natriuretic peptide is inversely related to metabolic cardiovascular risk factors and the metabolic syndrome. *Hypertension* **2005**, *46*, 660–666. [CrossRef] [PubMed]
13. Polak, J.; Kotrc, M.; Wedellova, Z.; Jabor, A.; Malek, I.; Kautzner, J.; Kazdova, L.; Melenovsky, V. Lipolytic effects of B-type natriuretic peptide 1-32 in adipose tissue of heart failure patients compared with healthy controls. *J. Am. Coll. Cardiol.* **2011**, *58*, 119–125. [CrossRef] [PubMed]
14. Birkenfeld, A.L.; Boschmann, M.; Moro, C.; Adams, F.; Heusser, K.; Tank, J.; Diedrich, A.; Schroeder, C.; Franke, G.; Berlan, M.; *et al.* Beta-adrenergic and atrial natriuretic peptide interactions on human cardiovascular and metabolic regulation. *J. Clin. Endocrinol. Metab.* **2006**, *91*, 5069–5075. [CrossRef] [PubMed]
15. Birkenfeld, A.L.; Budziarek, P.; Boschmann, M.; Moro, C.; Adams, F.; Franke, G.; Berlan, M.; Marques, M.A.; Sweep, F.C.; Luft, F.C.; *et al.* Atrial natriuretic peptide induces postprandial lipid oxidation in humans. *Diabetes* **2008**, *57*, 3199–3204. [CrossRef] [PubMed]
16. Engeli, S.; Birkenfeld, A.L.; Badin, P.M.; Bourlier, V.; Louche, K.; Viguerie, N.; Thalamas, C.; Montastier, E.; Larrouy, D.; Harant, I.; *et al.* Natriuretic peptides enhance the oxidative capacity of human skeletal muscle. *J. Clin. Investig.* **2012**, *122*, 4675–4679. [CrossRef] [PubMed]
17. Del Ry, S. C-type natriuretic peptide: A new cardiac mediator. *Peptides* **2013**, *40*, 93–98. [CrossRef] [PubMed]
18. Passino, C.; Del Ry, S.; Severino, S.; Gabutti, A.; Prontera, C.; Clerico, A.; Giannessi, D.; Emdin, M. C-type natriuretic peptide expression in patients with chronic heart failure: Effects of aerobic training. *Eur. J. Cardiovasc. Prev. Rehabil.* **2008**, *15*, 168–172. [CrossRef] [PubMed]
19. Gruden, G.; Landi, A.; Bruno, G. Natriuretic peptides, heart, and adipose tissue: New findings and future developments for diabetes research. *Diabetes Care.* **2014**, *37*, 2899–2908. [CrossRef] [PubMed]
20. Smart, N.A.; Steele, M. Systematic review of the effect of aerobic and resistance exercise training on systemic brain natriuretic peptide (BNP) and N-terminal BNP expression in heart failure patients. *Int. J. Cardiol.* **2010**, *140*, 260–265. [CrossRef] [PubMed]
21. Leers, M.P.; Schepers, R.; Baumgarten, R. Effects of a long-distance run on cardiac markers in healthy athletes. *Clin. Chem. Lab. Med.* **2006**, *44*, 999–1003. [CrossRef] [PubMed]
22. Neumayr, G.; Pfister, R.; Mitterbauer, G.; Eibl, G.; Hoertnagl, H. Effect of competitive marathon cycling on plasma N-terminal pro-brain natriuretic peptide and cardiac troponin T in healthy recreational cyclists. *Am. J. Cardiol.* **2005**, *96*, 732–735. [CrossRef] [PubMed]
23. Nielsen, H.B.; De Palo, E.F.; Meneghetti, M.; Madsen, P.L.; Ihlemann, N.; Secher, N.H. Circulating immunoreactive proANP1-30 and proANP31-67 responses to acute exercise. *Regul. Pept.* **2001**, *99*, 203–207. [CrossRef]
24. Barletta, G.; Stefani, L.; Del Bene, R.; Fronzaroli, C.; Vecchiarino, S.; Lazzeri, C.; Fantini, F.; La Villa, G. Effects of exercise on natriuretic peptides and cardiac function in man. *Int. J. Cardiol.* **1998**, *65*, 217–225. [CrossRef]
25. Hamasaki, H.; Yanai, H.; Kakei, M.; Noda, M.; Ezaki, O. The association between daily physical activity and plasma B-type natriuretic peptide in patients with glucose intolerance: A cross-sectional study. *BMJ Open* **2015**, *5*, e006276. [CrossRef] [PubMed]
26. Hamasaki, H.; Ezaki, O.; Yanai, H. Nonexercise Activity Thermogenesis is Significantly Lower in Type 2 Diabetic Patients With Mental Disorders Than in Those Without Mental Disorders: A Cross-sectional Study. *Medicine* **2016**, *95*, e2517. [CrossRef] [PubMed]
27. Yamashita, T.; Kohara, K.; Tabara, Y.; Ochi, M.; Nagai, T.; Okada, Y.; Igase, M.; Miki, T. Muscle mass, visceral fat, and plasma levels of B-type natriuretic peptide in healthy individuals (from the J-SHIPP Study). *Am. J. Cardiol.* **2014**, *114*, 635–640. [CrossRef] [PubMed]

28. Larsen, A.I.; Skadberg, Ø.; Aarsland, T.; Kvaløy, J.T.; Lindal, S.; Omland, T.; Dickstein, K. B-type natriuretic peptide is related to histological skeletal muscle abnormalities in patients with chronic heart failure. *Int. J. Cardiol.* **2009**, *136*, 358–362. [CrossRef] [PubMed]
29. Ohba, H.; Takada, H.; Musha, H.; Nagashima, J.; Mori, N.; Awaya, T.; Omiya, K.; Murayama, M. Effects of prolonged strenuous exercise on plasma levels of atrial natriuretic peptide and brain natriuretic peptide in healthy men. *Am. Heart J.* **2001**, *141*, 751–758. [CrossRef] [PubMed]
30. Freund, B.J.; Claybaugh, J.R.; Hashiro, G.M.; Buono, M.; Chrisney, S. Exaggerated ANF response to exercise in middle-aged *vs.* young runners. *J. Appl. Physiol* **1990**, *69*, 1607–1614. [PubMed]
31. Siegel, A.J.; Lewandrowski, E.L.; Chun, K.Y.; Sholar, M.B.; Fischman, A.J.; Lewandrowski, K.B. Changes in cardiac markers including B-natriuretic peptide in runners after the Boston marathon. *Am. J. Cardiol.* **2001**, *88*, 920–923. [CrossRef]
32. Scharhag, J.; Herrmann, M.; Urhausen, A.; Haschke, M.; Herrmann, W.; Kindermann, W. Independent elevations of N-terminal pro-brain natriuretic peptide and cardiac troponins in endurance athletes after prolonged strenuous exercise. *Am. Heart J.* **2005**, *150*, 1128–1134. [CrossRef] [PubMed]
33. D'Souza, S.P.; Baxter, G.F. B Type natriuretic peptide: A good omen in myocardial ischaemia? *Heart* **2003**, *89*, 707–709. [CrossRef] [PubMed]
34. D'Souza, S.P.; Yellon, D.M.; Martin, C.; Schulz, R.; Heusch, G.; Onody, A.; Ferdinandy, P.; Baxter, G.F. B-type natriuretic peptide limits infarct size in rat isolated hearts via KATP channel opening. *Am. J. Physiol. Heart Circ. Physiol.* **2003**, *284*, H1592–H1600. [CrossRef] [PubMed]
35. De Vito, P. Atrial natriuretic peptide: An old hormone or a new cytokine? *Peptides* **2014**, *58*, 108–116. [CrossRef] [PubMed]
36. De Vito, P.; Incerpi, S.; Pedersen, J.Z.; Luly, P. Atrial natriuretic peptide and oxidative stress. *Peptides* **2010**, *31*, 1412–1419. [CrossRef] [PubMed]
37. Scherr, J.; Braun, S.; Schuster, T.; Hartmann, C.; Moehlenkamp, S.; Wolfarth, B.; Pressler, A.; Halle, M. 72-h kinetics of high-sensitive troponin T and inflammatory markers after marathon. *Med. Sci. Sports Exerc.* **2011**, *43*, 1819–1827. [CrossRef] [PubMed]
38. Scharhag, J.; Urhausen, A.; Schneider, G.; Herrmann, M.; Schumacher, K.; Haschke, M.; Krieg, A.; Meyer, T.; Herrmann, W.; Kindermann, W. Reproducibility and clinical significance of exercise-induced increases in cardiac troponins and N-terminal pro brain natriuretic peptide in endurance athletes. *Eur. J. Cardiovasc. Prev. Rehabili.* **2006**, *13*, 388–397. [CrossRef]
39. Faviou, E.; Zachari, A.; Nounopoulos, C.; Agrafiotis, E.; Vourli, G.; Dionyssiou-Asteriou, A. Elevation of serum N-terminal pro-brain natriuretic peptide after exercise is an index of myocardial damage or a cytoprotective reflection? *J. Sports Med. Phys. Fitness.* **2008**, *48*, 90–96. [PubMed]
40. Clerico, A.; Recchia, F.A.; Passino, C.; Emdin, M. Cardiac endocrine function is an essential component of the homeostatic regulation network: Physiological and clinical implications. *Am. J. Physiol. Heart Circ. Physiol.* **2006**, *290*, H17–H29. [CrossRef] [PubMed]
41. Fuqua, J.S.; Rogol, A.D. Neuroendocrine alterations in the exercising human: Implications for energy homeostasis. *Metabolism* **2013**, *62*, 911–921. [CrossRef] [PubMed]
42. Popovic, D.; Popovic, B.; Plecas-Solarovic, B.; Pešić, V.; Markovic, V.; Stojiljkovic, S.; Vukcevic, V.; Petrovic, I.; Banovic, M.; Petrovic, M.; *et al.* The interface of hypothalamic-pituitary-adrenocortical axis and circulating brain natriuretic peptide in prediction of cardiopulmonary performance during physical stress. *Peptides* **2013**, *47*, 85–93. [CrossRef] [PubMed]
43. Wiesner, S.; Birkenfeld, A.L.; Engeli, S.; Haufe, S.; Brechtel, L.; Wein, J.; Hermsdorf, M.; Karnahl, B.; Berlan, M.; Lafontan, M.; *et al.* Neurohumoral and metabolic response to exercise in water. *Horm. Metab. Res.* **2010**, *42*, 334–339. [CrossRef] [PubMed]
44. Wilcock, I.M.; Cronin, J.B.; Hing, W.A. Physiological response to water immersion: A method for sport recovery? *Sports Med.* **2006**, *36*, 747–765. [CrossRef] [PubMed]
45. Engelmann, M.D.; Niemann, L.; Kanstrup, I.L.; Skagen, K.; Godtfredsen, J. Natriuretic peptide response to dynamic exercise in patients with atrial fibrillation. *Int. J. Cardiol.* **2005**, *105*, 31–39. [CrossRef] [PubMed]

46. Tanaka, M.; Ishizaka, Y.; Ishiyama, Y.; Kato, J.; Kida, O.; Kitamura, K.; Kangawa, K.; Matsuo, H.; Eto, T. Exercise-induced secretion of brain natriuretic peptide in essential hypertension and normal subjects. *Hypertens. Res.* **1995**, *18*, 159–166. [CrossRef] [PubMed]
47. Haufe, S.; Kaminski, J.; Utz, W.; Haas, V.; Mähler, A.; Daniels, M.A.; Birkenfeld, A.L.; Lichtinghagen, R.; Luft, F.C.; Schulz-Menger, J.; *et al.* Differential response of the natriuretic peptide system to weight loss and exercise in overweight or obese patients. *J. Hypertens.* **2015**, *33*, 1458–1464. [CrossRef] [PubMed]
48. Sengenès, C.; Berlan, M.; De Glisezinski, I.; Lafontan, M.; Galitzky, J. Natriuretic peptides: A new lipolytic pathway in human adipocytes. *FASEB J.* **2000**, *14*, 1345–1351. [CrossRef] [PubMed]
49. Tsukamoto, O.; Fujita, M.; Kato, M.; Yamazaki, S.; Asano, Y.; Ogai, A.; Okazaki, H.; Asai, M.; Nagamachi, Y.; Maeda, N.; *et al.* Natriuretic peptides enhance the production of adiponectin in human adipocytes and in patients with chronic heart failure. *J. Am. Coll. Cardiol.* **2009**, *53*, 2070–2077. [CrossRef] [PubMed]
50. Bordicchia, M.; Liu, D.; Amri, E.Z.; Ailhaud, G.; Dessì-Fulgheri, P.; Zhang, C.; Takahashi, N.; Sarzani, R.; Collins, S. Cardiac natriuretic peptides act via p38 MAPK to induce the brown fat thermogenic program in mouse and human adipocytes. *J. Clin. Investig.* **2012**, *122*, 1022–1036. [CrossRef] [PubMed]
51. Bordbar, S.; Bigi, M.A.; Aslani, A.; Rahimi, E.; Ahmadi, N. Effect of endurance and strength exercise on release of brain natriuretic peptide. *J. Cardiovasc. Dis. Res.* **2012**, *3*, 22–25. [CrossRef] [PubMed]
52. Beltran Valls, M.R.; Dimauro, I.; Brunelli, A.; Tranchita, E.; Ciminelli, E.; Caserotti, P.; Duranti, G.; Sabatini, S.; Parisi, P.; Parisi, A.; *et al.* Explosive type of moderate-resistance training induces functional, cardiovascular, and molecular adaptations in the elderly. *Age* **2014**, *36*, 759–772. [CrossRef] [PubMed]
53. Talha, S.; Bouitbir, J.; Charles, A.L.; Zoll, J.; Goette-Di Marco, P.; Meziani, F.; Piquard, F.; Geny, B. Pretreatment with brain natriuretic peptide reduces skeletal muscle mitochondrial dysfunction and oxidative stress after ischemia-reperfusion. *J. Appl. Phsiol.* **2013**, *114*, 172–179. [CrossRef] [PubMed]
54. Klenk, J.; Denkinger, M.; Nikolaus, T.; Peter, R.; Rothenbacher, D.; Koenig, W.; ActiFE Study Group. Association of objectively measured physical activity with established and novel cardiovascular biomarkers in elderly subjects: Every step counts. *J. Epidemiol. Community Health* **2013**, *67*, 194–197. [CrossRef] [PubMed]
55. Tanasescu, M.; Leitzmann, M.F.; Rimm, E.B.; Hu, F.B. Physical activity in relation to cardiovascular disease and total mortality among men with type 2 diabetes. *Circulation* **2003**, *107*, 2435–2439. [CrossRef] [PubMed]
56. Gregg, E.W.; Gerzoff, R.B.; Caspersen, C.J.; Williamson, D.F.; Narayan, K.M. Relationship of walking to mortality among US adults with diabetes. *Arch. Intern. Med.* **2003**, *163*, 1440–1447. [CrossRef] [PubMed]
57. Serrano-Ostáriz, E.; Legaz-Arrese, A.; Terreros-Blanco, J.L.; López-Ramón, M.; Cremades-Arroyos, D.; Carranza-García, L.E.; Izquierdo-Alvarez, S.; Bocos-Terraz, P. Cardiac biomarkers and exercise duration and intensity during a cycle-touring event. *Clin. J. Sport Med.* **2009**, *19*, 293–299. [CrossRef] [PubMed]
58. Legaz-Arrese, A.; George, K.; Carranza-García, L.E.; Munguía-Izquierdo, D.; Moros-García, T.; Serrano-Ostáriz, E. The impact of exercise intensity on the release of cardiac biomarkers in marathon runners. *Eur J. Appl. Physiol.* **2011**, *111*, 2961–2967. [CrossRef] [PubMed]
59. Serrano-Ostáriz, E.; Terreros-Blanco, J.L.; Legaz-Arrese, A.; George, K.; Shave, R.; Bocos-Terraz, P.; Izquierdo-Álvarez, S.; Bancalero, J.L.; Echavarri, J.M.; Quilez, J.; *et al.* The impact of exercise duration and intensity on the release of cardiac biomarkers. *Scand. J. Med. Sci. Sports.* **2011**, *21*, 244–249. [CrossRef] [PubMed]
60. Benda, N.M.; Eijsvogels, T.M.; Van Dijk, A.P.; Hopman, M.T.; Thijssen, D.H. Changes in BNP and cardiac troponin I after high-intensity interval and endurance exercise in heart failure patients and healthy controls. *Int. J. Cardiol.* **2015**, *184*, 426–427. [CrossRef] [PubMed]
61. Das, S.R.; Drazner, M.H.; Dries, D.L.; Vega, G.L.; Stanek, H.G.; Abdullah, S.M.; Canham, R.M.; Chung, A.K.; Leonard, D.; Wians, F.H., Jr.; *et al.* Impact of body mass and body composition on circulating levels of natriuretic peptides: Results from the Dallas Heart Study. *Circulation* **2005**, *112*, 2163–2168. [CrossRef] [PubMed]
62. Asferg, C.L.; Nielsen, S.J.; Andersen, U.B.; Linneberg, A.; Møller, D.V.; Hedley, P.L.; Christiansen, M.; Gøtze, J.P.; Jeppesen, J.L. Metabolic rather than body composition measurements are associated with lower serum natriuretic peptide concentrations in normal weight and obese men. *Am. J. Hypertens.* **2013**, *27*, 620–627. [CrossRef] [PubMed]

63. Asferg, C.L.; Nielsen, S.J.; Andersen, U.B.; Linneberg, A.; Møller, D.V.; Hedley, P.L.; Christiansen, M.; Gøtze, J.P.; Esler, M.; Jeppesen, J.L. Relative atrial natriuretic peptide deficiency and inadequate renin and angiotensin II suppression in obese hypertensive men. *Hypertension* **2013**, *62*, 147–153. [CrossRef] [PubMed]
64. Mizuno, Y.; Harada, E.; Katoh, D.; Kashiwagi, Y.; Morikawa, Y.; Nakagawa, H.; Yoshimura, M.; Saito, Y.; Yasue, H. Cardiac production of B-type natriuretic peptide is inversely related to the plasma level of free fatty acids in obese individuals-possible involvement of the insulin resistance-. *Endocr. J.* **2013**, *60*, 87–95. [CrossRef] [PubMed]

Type of Ground Surface during Plyometric Training Affects the Severity of Exercise-Induced Muscle Damage

Hamid Arazi [1,*], Roger Eston [2], Abbas Asadi [1,3], Behnam Roozbeh [1] and Alireza Saati Zarei [1]

[1] Department of Exercise Physiology, Faculty of Sport Sciences, University of Guilan, Rasht 1438, Iran; abbas_asadi1175@yahoo.com (A.A.); behnam.roozbeh@yahoo.com (B.R.); alisaati7@yahoo.com (A.S.Z.)

[2] Alliance for Research in Exercise, Nutrition and Activity; School of Health Sciences, University of South Australia, Adelaide 5000, Australia; Roger.Eston@unisa.edu.au

[3] Roudbar Branch, Islamic Azad University, Roudbar, Iran

* Correspondence: hamidarazi@yahoo.com

Academic Editor: Alessandro Pezzoli

Abstract: The purpose of this study was to compare the changes in the symptoms of exercise-induced muscle damage from a bout of plyometric exercise (PE; 10 × 10 vertical jumps) performed in aquatic, sand and firm conditions. Twenty-four healthy college-aged men were randomly assigned to one of three groups: Aquatic (AG, n = 8), Sand (SG, n = 8) and Firm (FG, n = 8). The AG performed PE in an aquatic setting with a depth of ~130 cm. The SG performed PE on a dry sand surface at a depth of 20 cm, and the FG performed PE on a 10-cm-thick wooden surface. Plasma creatine kinase (CK) activity, delayed onset muscle soreness (DOMS), knee range of motion (KROM), maximal isometric voluntary contraction (MIVC) of the knee extensors, vertical jump (VJ) and 10-m sprint were measured before and 24, 48 and 72 h after the PE. Compared to baseline values, FG showed significantly ($p < 0.05$) greater changes in CK, DOMS, and VJ at 24 until 48 h. The MIVC decreased significantly for the SG and FG at 24 until 48 h post-exercise in comparison to the pre-exercise values. There were no significant ($p > 0.05$) time or group by time interactions in KROM. In the 10-m sprint, all the treatment groups showed significant ($p < 0.05$) changes compared to pre-exercise values at 24 h, and there were no significant ($p > 0.05$) differences between groups. The results indicate that PE in an aquatic setting and on a sand surface induces less muscle damage than on a firm surface. Therefore, training in aquatic conditions and on sand may be beneficial for the improvement of performance, with a concurrently lower risk of muscle damage and soreness.

Keywords: plyometric exercise; aquatic setting; sand surface; muscle soreness

1. Introduction

Lower body plyometric training involves performing repeated consecutive jumping-type exercises with one's own body weight against gravity. Plyometric training is widely used to enhance the ability of skeletal muscles to generate power. The method involves a repeated series of bouts with each comprising a rapid deceleration of the body, followed immediately by a brief transition phase and rapid acceleration in the opposite direction [1–3]. This rapid combination of eccentric and concentric muscular activity involves the stretch-shortening cycle (SSC), which provides a physiological advantage in that the muscular force developed during the concentric phase is potentiated by the preceding eccentric contraction [1]. The use of plyometric training results in the improvement of vertical jumping ability (VJ) [2–4], strength [2,4], agility [3], sprint [3,4], balance [5] and running economy [6]. However, the eccentric contractions involved in plyometrics have been shown to induce skeletal-muscle trauma resulting in exercise-induced muscle damage (EIMD) [5–11]. Indeed, plyometric exercise (PE) in the form of vertical countermovement jumps on a solid surface is frequently used in studies as a means of inducing EIMD in the knee extensors [9–13]. Frequently observed symptoms of EIMD include muscle soreness [4,10,13], an increase in plasma creatine kinase activity (CK) [12,14,15], loss of strength [10,13] and power [5,14] and a reduction in joint range of motion (ROM) [15–19]. These effects begin approximately 6 h after exercise, peak at 24–72 h and subside four to seven days after exercise [11–14,19].

An important consideration regarding the impact of PE on EIMD is the nature of the training surface. Implementation of plyometric training in an aquatic setting has been observed to induce less EIMD and muscle soreness than plyometric training on a firm surface, but with the same improvements in muscular performance [4,20]. An aquatic setting provides a low-impact medium that produces less strain on muscles, bones and connective tissue. An aquatic environment also provides buoyancy which reduces weight-bearing stress on the limbs and thus reduces the impact forces and the potential trauma to the joints, thereby providing a therapeutic modality for reducing muscle soreness and pain [2,4,20]. Less EIMD is observed after similar plyometric activity on a sand surface compared to a firm, wooden surface. Robinson *et al.* [4] attributed the lower muscle soreness in the aquatic *versus* the land plyometric group to less strain on the musculoskeletal system. Similarly, as a sand surface is associated with a greater degree of shock absorbance and lower stress to soft tissue and bones of the lower limbs during PE [20,21]. The compliant nature of the sand surface plays a critical role for decreasing landing force and the absorptive qualities of sand are likely to decrease stress on the lower limbs, resulting in less muscle damage than that obtained on a firm surface [19,21,22].

Although several studies have explored how the impact of plyometric training on EIMD is affected by the nature of the landing and take-off surface, such as sand against grass [22], sand against wood [19] and aquatic against wood [4], no study has directly compared aquatic, sand and firm conditions in relation to muscle damage and the sense of effort in performing a similar number of plyometric jumps. It is important to understand the differences in response to PE among aquatic, sand and firm surfaces, since many assumptions have been made from studies using different surfaces that have reported the important effects of landing surface for reducing muscle damage with regard to the nature of surface. The present study used consecutive vertical jumps performed on aquatic, sand and firm surfaces as a model to investigate the influence of surface on EIMD. We hypothesized that PE would disturb indirect markers of muscle damage, increase muscle soreness and plasma creatine kinase activity for days after exercise and that this disturbance would be attenuated for the aquatic and sand surfaces.

2. Methods

2.1. Study Design

Three groups of male college students performed a series of vertical jumps (VJ) on either a dry sand surface, a dry wooden surface or a ceramic tiled surface in aquatic conditions. The aquatic group (AG) performed PE in a swimming pool with water at a depth of 130 cm (chest-deep) and a temperature of 28 °C; the sand group (SG) performed PE on a dry surface of 20-cm-deep sand and the firm surface group (FG) performed PE on a 10-cm-thick wood surface. Indirect markers of muscle damage (plasma creatine kinase activity, range of motion, isometric strength, muscle soreness, vertical jump height and sprint speed) were assessed at baseline, and 24, 48 and 72 h after the PE protocol. All risks associated with the experimental procedures were explained prior to involvement in the study and each participant was asked to complete a written informed consent form and a medical health questionnaire before assessment. Procedures and the study were conducted in accordance with ethical standards in sport and exercise science research [23] and approved by the Local Ethics Committee.

2.2. Participants

Twenty-four healthy untrained young men, who were familiar with plyometric exercise training but who had not performed this type of exercises for at least six months prior to the study, volunteered for the study. All participants were free from injury. Prior to recruitment, participants were asked about their activity levels. Those who performed any lower extremity resistive exercise/eccentric resistive exercise were excluded from the study. Prior to the initial testing, each participant was familiarized with the testing protocol and completed a full practice testing session and plyometric exercise. After this familiarization session, each participant was tested on four separate occasions using identical protocols at 24 h before starting exercise, and 24, 48 and 72 h post plyometric exercise. After baseline testing, participants were randomly assigned to three treatment groups; AG ($N = 8$, age 20.2 ± 0.4 y, height 180.5 ± 4.2 cm, body mass 73.3 ± 7.1 kg), SG ($N = 8$, age 20.3 ± 0.7 y, height 177.8 ± 6.6 cm, body mass 67.8 ± 9.5 kg), and FG ($N = 8$, age 20.7 ± 0.4 y, height 180.1 ± 5.5 cm, body mass 71.7 ± 9.6 kg). *A priori* calculations of statistical power indicated that this sample size was appropriate to satisfy power at or above 80% [24]. Participants performed PE barefoot, because (a) most sports activities on sand and in aquatic setting are performed without shoes, and (b) it is easier to compare differences in responses among conditions by eliminating the effect of shoes. The investigators carefully supervised the exercise to eliminate the risks of unexpected injury. Participants abstained from any strenuous physical activity for at least 15 days before and after the experimental period. Participants were instructed to maintain their normal eating pattern for two weeks before data collection and during the investigation. Participants were not taking any medication or dietary supplements with anti-inflammatory action for six months before the study.

2.3. Plyometric Exercise Protocol

All participants performed 10 sets of 10 maximal vertical jumps, interspersed with a one-minute recovery between each set. Immediately prior to starting the exercise, a maximal vertical jump was performed with a chalk mark made by the fingertips at the highest point of the jump. The participants were instructed to perform each jump with maximal effort to reach the target height and the authors encouraged the participants to reach the mark. On landing, participants were instructed to adopt a knee joint angle of ~90°. This protocol has been used successfully to induce EIMD in previous studies [11,12].

2.4. Dependent Variables

Indirect markers of muscle damage were plasma creatine kinase (CK) activity, delayed onset muscle soreness (DOMS), knee flexion range of motion (KROM), maximal isometric voluntary contraction (MIVC) of the knee extensors, vertical jump height (VJ) and 10-m sprint time. The rating of perceived exertion (RPE) was also assessed after each set of the plyometric exercise. One week prior to commencement of the study, the participants attended the laboratory for the familiarization of testing procedures. During this session the participants performed three to four trials of each test to eliminate any potential learning effect.

2.5. Plasma Creatine Kinase Activity (CK)

Blood samples were drawn (10 mL) from the antecubital vein into plain evacuated test tubes. The blood was allowed to clot at room temperature for 30 min and centrifuged at 1500× g for 10 min. The serum layer was removed and frozen at −20 °C in multiple aliquots for further analyses. Plasma CK activity was determined spectrophotometrically (Milton Roy, Spectronic 401, Rochester, NY, USA) in duplicates using a commercially available kit (Autoanalyzer, Technicon RA-1000, Clackamas, OR, USA). The normal reference range of CK activity for men using this method is 40–195 U/L. The intra-assay coefficient of variation was 8.5% for CK.

2.6. Delayed Onset Muscle Soreness (DOMS)

Each participant was asked to indicate muscle soreness (DOMS) of the knee extensors using a visual analogue scale. The scale was numbered from 1 to 10 (on the reverse side of the sliding scale) with 1 indicating no muscle soreness and 10 signifying that the muscle was very, very sore to move. With hands on hips and squatting to an approximate knee angle of 90°, volunteers were asked to indicate the level of perceived soreness based on the rating scale. This corresponded to the location of perceived muscle soreness on the continuum. This technique has been used successfully in previous studies [11,16]. The reliability coefficient for a repetitive measurement in DOMS was 0.98.

2.7. Knee Flexion Range of Motion (KROM)

The knee flexion range of motion (KROM) testing protocol has been previously described by Clarkson [25]. From a prone-lying position, participants were asked to perform full active flexion of the knee of the right leg. The knee joint angle was measured between the lateral epicondyle of the femur, lateral malleous of the fibula and greater trochanter using a goniometer (Lafayette Instrument Company, Lafayette, IN, USA). These bony landmarks were marked on the initial day of testing with a semi-permanent pen to ensure consistency on subsequent days. The mean of two measurements was used for data analysis. Reliability coefficient for repetitive measurements in KROM was 0.99.

2.8. Maximal Isometric Voluntary Contraction (MIVC)

Maximal isometric voluntary contraction (MIVC) of the quadriceps was assessed at a joint angle of 70° of flexion using a JAMAR® dynamometer (Back-Leg-Chest Dynamometer, Model 68815, Gays Mills, WI, USA) because Byrne *et al.* [26] suggest the optimal knee angle for isometric knee extensor torque is 60°–80°. The joint position was marked on the initial day of testing with a semi-permanent pen to ensure consistency during subsequent testing sessions. Participants were given a total of two trials with maximal effort and each repetition lasted 3 s and was interspersed with 60 s of rest. The best value was collected for the further analyses [15,19]. Reliability coefficient for repetitive measurements in MIVC was 0.93.

2.9. Vertical Jump (VJ)

The vertical jump (VJ) was assessed using a Vertec (Power Systems, Knoxville, Tennessee, TN, USA). The Vertec was adjusted to match the height of the individual participant by having him stand with the dominant side to the base of the testing device. The dominant hand was raised and the Vertec was adjusted so that the hand was the appropriate distance away from the marker based on markings on the device itself. VJ was performed from a squatting position with a knee joint angle of ~90°. Participants were asked to hold this position for three seconds, then jump upward in an attempt to reach the maximal height with no countermovement after a verbal command of "Go". Each test was performed twice, and the best value of the two measurements was used for the analysis [9]. Reliability coefficient for repetitive measurements in VJ was 0.95.

2.10. The 10-m Sprint

Participants performed two sets of a single 10-m sprint from a standing start on an indoor track with a 3-min recovery. Prior to commencing the test, participants performed two sub-maximal jogs. Sprint time was recorded using two electronic photo cells positioned at 0 (start) and 10 m (JBL Systems, Oslo, Norway). Time for sprint performance was recorded to the nearest 0.01 s via telemetry to a handheld system. The fastest time recorded was used for analysis [11]. Reliability coefficient for repetitive measurements in 10-m sprint was 0.96.

2.11. *Rating of Perceived Exertion (RPE)*

The rating of perceived exertion (RPE) using the Borg 6-20 RPE Scale [27] was recorded immediately following each set of jumps. After the final repetition of each set, participants were reminded to think about feelings of exertion in the active muscle group, in accordance with previous procedures [28].

2.12. *Statistical Analysis*

Data are presented as mean ± SD. Data normality was checked and verified with the Shapiro-Wilk test. As the CK activity data were found not to be normally distributed, the values were log-transformed before statistical analysis [11,18,29]. Following transformation the CK activity data were normally distributed. A repeated-measures ANOVA (3 × 4, group × time) was used to analyze data (SPSS 16.0). Assumptions of sphericity were assessed using Mauchly's test of sphericity, with any violations adjusted by use of the Greenhouse-Geisser(GG) correction. To assess changes in RPE between sets, a 3 (group) × 10 (set) ANOVA was applied to the data. When a significant F value was achieved, a Tukey *post hoc* test was used to detect differences in the measures. Significance was set at $p \leqslant 0.05$.

3. Results

3.1. *CK Activity*

There was a significant increase in CK activity after the plyometric exercise protocol for all groups, with CK values peaking at 24 h for each group ($p < 0.01$). There was a significant group × time interaction, which indicated a greater increase in CK for FG than for SG and AG ($p \leqslant 0.05$) at 24 h, which remained higher than baseline at 72 h (Figure 1A).

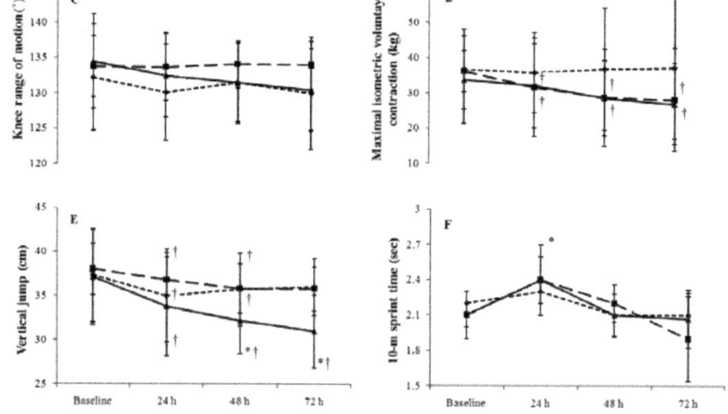

Figure 1. Mean ± SD for creatine kinase (CK) activity (**A**), delayed onset muscle soreness (DOMS) (**B**), knee flexion range of motion (**C**), maximal isometric voluntary contraction (**D**), vertical jump (**E**) and 10-m sprint (**F**) at baseline and 24–72 h following 100 plyometric jumps. AG: Aquatic group; SG: Sand group; FG: Firm group. *: Significant difference compared to AG and SG ($p \leqslant 0.05$); †: Significant difference compared to baseline ($p \leqslant 0.05$).

3.2. *Muscle Soreness*

There was a significant group × time interaction which indicated significantly greater soreness in the FG compared to the AG and SG at 24 and 48 h post-exercise ($p \leqslant 0.05$). Compared with baseline data, muscle soreness was greater at 24 and 48 h for FG and at 24 h for SG. There was no significant change in soreness for the AG (Figure 1B).

3.3. *Knee Range of Motion (KROM)*

No statistically significant changes in knee range of motion were observed after plyometric exercises in the experimental groups ($p > 0.05$) (Figure 1C).

3.4. *Maximal Isometric Voluntary Contraction (MIVC)*

No statistically significant group × time interactions in muscle strength were observed after plyometric exercises, although changes across time were significance for the FG and SG ($p \leqslant 0.05$) (Figure 1D).

3.5. *Vertical Jump*

All treatment groups showed a significant decrease in VJ at 24 and 48 h post-exercise ($p < 0.01$). There was also a significant group × time interaction ($p < 0.01$). Follow-up analysis indicated that the decrease in vertical jump height was similar for the AG and SG, whereas the decrease in VJ was greater for the FG at 48 h and remained lower at 72 h following the plyometric exercise protocol (Figure 1E).

3.6. *10-m Sprint Times*

The peak running time over 10 m was significantly higher following plyometric exercises in all groups ($p < 0.01$). There was no significant group × time interaction. *Post hoc* analysis showed that the sprint time at 24 hours was significantly higher than baseline values before returning to baseline levels at 48 h (Figure 1F).

4. Rating of Perceived Exertion (RPE)

Table 1 shows the changes in RPE following each set of VJ exercises. The RPE increased progressively throughout the plyometric VJ testing ($p < 0.01$). There was no significant group main effect, and no group × set interaction. *Post hoc* analysis showed that set 4 was perceived to be harder than set 1, and set 5 harder than set 2, and sets 9 and 10 were harder than set 7.

Table 1. Mean ± SD for rating of perceived exertion after each set of VJ exercise.

Group	Sets									
	1	2	3	4 *	5 †	6	7	8	9 ‡	10 ‡
AG	8.25 ± 2.3	9 ± 2.3	9.1 ± 2.1	9.7 ± 2	10.8 ± 2.2	10.6 ± 2	11.2 ± 2.1	11.8 ± 1.8	12.7 ± 2.1	13.5 ± 2.1
SG	7.5 ± 0.9	8.5 ± 0.7	9.3 ± 1.1	10.3 ± 1.9	10.8 ± 2.1	11.7 ± 2.6	12.3 ± 2.6	12.8 ± 2.9	13.3 ± 2	14.1 ± 2
FG	7.1 ± 0.8	7 ± 1.4	8.62 ± 1.8	8.8 ± 2.1	9.1 ± 2.4	9.8 ± 2.8	10.5 ± 2.8	11 ± 3	11.2 ± 3.4	12 ± 3.8

AG: Aquatic group; SG: Sand group; FG: Firm group. *: Significant difference compared to set 1 ($p \leqslant 0.05$); †: Significant difference compared to set 2 ($p \leqslant 0.05$); ‡: Significant difference compared to set 7 ($p \leqslant 0.05$).

5. Discussion

Plyometrics is a form of explosive physical training that is used to enhance power output, force production and velocity [2–4]. This type of training has been shown to induce skeletal-muscle damage [7–14]. Although a number of studies have assessed the effects of plyometric exercise on indirect indices of muscle damage (*i.e.*, VJ, strength, sprint, ROM and agility) [7–14,16,18,19], limited knowledge exists regarding how the extent of damage and post-exercise recovery is moderated by the type of surface. To the authors' knowledge, this is the first study that has directly compared the symptoms of EIMD between aquatic, sand and firm surface conditions. Overall, we found that the symptoms of EIMD were greater for the participants in the firm surface group (FG), while the changes in indices of muscle damage were generally significantly smaller for the AG.

6. Evidence of Muscle Damage

This research has shown that an intense, acute bout of PE (10 × 10 VJs) increased plasma CK activity and DOMS at 24–72 h post-exercise for the FG and the SG. The changes in CK were consistent with those observed following plyometric exercises with values peaking at 24 h after the damaging exercise in the firm and sand conditions [17,30,31]. Perceived soreness (DOMS) was also increased above the baseline value following muscle-damaging exercise, with peak values occurring at 48 h for participants in the SG and at 24 h for the FG. These findings mirror those of previous research, which has demonstrated increases in muscle soreness peaking between 24 and 48 h [9,12,14,30,31]. Previous investigations have suggested that PE on a firm wooden surface may induce muscle damage because of the forces produced during ground impact and the associated eccentric contractions [14,16] and this damage is greater in the type II muscle and Z-line [30,31]. To resist the impact of landing, the quadriceps muscles perform an eccentric action that involves a counter-extension movement to absorb kinetic energy. During the negative phase of PE, eccentric activation produces higher tension per cross-sectional area of active muscle mass compared with concentric actions, resulting in significant structural muscle damage [16]. Compared with the aquatic group, the FG indicated higher perception of muscle soreness (~4 *vs.* 1) and a greater level of plasma CK activity. These results provide further confirmation that PE in waist-deep water provides a safer environment and reduces impact on the joints and muscles due to the buoyancy effect which appears to reduce the extent of musculoskeletal trauma and damage [4,19].

In addition, we observed a limited development of muscle soreness for the SG at 48 h. The lack of change in muscle soreness may be associated with the execution of the PE on a soft surface (sand and/or aquatic) because it is known that performing plyometrics on a soft surface induces less muscle damage than a firm surface [4,19]. The compliance and instability of the sand results in a reduction of maximum force and landing force during plyometrics, resulting in less muscle damage and soreness compared to the firm surface condition [21,22]. On the other hand, performing PE in an aquatic setting could provide a non-impact medium that reduces stress on the lower limbs, providing a therapeutic modality for reducing muscle soreness and damage [2,4,20]. Similarly, the absorptive qualities of the sand surface during PE decreased stress on the lower limbs, resulting in less muscle damage than that on firm surface [19,21,22].

7. Muscle Function during Recovery from Plyometric Exercise

Although several studies have examined the effects of PE on muscle function, to our knowledge, this is the first attempt to examine the effects of different surfaces during plyometrics on muscle function. In this study, we measured muscle function using knee range of motion (KROM), maximal isometric voluntary contraction (MIVC), vertical jump (VJ) and 10-m sprint time. The decreases in MIVC and VJ height and increase in sprint time after PE are supported by previous investigations [9,14,29]. In our study, one of the indices of muscle performance (KROM) did not change. In contrast to our finding which indicates no statistically significant changes in KROM, Chatzinikolaou *et al.* [16] reported KROM decline for 48 h after PE. However, in accordance with this finding, Tofas *et al.* [14] did not find any significant changes in the KROM following PE. Since the muscle soreness (DOMS) and edema increase after PE [16] and this condition led to a decrease KROM, this limited DOMS (between 1 and 4, Figure 1B) response coincides with the lack of changes in KROM. However, the possible explanation for these discrepancies may be attributed to different modes of KROM assessment.

Strength performance loss after EIMD is one of the common indicators of muscle trauma [7,8,19]. In this study, we measured isometric strength and found incremental decreases in MIVC for the FG and SG. In the previous studies by Tofas *et al.* [14] and Chatzinikolaou *et al.* [16], the authors reported no significant changes in the isometric and isokinetic torque at knee extensors after the PE protocol. The variation in results between these studies could be different modes and knee angles in leg strength assessment. It has been suggested that following PE, voluntary activation might be impaired as a result of increased muscle pain and tenderness, leading to a reduction in neural drive to the muscle [32]. Hence, it is possible that a reduced voluntary effort was manifested as a reduction in maximal strength. In addition, several researchers reported the loss of concentric, isometric and eccentric strength after EIMD [33,34], which would undoubtedly exacerbate the stretch-shortening capabilities of the muscle and result in an increased contact time. The observations in this further confirm that EIMD not only impairs maximal strength but also impairs VJ height.

With regard to VJ height following the PE protocol, it is notable that the AG and SG returned to baseline level at 72 h post-exercise, whereas VJ height remained significantly lower at 72 h for the FG. A number of studies have observed that EIMD causes prolonged reductions in jump performance [6,10,12,16]. The decline in VJ performance is attributed to the inflammatory response to muscle damage [16]. This suggests that damaged muscle has a reduced tolerance to impact forces during movements involving the stretch-shortening cycle, resulting in decreases in VJ height. Impaired muscle glycogen resynthesis following EIMD is also well documented [35]. It is therefore possible that a reduced glycogen content in the knee extensors may have contributed to the decrease in muscle function and power output observed by the decrease in VJ performance. Another possible explanation for the decrement in VJ height after muscle-damaging exercise could be muscle soreness [33], muscular pain experienced as a result of the EIMD-reduced participant's tolerance to exercise, protecting the muscle against further injury with a reduced neural drive to the muscle [36–38]. The disruption of normal neural function following muscle damage has been associated with the subsequent inhibition of muscle function and it has previously been considered that perceptions of soreness may serve as a protective mechanism following damaging exercise to prevent full muscle activation from exacerbating damage and this consequently leads to VJ height decrement [19,37,38].

Studies have also shown a reduced excitation-contraction (E-C) coupling efficiency due to a reduction in calcium release per action potential, which has been associated with a decrease in maximal force production for several days following PE [35,38]. Therefore, a reduction in the force-generating capability due to E-C coupling failure would reduce the ability of the muscle to produce power. It is plausible that repeated stretching of the quadriceps during plyometric jumping may have led to preferential disruption of type II muscle fibers, as a result of early fatigue and temporary increases in muscle stiffness caused within these fibers by the eccentric component of the plyometric exercise [39].

Sprint times in the SG and FG significantly increased at 24 h and recovered to baseline completely at 72 h after PE, whereas no significant change was observed for the AG. These findings are consistent with previous studies [11,40] which reported that linear sprint running time over 10 m was significantly reduced by ~3% following 100 VJs on a rigid surface. In contrast, Semark and coworkers [41] reported that completing 70 drop jumps did not significantly impair 10-m sprint running performance, although evidence of greater muscle damage is presented in the present study. There was no significant change in 10-m sprint time for the AG. It appears that plyometric exercises in an aquatic setting do not seem to impair sprint performance, which may be attributed to the lower-impact forces experienced within the buoyant environment of the aquatic condition.

Overall, the results of this study indicated that PE in water provided a low-impact medium that produced less stress in the lower limbs and the buoyancy properties of the water reduced weight-bearing stress on the limbs and consequently reduced the muscle soreness and damage in addition to lesser decrements in performance capacity [2,4]. Furthermore, the high-shock absorptive qualities of sand could decrease the impact forces experienced during PE, potentially to reduce muscle damage and soreness, in addition to lesser decreases in maximal-intensity exercise performance tests [21,22,42,43]. Therefore, aquatic and sand environments might be considered as viable options for recovery and rehabilitation for the plyometric training sessions.

In contrast to the positive effects of sand and aquatic conditions in reducing muscle damage and soreness following PE, it appears that training on these surfaces has negative effects on SSC [44]. On the other hand, the friction and instability of sand may induce negative effects on SSC, decreases in myotatic reflex, degradation of elastic energy potentiation and an increase in the amortization phase, resulting performance decrements [21,44]. Similarly, water resistance plays an important role in decreasing the properties of SSC by increasing the time period between eccentric-to-concentric muscle action, deficits in SSC capability, and loss of elastic energy resulting in decreases in performance [20]. However, future studies should investigate the safety of prolonged plyometric training on sand and in water, because joint injury and overuse may occur after longitudinal plyometric training. Although the magnitude of muscle damage is less for PE performed on sand and in water than for that on wood surfaces, it does not necessarily mean that sand and aquatic surfaces are preferable for training. Although the preliminary results of the present study suggest that plyometric training on sand and in water may be potentially useful, the biomechanical characteristics of jumping may increase the risk of overuse injuries to the low back. Also, consideration should be given to how the difference in surface affects the training effect. The specific type of exercise being performed should be considered when choosing a training surface, remembering that plyometric drills may require a firm surface.

8. Perceived Exertion

The RPE increased progressively from set 1 to set 10 for all treatment groups, These findings are in line with Brown and coworkers [28], who examined the effects of eight sets of 10 repetitions of depth jumps from an 80-cm box on RPE and reported progressive increases in RPE during PE from ~11 to ~17 for college-aged men. In the present study, it is interesting to note that there was no statistical difference between groups in the rate of increase in the RPE, which indicates that the degree of exertion and fatigue experienced within the three conditions was similar.

The current study compared aquatic, sand and firm (wood) surfaces for the development of muscle damage and soreness following EIMD (10 × 10 VJs). Changes in the indirect markers of muscle damage (*i.e.*, CK activity, VJ, sprint, KROM and strength) were generally smaller following the PE in the aquatic setting and sand when compared with that performed on the firm surface. High-impact forces in the order of three to four times the body weight can occur during PE on a rigid surface. These high, transient forces impact the musculoskeletal system and can induce acute muscle soreness, muscle damage and even musculoskeletal injuries. Landing on a compliant sand surface will increase the extent of shock absorbance, and consequently decrease the stress to soft tissues and bones of the lower limbs during PE, compared to the same exercise on rigid surface. An aquatic setting can provide a safer environment in which impact is minimized, but the sense of effort experienced is similar to that experienced doing plyometric activity on dry land. The limitations of this study include the low number of subjects, which prevents generalization of the results. Additionally, the results of the current investigation are based on a non-sporting population, and further research is needed to determine if similar effects are obtained in the sporting population. The results of this investigation therefore suggest that PE performed in an aquatic setting and on a sand surface is less stressful to the muscle-tendon complex than when compared to a firm surface, and this may have implications for rehabilitation and in the prevention of musculoskeletal injury. Thus, it can be recommend that coaches and strength and conditioning professionals use safe surfaces for plyometric exercises and training to decrease symptoms of muscle damage; however, they must remember that plyometric drills may require a firm surface. Moreover, there is no financial support for this project and we did not measure some of the blood indicators of muscle damage, biopsy and MRI, which can be a subject for further research.

Acknowledgments: We gratefully acknowledge the participants involved in this study.

Author Contributions: H.A. conceived and designed the experiments; B.R. and A.S.Z performed the experiments; A.A. analyzed the data and R.E. helped for the statistical analysis; B.R. and A.S.Z. contributed reagents/materials/analysis tools; H.A., A.A. and R.E. wrote the paper and responses to reviewers' comments.

Conflicts of Interest: The authors declare no conflict of interest.

References

1. Potach, D.; Chu, D.A. Plyometric training. In *Essential of Strength and Conditioning*; Bachle, T., Erale, R., Eds.; Human Kinetic: Champaign, IL, USA, 2000; pp. 135–141.
2. Arazi, H.; Asadi, A. The effect of aquatic and land plyometric training on strength, sprint, and balance in young basketball players. *J. Hum. Sport Exerc.* **2011**, *6*, 101–111. [CrossRef]
3. Asadi, A.; Arazi, H. Effects of high-intensity plyometric training on dynamic balance, agility, vertical jump and sprint performance in young male basketball players. *J. Sport Health Res.* **2012**, *4*, 34–44.
4. Robinson, L.E.; Décor, S.T.; Merrick, M.A.; Buckworth, J. The effects of land *vs.* aquatic plyometrics on power, torque, velocity, and muscle soreness in women. *J. Strength Cond. Res.* **2004**, *18*, 84–91. [PubMed]
5. Asadi, A.; Saez de Villarreal, E.; Arazi, H. The effects of plyometric type neuromuscular training on postural control performance of male team basketball players. *J. Strength Cond. Res.* **2015**, *29*, 1870–1875. [CrossRef] [PubMed]
6. Turner, A.M.; Owings, M.; Schwane, J.A. Improvement in running economy after 6 weeks of plyometric training. *J. Strength Cond. Res.* **2003**, *17*, 60–67. [PubMed]
7. Byrne, C.; Twist, C.; Eston, R.G. Neuromuscular function after exercise-induced muscle damage: Theoretical and applied implications. *Sports Med.* **2004**, *34*, 49–69. [CrossRef] [PubMed]
8. Eston, R.G.; Byrne, C.; Twist, C. Muscle function after exercise-induced muscle damage: Considerations for athletic performance in children and adults. *J. Exerc. Sci. Fit.* **2003**, *1*, 85–96.
9. Jakeman, J.R.; Byrne, C.; Eston, R.G. Lower limb compression garment improves recovery from exercise-induced muscle damage in young, active females. *Eur. J. Appl. Physiol.* **2010**, *109*, 1137–1144. [CrossRef] [PubMed]
10. Marginson, V.; Rowland, A.V.; Gleeson, N.P.; Eston, R.G. Comparison of the symptoms of exercise-induced muscle damage after an initial and repeated bout of plyometric exercise in men and boys. *J. Appl. Physiol.* **2005**, *99*, 1174–1181. [CrossRef] [PubMed]
11. Twist, C.; Eston, R.G. The effects of exercise-induced muscle damage on maximal intensity intermittent exercise performance. *Eur. J. Appl. Physiol.* **2005**, *94*, 652–658. [CrossRef] [PubMed]
12. Twist, C.; Eston, R.G. The effect of muscle-damaging exercise on maximal intensity cycling and drop jump performance. *J. Exerc. Sci. Fit* **2007**, *5*, 79–87.
13. Twist, C.; Eston, R.G. The effect of exercise-induced muscle damage on perceived exertion and cycling endurance performance. *Eur. J. Appl. Physiol.* **2009**, *105*, 559–567. [CrossRef] [PubMed]
14. Tofas, T.; Jumurtas, A.Z.; Fatouros, I.; Nikolaidis, M.G.; Koutedakis, Y.; Sinouris, E.A.; Papageorgakopoulou, N.; Theochathios, D.A. Plyometric exercise increases serum indices of muscle damage and collagen breakdown. *J. Strength Cond. Res.* **2008**, *22*, 490–496. [CrossRef] [PubMed]
15. Byrne, C.; Eston, R.G. The effects of exercise-induced muscle damage on isometric and dynamic knee extensor strength and vertical jump performance. *J. Sports Sci.* **2002**, *20*, 417–425. [CrossRef] [PubMed]
16. Chatzinikolaou, A.; Fatouros, I.G.; Gourgoulis, V.; Avloniti, A.; Jamurtas, A.Z.; Nikolaidis, M.G.; Douroudos, I.; Michailidis, Y.; Beneka, A.; Malliou, P.; *et al.* Time course of changes in performance and inflammatory responses after acute plyometric exercise. *J. Strength Cond. Res.* **2010**, *24*, 1389–1398. [CrossRef] [PubMed]
17. Chen, T.C.; Chen, H.-L.; Wu, C.-J.; Lin, M.-R.; Chen, C.-H.; Wang, L.-L.; Wang, S.-Y.; Tu, J.-H. Changes in running economy following a repeated bout of downhill running. *J. Exerc. Sci. Fit.* **2007**, *5*, 109–117. [CrossRef]
18. Eston, R.G.; Peters, D. Effects of cold water immersion on the symptoms of exercise-induced muscle damage. *J. Sports Sci.* **1999**, *17*, 231–238. [CrossRef] [PubMed]
19. Miyama, M.; Nosaka, K. Influence of surface on muscle damage and soreness induced by consecutive drop jumps. *J. Strength Cond. Res.* **2004**, *18*, 206–211. [PubMed]
20. Martel, G.F.; Harmer, M.L.; Logan, J.M.; Parker, C.B. Aquatic plyometric training increases vertical jump in female volleyball players. *Med. Sci. Sports Exerc.* **2005**, *37*, 1814–1819. [CrossRef] [PubMed]
21. Barrett, R.S.; Neal, R.J.; Roberts, L.J. The dynamic loading response of surfaces encountered in beach running. *J. Sci. Med. Sport* **1997**, *1*, 1–11. [CrossRef]

22. Impellizzeri, F.M.; Rampinini, E.; Castagna, C.; Martino, F.; Fiorini, S.; Wisloff, U. Effect of plyometric training on sand *versus* grass on muscle soreness and jumping and sprinting ability in soccer players. *Br. J. Sports Med.* **2008**, *42*, 42–46. [CrossRef] [PubMed]
23. Harriss, D.J.; Atkinson, G. Ethical standards in sport and exercise science research. *Int. J. Sports Med.* **2011**, *32*, 819–821. [CrossRef] [PubMed]
24. Faul, F.; Erdfelder, E.; Lang, A.G.; Buchner, A. G*Power 3, a flexible statistical power analysis program for the social, behavioural and biomedical sciences. *Behav. Res. Methods* **2007**, *39*, 175–191. [CrossRef] [PubMed]
25. Clarkson, H.M. *Joint Motion and Function Assessment*; Lippincott Williams & Wilkins: Philadelphia, PA, USA, 2005; pp. 177–178.
26. Byrne, C.; Eston, R.G.; Edwards, R.H.T. Characteristics of isometric and dynamic strength loss following eccentric exercise-induced muscle damage. *Scan. J. Med. Sci. Sports* **2003**, *11*, 134–140. [CrossRef]
27. Borg, G. *Borg's Perceived Exertion and Pain Scales*; Human Kinetics: Leeds, UK, 1998.
28. Brown, A.G.; Ray, M.W.; Abbey, B.M.; Shaw, B.S.; Shaw, I. Oxygen consumption, heart rate, and blood lactate responses to an acute bout of plyometric depth jumps in college-aged men and women. *J. Strength Cond. Res.* **2010**, *24*, 2475–2482. [CrossRef] [PubMed]
29. Davies, R.C.; Eston, R.G.; Poole, D.C.; Rowlands, A.V.; Dimenna, F.; Wilkerson, D.P.; Jones, A.M. The effect of eccentric exercise induced muscle damage on the dynamics of muscle oxygenation and pulmonary oxygen uptake. *J. Appl. Physiol.* **2008**, *105*, 1413–1421. [CrossRef] [PubMed]
30. Macaluso, F.; Isaacs, A.W.; Myburgh, K.H. Preferntial type II muscle fiber damage from plyometric exercise. *J. Athl. Train.* **2012**, *47*, 414–420. [PubMed]
31. Macaluso, F.; Isaacs, A.W.; di Felice, V.; Myburgh, K.H. Acute change of titin at mid-sarcomer remains despite 8 wk of plyometric training. *J. Appl. Physiol.* **2014**, *116*, 1512–1519. [CrossRef] [PubMed]
32. Byrne, C.; Eston, R.G. Maximal-intensity isometric and dynamic exercise performance after eccentric muscle actions. *J. Sports Sci.* **2002**, *20*, 951–959. [CrossRef] [PubMed]
33. Hortobágyi, T.; Houmard, J.; Fraser, D.; Dudek, R.; Lambert, J.; Tracy, J. Normal forces and myofibrillar disruption after repeated eccentric exercise. *J. Appl. Physiol.* **1998**, *84*, 492–498. [PubMed]
34. Costill, D.L.; Pascoe, D.D.; Fink, W.J. Impaired muscle glycogen synthesis after eccentric exercise. *J. Appl. Physiol.* **1990**, *69*, 46–50. [PubMed]
35. Ingalls, C.P.; Warren, G.L.; Williams, J.H.; Ward, C.W.; Armstrong, R.B. E-C coupling failure in mouse EDL muscle after *in vivo* eccentric contractions. *J. Appl. Physiol.* **1999**, *85*, 58–67.
36. Avela, J.; Kyrolainen, H.; Komi, P.V.; Rama, D. Reduced reflex sensivity persists several days after long-lasting stretch-shortening cycle exercise. *J. Appl. Physiol.* **1999**, *86*, 1292–1300. [PubMed]
37. Komi, P.V. Stretch-shortening cycle: A powerful model to study normal and fatigued muscle. *J. Biomech.* **2000**, *33*, 1197–1206. [CrossRef]
38. Warren, G.L.; Lowe, D.A.; Hayes, D.A.; Farmer, M.A.; Armstrong, R.B. Excitation failure in eccentric contraction-induced injury of mouse soleus muscle. *J. Appl. Physiol.* **1993**, *68*, 487–490. [CrossRef]
39. Brockett, C.L.; Morgan, D.L.; Gregory, J.E.; Proske, U. Damage in different types of motor units following repeated active lengthening of the medial gastrocnemius muscle of the cat. *J. Appl. Physiol.* **2002**, *92*, 1104–1110. [CrossRef] [PubMed]
40. Highton, J.M.; Twist, C.; Eston, R.G. The effects of exercise-induced muscle damage on agility and sprint running performance. *J. Exerc. Sci. Fit.* **2009**, *7*, 24–30. [CrossRef]
41. Semark, A.; Noakes, T.D.; St Clair Gibson, A.; Lambert, M.I. The effect of a prophylactic dose of flurbiprofen on muscle soreness and sprinting performance in trained subjects. *J. Sports Sci.* **1999**, *17*, 197–203. [CrossRef] [PubMed]
42. Binnie, M.J.; Dawson, B.; Pinnington, H.; Landers, G.; Peeling, P. Sand training: A review of current research and practical applications. *J. Sports Sci.* **2014**, *32*, 8–15. [CrossRef] [PubMed]

43. Binnie, M.J.; Dawson, B.; Arnot, M.A.; Pinnington, H.; Landers, G.; Peeling, P. Effect of sand *versus* grass training syrfaces during an 8-week pre-season conditioning programme in team sport athletes. *J. Sports Sci.* **2014**, *32*, 1001–1012. [CrossRef] [PubMed]
44. Mirzaei, B.; Norasteh, A.; Saez de Villarreal, E.; Asadi, A. Effects of 6 weeks of depth jump *vs.* countermovement jump training on sand on muscle soreness and performance. *Kinesiology* **2014**, *46*, 97–108.

5

Physical and Physiological Characteristics of Judo Athletes

Gema Torres-Luque [1,*], Raquel Hernández-García [2], Raquel Escobar-Molina [3], Nuria Garatachea [4] and Pantelis T. Nikolaidis [5,6]

1 Faculty of Humanities and Science Education, University of Jaen, Jaen 23071, Spain
2 Faculty of Sport Science, University of Murcia, Murcia 30720, Spain; raquelhgarcia@gmail.com
3 Faculty of Sport Science, University of Granada, Granada 18001, Spain; rescobar@ugr.es
4 Faculty of Health and Sport Science, University of Zaragoza, Zaragoza 22002, Spain; nugarata@unizar.es
5 Department of Physical and Cultural Education, Hellenic Army Academy, Athens 16673, Greece; pademil@hotmail.com
6 Exercise Physiology Laboratory, Nikaia 18450, Greece
* Correspondence: gtluque@ujaen.es

Academic Editor: Eling Douwe de Bruin

Abstract: Judo competition is characterized structurally by weight category, which raises the importance of physiological control training in judo. The aim of the present review was to examine scientific papers on the physiological profile of the judokas, maintenance or loss of weight, framing issues, such as anthropometric parameters (body fat percentage), heart rate responses to training and combat, maximal oxygen uptake, hematological, biological and hormones indicators. The values shown in this review should be used as a reference for the evaluation of physical fitness and the effectiveness of training programs. Hence, this information is expected to contribute to the development of optimal training interventions aiming to achieve maximum athletic performance and to maintain the health of judokas.

Keywords: anthropometry; evaluation; judo; physiology; training

1. Introduction

Judo became an official sport event in the Olympic Games of Munich in 1972 for men and in the 1992 Games (Barcelona) for women (International Judo Federation). In the 1964 Games, judo was invited in Tokyo for men, whereas the same happened for women in the 1988 Games (Seoul). In 1961, there were world championships in Paris. The first competition with weight categories took place in the 1964 Games (Tokyo), including three categories and an open, while in 1965 (Rio de Janeiro), five categories and an open were included in the program.

Competitive judo demands high-intensity intermittent actions, in which optimal physical attributes are necessary in order to achieve technical-tactical development and success in combat [1,2]. Actually, high training loads, which require successful and coordinated actions, are applied to judokas in order to achieve high sport's performance. Since judo is a sport including weight categories [3], a major training goal is the achievement of an optimal weight through the combination of restricted diet and aerobic training, usually aiming to decrease fat mass rapidly [4]. According to several studies, there are judokas who can lose between 3% and 6% fat mass during the last weeks before the competition [5–10]. This decrease might reach even 10% of body mass [11] in an attempt to get an advantage by competing against lighter, smaller and weaker opponents [12].

Judo trainers and judokas should have a solid knowledge about physiological responses to competitions and physiological adaptations to training in order to design an adequate training session and season [13]. A combination of high demands of training and rapid weight loss before competition could induce muscle damage and increase the risk of damage in other tissue [14]. The cumulative effect of weight changes along a complete season together with intense training load could be even more harmful and put judokas' health at risk.

There are many authors who have written about the variation of physical and physiological profile of judokas during the training season [9,15], as well as other studies that have monitored this profile in the competitive time [5,7,16]. One of the most studied aspects is the effects of rapid weight loss on performance, where it has been reported that even in the case of "weight cycling" (down periodically), the body seems to suffer from physiological adaptation to these cycles [12]. For example, senior judokas presented higher use of weight loss methods, especially in the period one week before competitions compared to their junior counterparts. Judokas were involved in their diets and reduced more weight to a greater extent as they were getting older [17]. This review aimed to bring together all of those studies that have framed the physical and physiological characteristics of judokas.

2. Body Composition

Judo is a combat sport with strict competitive weight categories. In 1964, when judo became an official Olympic event, a competitive weight class system was adopted. Judokas should optimally select the weight class that is appropriate to their height and physique. However, many of them often undergo severe weight reduction through calorie restriction in order to select a lower-weight class and, in this way, to gain an advantage over other judokas in a particular weight class. In order to achieve the weight that would allow them to participate in a specific class, many contestants undergo drastic food restriction, especially during the week preceding the competition. The amount of weight loss is subsequently regained as the athletes compensate for the sustained energy drain by excess food intake during the post-competition period [18]. This rapid alternation between weight loss and regain is known as "weight cycling". Artioli and his colleagues [3] highlighted the need to assess the importance of maintaining weight in judo after learning that 80% of judokas performed fast weight descents. Ebine and colleagues have described anthropometric characteristics and weight in high-level judokas distinguished by sex and weight category [19].

Body mass and body fat percentage are essential measurements that could change largely according to sex, age, weight category and training. With regards to sex, it has been established that body fat percentage for elite female judokas is about 10% higher than for male judokas [20]. A study indicated that male judokas were heavier, taller, had lower body fat and higher percentage and absolute values of muscle mass, higher circumferences and bone diameters, lower endomorphic and higher mesomorphic components than females [21].

With regards to age, it has been noticed that in young judokas (14–18 years old), the body fat percentage is between 10% and 16%, whereas in older judokas (19–24 years old), it was 8%–10% in the case of the international level and 8%–15% in the case of the national level [22]. Female judokas of 15–16 years old presented body fat percentage from 16%–23% [23], and female college judokas aged 19–20 years old had 19.3% [24]. These data were very close those found by Franchini *et al.* [21] in the assessment of the Spanish judo team from cadets to seniors. The latter authors reported values as follows: in females, cadet category (16 years old), 19.5% body fat, junior category (20 years old), 24.0% body fat and in senior category (22 years old), 19.9%; in males, of the cadet category, 12.1% body fat, in the junior category, 10.6% body fat, and the senior category, 8% body fat; as for the values of muscle mass, in females, 44%, 41.5% and 44.7% in the cadet, junior and senior category, respectively; in males, 48.5%, 50.3% and 53.2% of muscle body mass.

Various studies have compared body fat percentage among groups differing for competitive level (e.g., international *vs.* national level). It was well documented that national-level judokas had a higher body fat percentage than international level [4,20,25]. A study [26] demonstrated that judokas who participated in the Olympic Games or Asian Games (international level) had significantly higher fat-free mass than university judokas (university level) who did not participate in intercollegiate competitions.

In fact, the muscle density normalized to the height of the individual was larger in judokas at the international level than in those at the university level. World- and Olympic-level male judokas usually had lower than 10% body fat [16]. Nevertheless, caution was needed when using this value as a reference, because most studies predicted body fat by skinfold thickness measurements, and therefore, the specific mean error of the estimate of each equation should be taken into consideration [21]. To sum up, the abovementioned studies showed that body fat percentage decreased as competition level increased.

With regards to the association between competition level and body fat percentage, an alternative research approach to the comparison between groups differing for competition level was to examine correlations. These fat mass differences between competitive levels had an important repercussion in sport's performance [16]. Franchini *et al.* [16] compared the morphological characteristics of the male judokas of the Brazilian Team A with the judokas of Teams B and C (reserves). These authors concluded that a higher body fat percentage was negatively correlated with performance in activities with body mass locomotion. However, the aforementioned correlation was not statistically significant in adolescent judokas [27].

Another study found that judokas in the heaviest weight categories were stronger (relative to lean body mass values) than those in the lightest categories [28]. Some other studies compared weight categories concerning the body fat percentage, and they found a linear increase from the under-60 kg to the 81–90 kg category and a large increase in the half-heavy-weight (100 kg) and heavy-weight (more than 100 kg) categories [28].

Because judo is a weight-classified sport, the body mass changes along the sport, season especially when judokas are preparing for a competition. A decrease of body fat percentage (3%–6%) during the last weeks before competition has been described [5–10,29] and even 10% in another case [11]. It was recommended to assess body composition in different periods of the season, at least on three or four occasions [7–9,29,30]. Several studies reported that fat mass percentage during the competition period was lower than during rest or pre-competition periods [7,27,29,31]. For this reason, Artioli *et al.* [3] proposed six basic rules for the control of the judoka weight and the prevention of the negative effects of the sudden loss of weight in this sport's performance: (1) the combats begin no more than 1 h after the weigh-in; (2) each athlete is allowed to weigh-in only on time; (3) rapid weight loss methods and artificial rehydration methods are prohibited in the days of the competition; (4) athletes must pass the hydration test to get the weigh-in validated; (5) an individual minimum competitive weight is determined at the beginning of each season; and (6) no athletes are allowed to compete in a weight class that would require weight loss greater than 1.5% of body weight per week. Moreover, the fat mass percentage of high level judokas was usually lower than the sedentary population [32] (Tables 1 and 2).

Table 1. Body mass, height and body mass index in judokas.

Sample	Age (years)	Body Mass (kg)	Height (cm)	BMI (kg·m^{-2})	Reference
			Males		
Spanish (*n* = 74)	14.7 ± 1.1	60.8 ± 13.8	168 ± 10	21.4 ± 3.0	(Torres-Luque *et al.*, 2015) [33]
Koreans (*n* = 28)	16.0 ± 0.9	67.0 ± 9.7	175 ± 6	21.9 ^{a}	(Kim *et al.*, 2011) [34]
French national (*n* = 10)	17 ± 1	71.4			(Koral and Dosseville, 2009) [35]
Tunisians national (*n* = 15)	18 ± 1	68.1 ± 8	1.74 ^{a}	22.4 ± 1.8	(Chaouachi *et al.*, 2009) [36]
Tunisians regional (*n* = 10)	18.1 ± 1.7	77.2 ± 11.7	176 ± 5	24.9 ^{a}	(El Abed *et al.*, 2009) [37]
Tunisians national (*n* = 12)	18.6 ± 2.4	77.1 ± 10.7	178 ± 6	24.3 ^{a}	(Souissi *et al.*, 2013) [38]
Japans collegiate (*n* = 14)	19.9 ± 1.1	68.9 ± 5.0	169 ± 3	24.1 ^{a}	(Iwai *et al.*, 2008) [39]
Cypriots competitive (*n* = 11)	20 ± 6	74.9 ± 12.1	172 ± 4	25.3 ^{a}	(Papacosta *et al.*, 2013) [40]
Koreans collegiate (*n* = 26)	20.4 ± 0.7	78.6 ± 15.2	174 ± 7	26.0 ^{a}	(Kim *et al.*, 2011) [34]
Brazilian professional (*n* = 39)	20.4	73.7	170	25.5	(Saraiva *et al.*, 2014) [41]
Brazilian national (*n* = 20)	20.7 ± 4.6	72.8 ± 12.6	174 ± 9	24.0 ^{a}	(Detanico *et al.*, 2015) [42]
Spanish national (*n* = 12)	22.0 ± 3.2	76.3 ± 12.7	176 ± 7	24.6 ^{a}	(Bonitch-Góngora *et al.*, 2012) [43]
Polish competitive (n = 22)	22.2 ± 3.6	87.5 ± 24.9	180 ± 8	26.8 ± 5.2	(Sterkowicz-Przybycień and Almansba, 2011) [44]
Brazilian competitive (*n* = 22)	22.5 ± 3.9	76.9 ± 9.1	176 ± 5	24.8 ^{a}	(Ache Dias *et al.*, 2012) [45]
French national (*n* = 10)	22.6 ± 2.1	85.8 ± 10.2	180 ± 7	26.5 ^{a}	(Cottin *et al.*, 2001) [46]

Table 1. *Cont.*

Sample	Age (years)	Body Mass (kg)	Height (cm)	BMI (kg· m^{-2})	Reference
Spanish national (*n* = 14)	22.9	76.9	174	25.4 [a]	(Morales *et al.*, 2014) [47]
Portuguese national (*n* = 27)	23.2 ± 2.8	72.8 ± 7.1	176 ± 5	23.6 ± 2.3	(Silva *et al.*, 2010) [48] (Silva *et al.*, 2011) [49]
Portuguese national (*n* = 32)	23.2 ± 3.3	73.4 ± 8.3	174 ± 5	24.2 [a]	(Gonçalves *et al.*, 2015) [50]
Korean national (*n* = 10)	24.3 ± 3.3	81.4 ± 14.3	174 ± 8	26.9 [a]	(Kim *et al.*, 2011) [34]
Europeans elite (*n* = 10)	25.6	100.7	186	29.1 [a]	(Drid *et al.*, 2015) [51]
Brazilian recreational (*n* = 180)	25.7 ± 4.9	78.3 ± 15.1	~174	25.9 ± 4.0	(Schwart *et al.*, 2015) [52]
French competitive (*n* = 13)	adults	78.7	173	26.3 [a]	(Franchini *et al.*, 2015) [53]
			Females		
Spanish (*n* = 72)	14.5 ± 1.2	56.4 ± 13.1	162 ± 7	21.4 ± 4.2	(Torres-Luque *et al.*, 2015) [33]
French national (*n* = 10)	17 ± 1	69.6			(Koral and Dosseville, 2009) [35]
Polish competitive (*n* = 12)	23.1 ± 1.7	74.9 ± 24.0	169 ± 8	25.7 ± 5.6	(Sterkowicz-Przybycień and Almansba, 2011) [44]

BMI = body mass index. [a] Calculated by the authors of the present study.

Table 2. Body composition in judokas.

Sample	Age (years)	BF (%)	Assessment Method	Reference
		Males		
Spanish (*n* = 74)	14.7 ± 1.1	12.7 ± 4.5	BIA	(Torres-Luque *et al.*, 2015) [33]
Koreans (*n* = 28)	16.0 ± 0.9	12.9 ± 2.8	BIA	(Kim *et al.*, 2011) [34]
French national (*n* = 10)	17 ± 1	12.7	4 skinfolds	(Koral and Dosseville, 2009) [35]
Cypriots competitive (*n* = 11)	20 ± 6	8.1 ± 1.9	skinfolds	(Papacosta *et al.*, 2013) [40]
Koreans collegiate (*n* = 26)	20.4 ± 0.7	14.1 ± 2.5	BIA	(Kim *et al.*, 2011) [34]
Brazilian national (*n* = 20)	20.7 ± 4.6	13.9 ± 3.1	-	(Detanico *et al.*, 2015) [42]
Spanish national (*n* = 12)	22.0 ± 3.2	15.3	skinfolds	(Bonitch-Góngora *et al.*, 2012) [43]
Polish competitive (*n* = 22)	22.2 ± 3.6	14.3 ± 4.3	2 skinfolds	(Sterkowicz-Przybycień and Almansba, 2011) [44]
Portuguese national (*n* = 27)	23.2 ± 2.8	12.1 ± 3.1	DEXA	(Silva *et al.*, 2010, 2011) [48,49]
Portuguese national (*n* = 32)	23.2 ± 3.3	12.1	DEXA	(Gonçalves *et al.*, 2015) [50]
Korean national (*n* = 10)	24.3 ± 3.3	12.5 ± 3.1	BIA	(Kim *et al.*, 2011) [34]
Brazilian recreational (*n* = 180)	25.7 ± 4.9	15.7 ± 7.6	3 skinfolds	(Schwartz *et al.*, 2015) [52]
		Females		
Spanish (*n* = 72)	14.5 ± 1.2	24.6 ± 7.5	BIA	(Torres-Luque *et al.*, 2015) [33]
French national (*n* = 10)	17 ± 1	23.1	4 skinfolds	(Koral and Dosseville, 2009) [35]
Polish competitive (*n* = 12)	23.1 ± 1.7	23.3 ± 3.7	2 skinfolds	(Sterkowicz-Przybycień and Almansba, 2011) [44]

BF = body fat percentage; BIA = bioelectrical impedance analysis; DEXA = dual-energy X-ray absorptiometry.

3. Physical Fitness

Maximal oxygen uptake (VO_2max) has been used as a measure of aerobic capacity in male and female judokas. The literature has reported VO_2max values between 43 and 65 mL· kg^{-1}· min^{-1} [54] (Table 3). Male judokas had higher VO_2max values (from 44–64 mL· kg^{-1}· min^{-1}) than females (from 43–53 mL· kg^{-1}· min^{-1}) [4,15,28,55]. Considering VO_2max by weight categories, values from 39–57 mL· kg^{-1}· min^{-1} were reported for lightweight, from 42–59.5 mL· kg^{-1}· min^{-1} for medium weight and from 42–59.5 mL· kg^{-1}· min^{-1} for the heavy weight category [4,15,28,55].

Table 3. Flexibility in judokas.

Sample	Age (years)	Flexibility (cm)	Assessment Method	Reference
		Males		
Spanish (*n* = 74)	14.7 ± 1.1	2.0 ± 7.9	SAR	(Torres-Luque *et al.*, 2015) [33]
Brazilian recreational (*n* = 180)	25.7 ± 4.9	37.7 ± 11.9	SAR [a]	(Schwartz *et al.*, 2015) [52]
		Females		
Spanish (*n* = 72)	14.5 ± 1.2	4.9 ± 7.8	SAR	(Torres-Luque *et al.*, 2015) [33]

SAR = sit-and-reach test; [a] equipment provides an advantage of 26 cm.

Although the aerobic profile of judokas has been well documented by the aforementioned studies, the chronic adaptations of aerobic capacity to judo training were less studied [4,28,56]. There was a study supporting that judo training might induce an increase of VO_2max, where De Cree *et al.* [4] reported a significant increase of VO_2max after six weeks of judo training in woman around 17–29 years. In contrast, Callister *et al.* [28] did not find changes in VO_2max after 10 weeks in elite judokas. An interpretation for the lack of changes in the latter study might be the level of judokas; since they were elite, they would be expected to possess a high level of VO_2max at baseline, which would be difficult to improve further. On the other side, such a lack of changes might be due to the nature of judo training, which is more anaerobic rather than aerobic and does not consist of an exercise stimulus for improvement of the high level of VO_2max. Thus, it is necessary to conduct more research on the effects of judo training on VO_2max. Franchini *et al.* [56] showed the values of VO_2 in males judokas of 25 years old while performing nine intermittent series of uchikomis for one minute: VO_2 differed over time during activity with lower values during the first minute (32 $mL \cdot kg^{-1} \cdot min^{-1}$).

In addition to the abovementioned research that focused on aerobic capacity, several studies have profiled other parameters of physical fitness, such as flexibility, handgrip muscle strength and vertical jump of judokas [33,35,36,40,47,51,52] (Tables 4–6). The data presented by these studies provided valuable reference values of physical fitness in other judo practitioners (e.g., coaches, fitness trainers) to evaluate and monitor their judokas.

Table 4. Handgrip muscle strength in judokas.

Sample	Age (years)	Right Hand (kg)	Left Hand (kg)	Sum of Two Hands (kg)	Reference
			Males		
Spanish (*n* = 74)	14.7 ± 1.1	37.7 ± 11.9			(Torres-Luque *et al.*, 2015) [33]
Tunisians national (*n* = 12)	18.6 ± 2.4	~54			(Souissi *et al.*, 2013) [38]
Cypriots competitive (*n* = 11)	20 ± 6	46.5 ± 8.8	42.0 ± 8.8	88.5 [a]	(Papacosta *et al.*, 2013) [40]
Spanish national (*n* = 12)	22.0 ± 3.2	57.6 ± 6.9	55.4 ± 7.4	113 [a]	(Bonitch-Góngora *et al.*, 2012) [43]
Spanish national (*n* = 14)	22.9	48.4	46.5	94.9	(Morales *et al.*, 2014) [47]
Portuguese national (*n* = 27)	23.2 ± 2.8	50.8 ± 7.4 [b]			(Silva *et al.*, 2011) [49]
Europeans elite (*n* = 10)	25.6 ± 3.6	64.3	69.0	133.3 [a]	(Drid *et al.*, 2015) [51]
Brazilian recreational (*n* = 180)	25.7 ± 4.9			101 ± 15	(Schwartz *et al.*, 2015) [52]
Brazilian competitive (*n* = 22)	22.5 ± 3.9	51.4 ± 8.2 [c]	51.4 ± 7.9	102.8 [a]	(Ache Dias *et al.*, 2012) [45]
French competitive (*n* = 13)	adults	50.0	49.6	99.6 [a]	(Franchini *et al.*, 2015) [53]
			Females		
Spanish (*n* = 72)	14.5 ± 1.2	26.6 ± 7.4			(Torres-Luque *et al.*, 2015) [33]

[a] Calculated by the authors of the present study; [b] dominant hand; [c] dominant and non-dominant hand.

Table 5. Vertical jump ability in judokas.

Sample	Age (years)	Jump (cm)	Assessment Method	Reference
		Males		
Spanish (*n* = 74)	14.7 ± 1.1	30.8 ± 10.5	CMJ	(Torres-Luque *et al.*, 2015) [33]
French national (*n* = 10)	17 ± 1	57.3	SJ	(Koral and Dosseville, 2009) [35]
French national (*n* = 10)	17 ± 1	58.7	CMJ	(Koral and Dosseville, 2009) [35]
Tunisians national (*n* = 15)	18 ± 1	42.0 ± 3.2	SJ	(Chaouachi *et al.*, 2009) [36]
Tunisians national (*n* = 15)	18 ± 1	45.6 ± 4.2	CMJ	(Chaouachi *et al.*, 2009) [36]
Cypriots competitive (*n* = 11)	20 ± 6	41.7 ± 5.3	CMJ	(Papacosta *et al.*, 2013) [40]
Brazilian national (*n* = 20)	20.7 ± 4.6	45.4 ± 5.2	CMJ	(Detanico *et al.*, 2015) [42]
		Females		
Spanish (*n* = 72)	14.5 ± 1.2	27.7 ± 13.5	CMJ	(Torres-Luque *et al.*, 2015) [33]
French national (*n* = 10)	17 ± 1	44.3	SJ	(Koral and Dosseville, 2009) [35]
French national (*n* = 10)	17 ± 1	45.3	CMJ	(Koral and Dosseville, 2009) [35]

CMJ = countermovement jump; SJ = squat jump.

Table 6. Aerobic capacity in judokas.

Sample	Age (years)	Aerobic Capacity	Assessment Method	Reference
		Males		
Tunisians national (*n* = 15)	18 ± 1	53.3 ± 3.9	SRT	(Chaouachi *et al.*, 2009) [36]
Cypriots competitive (*n* = 11)	20 ± 6	57.2 ± 7.2	GXT [b]	(Papacosta *et al.*, 2013) [40]
French national (*n* = 10)	22.6 ± 2.1	44.5 ± 6	GXT [a]	(Cottin *et al.*, 2001) [46]
Europeans elite (*n* = 10)	25.6	56.0	GXT [b]	(Drid *et al.*, 2015) [51]
Brazilian recreational (*n* = 180)	25.7 ± 4.9	52.2 ± 7.9	Queen's College step test	(Schwartz *et al.*, 2015) [52]

SRT = 20-m shuttle run test; GXT = graded exercise test; [a] cycle ergometer; [b] treadmill.

4. Heart Rate

The assessment of heart rate (HR) at rest (HR_{rest} submaximal and maximal intensities (HR_{max}) contributes to monitoring of aerobic capacity and exercise intensity. HRrest in male judokas ranged from 54–65 bpm and was slightly lower than in female judokas (65–71 bpm) [15,19,55]. During judo contests, several studies have reported mean HR in male judokas of 180–182 bpm, which corresponded to 85%–90% of HR_{max} [15,55,57,58]. HRmax during judo contests was 190–200 bpm in male and slightly lower in female judokas [4,58].

HR has been also used to quantify exercise intensity during judo training. For instance, a study [59] classified the intensity of the different efforts of judo training. The most common efforts of judo training were put in order from the highest to lowest intensity as follows: *randori* (4 min and 30 s), *randori* (5 min 30 s), *uchi-komi* once each every 3 s, *nage-komi* every 3 s during 1 min 30 s, *uchi-komi* once each every 4 s and *nage-komi* every 4 s during 1 min 30 s. Moreover, Franchini *et al.* [56] in a more recent study evaluated the performance and physiological responses in intermittent training uchikomi and showed HR scores during execution of 183 bpm and during rest of 95 bpm, with lower values observed in the first minute compared to the second and third minute.

5. Blood Lactate

The concentration of lactate in blood $[La^-]$ has been extensively studied in judo, both in real competition, simulations of competition and training. $[La^-]$ values have ranged 7–10 $mmol \cdot L^{-1}$ after combat simulations [15,55,58,60]. In simulated judo contests, differences in $[La^-]$ have not been found, either between competition levels [2] or sexes [58]. Callister *et al.* [28] reported $[La^-]$ of 9.1 ± 1.1 $mmol \cdot L^{-1}$ after a specific training judo (*uchikomis, ne waza* and 3–7 *randori*). In addition, Franchini *et al.* [61] found significant increments after a simulated contest. In a recent review [56], there were variations in $[La^-]$ after combats, at least in simulated combat. In these studies, it was found that peak $[La^-]$ was higher after the first combat compared to the second, third and fourth combat, about 2 $mmol \cdot L^{-1}$ [22,62]. Taken together, these studies suggested a decrease in anaerobic lactic contribution as the judokas performed consecutive combats [56]. Serrano *et al.* [60] found a positive correlation between the rate of perceived exertion and maximal $[La^-]$ during competition in regional-level male judokas.

6. Hematological Evaluation

Hematological evaluation in judokas has focused on concentrations of total erythrocytes and leukocytes, as well as quantification of hemoglobin (Hb) and hematocrit (Hct). Malczewska *et al.* [63] reported total erythrocyte and leukocyte levels in male high level judokas of 4.82×10^{12} L^{-1} and 5.8×10^9 L^{-1}, respectively. These authors reported values of Hb of 15.5 $g \cdot L^{-1}$ and Hct of 43% for the same group of judokas. In female high level judokas, Hb was 12.5 $g \cdot dL^{-1}$ and 38% for Hct [64]. In the case of young judokas (16 years old), Hb and Hct have been reported a bit lower (137 $g \cdot L^{-1}$ and 42%, respectively) than in adult judokas [65].

Hb and Hct did not change significantly during a 20-day rapid weight loss period before competition [7,29]. A study [66] has found similar results in junior male judokas; in this study, Hb and Htc did not change after training. In contrast, Su *et al.* [65] found a significant decrement in Hb (from 137 down to 128 g$\cdot$ L^{-1}) and Htc (from 42% down to 39%) after a five-week training period in young judokas (16 years old). This finding was in agreement with that of Umeda *et al.* [24], who showed that the effect of a training round for seven days resulted in a significant decrease in leukocytes and Hb levels in a group of female judokas (19 years old). Furthermore, another study investigated the combined effects of dietary restriction and weight reduction through exercise on markers of immune function in college judokas before and after a single competition [29]. These authors found that the weight reduction group exhibited significant decreases in concentrations of serum immunoglobulins and complements (IgG, IgM and C3) at seven days after the competition. In the dietary restriction group, significant decreases in IgM and C3 were observed at seven days after the competition, though to a lesser degree than in the weight reduction group. Moreover, the authors of this study observed a significant decrease in total leukocytes one day before competition (from 6329 down to 5497 cel$\cdot$ mm^2). This study concluded that energy restriction seemed to exacerbate alterations in immune markers, such as immunoglobulin, and complements induced by vigorous exercise at seven days after a competition. Although the changed values were still within normal limits, the authors hypothesized that the potential cumulative effect of these changes over many competitions in one year might well induce abnormal levels with a possibly harmful clinical effect on judokas. In contrast, the study of Kowatari *et al.* [5] failed to find changes in leukocytes, lymphocytes and neutrophils after a combined weight reduction and training program.

On the other hand, white blood cells and neutrophils in the blood values showed a significant increase after training judo, $\pm$1.2–10.7 $\pm$ 1.8 $\times$ 10^3/µL and 2.98 $\pm$ 0.82–7.95 $\pm$1.8 $\times$ 10^3/µL, respectively, in 18 male judokas [66]. Another study evaluating the effects of an intense training camp of seven days in female judokas of 19 years old showed a decreased in immunoglobulin after training compared with baseline values, suggesting the appearance and accumulation of physical fatigue [24].

Ohta *et al.* [7] and Umeda *et al.* [29] controlled IgG, IgA and IgM variability four times (Days 20 and 7, one day before the competition and five days later) in judokas depending on the range of weight loss. Ohta *et al.* [7] showed a significant reduction in the three types of immunoglobulins in the group with a high reduction of weight; however, in Umeda *et al.* [29] only was a decrease in IgG and IgM in the group of normal weight reduction observed. Concerning weight maintenance, group values remain constant in both works during the period of the study; coinciding with some of the above authors claiming that a sharp reduction of body weight along with the practice of intense training may induce a decreased ability of the immune system of athletes [7,29].

Kim *et al.* [32] pointed out that studies focused on the immune system of female judokas are limited. They found that the level of immunoglobulins (IgG and IgM) in female judokas was lower than in sedentary females. These results reinforced the fact that high demands of training linked with imbalanced nutrition in female judokas could induce a low immune function and impairments in sport's performance and health status.

7. Free Fatty Acids and Glycerol

Among sports where athletes are categorized by weight, judo is characterized by relatively short duration, high intensity and intermittent exercise with a combat lasting ~7.18 min in males. It has been shown that a single judo combat is able to induce mobilization of both protein and lipid metabolism [55].

Finaud *et al.* [8] observed in national judokas that after a week of weight loss, the triglyceride concentration decreases significantly compared to the initial values, and also, triglycerides in the blood after the competition levels are lower than before they compete. However, free fatty acids, after having increased significantly after a week of reduction of body weight, return to the initial values after the competition. With respect to glycerol, a significant increase in blood concentration occurs the day before a competition, and then continues after the championship, but not significantly. In the control group, only statistically significant differences in the levels of glycerol appear after the competition. These results were similar to other studies [7,30].

On the contrary, Filaire *et al.* [67] observed a significant increase in the concentration of triglycerides in blood after a week of male judokas of −73 kg on food restriction. With regards to glycerol concentrations, they decreased after a week of strict diet, but without reaching statistically significant differences (0.12–0.17 mmol$\cdot$ L^{-1}).

A study [15] about the contribution of protein metabolism during judo combat and recovery showed significant increments in triglycerides, free fatty acids and glycerol 3 min after judo combat; similarly, there was a significant increase in free fatty acids and glycerol 60 min after combat. Glycerol levels obtained 3 and 60 min after the end of the combat are above the rank of normality (50–100 μmol$\cdot$ L^{-1}). Therefore, the authors hypothesize that since the judoka study was carried out with the misleading use of lipid metabolism (lipolysis), bringing with it the increase in free fatty acids and glycerol after the effort, characterized by an intake of a carbohydrate diet rather than that recommended, this can be the case.

8. Testosterone and Cortisol

Stress management before a competition for athletes is very important, especially for those who reduce their weight, such as judokas. In general, adrenocortical hormone is well known as a stress marker, and cortisol (C) is representative of it. Nowadays, the ratio of testosterone (T) to C (T/C) is a good marker of overtraining diagnosis [68]. In a study aiming to investigate the salivary T and C and the mental state responses to a real judo championship [69], C response to competition was shown, which was especially characterized by an anticipatory rise, which was confirmed later by Salvador *et al.* [70] and Obminski [71], suggesting that increased levels of C on judokas' competition day predisposed them to success. Depending on the outcome, the results did not show significant differences in C responses. T values recorded after the last fight were significantly greater in the losers than those in the winners. Hormonal response did not show a relationship with psychological variables depending on the outcome. Finally, even if no relationship between hormonal and psychological variables depending on the outcome was found, the results showed that state and trait psychological variables, as well as the coping strategies, must be taken into account to better understand the response to competitive situations.

Salvador *et al.* [70] compared the anticipatory hormonal and psychological responses of 17 male judokas in the resting sessions and before competition sessions along the official competition. C levels and anxiety scores were concurrently higher before the contest than in resting conditions. Their results showed that one group of subjects did display T increases, higher C levels and higher motivation to win scores than the other group, indicating that this hormonal pattern and its relationships with psychological variables suggested an adaptive psychobiological response to a competition.

The relationships between psychophysiological variables have been investigated at two levels (regional *vs.* interregional) by comparing physiological responses (salivary C and T concentrations) and psychological responses prior to judo competitions [69]. C levels increased sharply (about 2.5-fold resting levels) throughout both competitions with no changes in T levels. Positive relationships between anxiety components (somatic and cognitive anxiety) and C were noted in both competitions. The study concluded that salivary C, together with anxiety components, may provide a better sensitivity index of physiological stress than T concentrations.

Correlations between T levels and fighting in male participants in judo contests have been studied [72]. A positive relation between T and offensive behaviors was obtained in the sense that the greater the hormonal titer, the greater the number of threats, fights and attacks. These findings coincide with the pattern of relationships found using observational scales. Conversely, C also presented positive correlations with some of these behavioral categories, but did not moderate the relationship between T and competitive behavior. These results give support to the view that T can be linked to the expression of competitive aggression in judo.

Toda *et al.* [6] investigated the effect of weight reduction prior to a competition on the salivary C level of judokas varying for the reduction rate (WRR, %). In this study, participants were divided into three groups depending on their WRR: the no-weight reduction group (WRR < 3%), the low-weight reduction group ($3 \leqslant$ WRR $< 6\%$) and the high-weight reduction group. The collection of the measurements was carried out on three different days: 20 days before the competition (before weight reduction), the day before the competition (the peak of weight reduction) and seven days after the competition. There was no significant change in the salivary C levels during the weight reduction. On the day before the competition, however, those of the low- and high-weight reduction groups showed a tendency to decrease and were significantly lower than that of the no-weight reduction group. In addition, their recovery was observed at seven days after the competition. These findings suggested that the HPA axis is affected during the relatively early stage of weight reduction.

Degoutte *et al.* [30] examined the effects of weight loss induced by restricting energy and fluid intake on the physiology, psychology and physical performance of judo athletes. These authors observed that the plasma level of C, after a significant weight reduction, increased significantly, whereas the T and T/C ratio decreased significantly. These results suggested that the combination of energy restriction and intense exercise training, resulting in weight reduction before a competition, adversely affected the physiology and psychology of judo athletes and impaired physical performance before the competition. The results of another study [9], in line with those of Degoutte *et al.* [30], showed an 81% increment in C level compared to the baseline value, although when the normal weight was recovered again, the C decreased 27%, indicating that catabolic processes were augmented after weight reduction.

This study has a something's limitations. It discussed a compendium of studies related to the functional and physiological characteristics judo athlete. However, it is not a systematic review of these aspects. Coaches can consider directions and guidelines; and can serve as support for their workouts. Therefore, data must be taken with caution.

9. Conclusions

The values shown in this review are vital for training control. It collaborates with the planning of training and maintaining the health of judokas.

Conflicts of Interest: The authors declare no conflict of interest.

References

1. Bohannon, J. The science of judo. *Science* **2012**, *335*, 1552.
2. Franchini, E.; Takito, M.Y.; Mapdm, K.; Strerkowicz, S. Physical fitness and anthropometric differences between elite and nonelite judo players. In Proceedings of the 2nd International Judo Federation World Judo Conference Scientific Studies on Judo, Osaka, Japan, 24 July 2001.
3. Artioli, G.; Franchini, E.; Nicastro, H.; Sterkowicz, S.; Solis, M.Y.; Lancha, A.H. The need of a weight management control program in judo: A proposal based on the successful case of wrestling. *J. Int. Soc. Sports Nutr.* **2010**, *7*, 1–5. [CrossRef] [PubMed]
4. De Cree, C.; Lewin, R.; Barros, A. Hypoestrogenemia and rhabdomyelysis (myoglobinuria) in the female judoist: A new worrying phenomenon? *J. Clin. Endocrinol. Metab.* **1995**, *80*, 3639–3646. [CrossRef] [PubMed]
5. Kowatari, K.; Umeda, T.; Shimoyama, T.; Nakaji, S.; Yamamoto, Y.; Sugawara, K. Exercise training and energy restriction decrease neutrophil phagocytic activity in judoists. *Med. Sci. Sports Exerc.* **2001**, *33*, 519–524. [CrossRef] [PubMed]
6. Toda, M.; Morimoto, K.; Fukuda, S.; Umeda, T.; Nakaji, S.; Sugawara, K. The effect of the weight reduction on the salivary cortisol levels of judo players. *Environ. Health Prev. Med.* **2001**, *6*, 113–116. [CrossRef] [PubMed]
7. Ohta, S.; Nakaji, S.; Suzuki, K.; Totsuka, M.; Umeda, T.; Sugawara, K. Depressed humoral immunity after weight reduction in competitive judoists. *Luminescence* **2002**, *17*, 150–157. [CrossRef] [PubMed]

8. Finaud, J.; Degoutte, F.; Scislowski, V.; Rouveix, M.; Durand, D.; Filaire, E. Competition and food restriction effects on oxidative stress in judo. *Int. J. Sports Med.* **2006**, *27*, 834–841. [CrossRef] [PubMed]
9. Prouteau, S.; Benhamou, L.; Courteix, D. Relationships between serum leptin and bone markers during stable weight, weight reduction and weight regain in male and female judoists. *Eur. J. Endocrinol.* **2006**, *154*, 389–395. [CrossRef] [PubMed]
10. Yoshioka, Y.; Umeda, T.; Nakaji, S.; Kojima, A.; Tanabe, M.; Mochida, N.; Sugawara, K. Gender differences in the psychological response to weight reduction in judoists. *Int. J. Sports Nutr. Exerc. Metab.* **2006**, *16*, 187–198.
11. Steen, S.N.; Brownell, K.D. Patterns of weight loss and regain in wrestlers: Has the tradition changed? *Med. Sci. Sports Exerc.* **1990**, *22*, 762–768. [CrossRef] [PubMed]
12. Franchini, E.; Brito, C.J.; Artiolo, G.G. Weight loss in combats sports: Physiological, psychological and performance effects. *J. Int. Soc. Sports Nutr.* **2012**, *9*. [CrossRef] [PubMed]
13. Sterkowicz, D.; Franchini, E. Specific fitness of elite and novice judoists. *J. Hum. Kinet.* **2001**, *6*, 81–98.
14. Cavas, L. Does underwater rugby stimulate the over-production of reactive oxygen species? *Cell. Biochem. Funct.* **2005**, *23*, 59–63. [CrossRef] [PubMed]
15. Degoutte, F.; Jouanel, P.; Filaire, E. Solicitation of protein metabolism during a judo match and recovery. *Sci. Sports* **2004**, *19*, 28–33. [CrossRef]
16. Franchini, E.; Velly Nunes, A.; Morrison, J.; Boscoso, F. Physical fitness and anthropometrical profile of the Brazilian male judo team. *J. Physiol. Anthropol.* **2007**, *26*, 59–67. [CrossRef] [PubMed]
17. Escobar-Molina, R.; Rodríguez-Ruiz, S.; Gutierrez-García, C.; Franchini, E. Weight loss and psychological-related states in high-level judo athletes. *Int. J. Sport Nutr. Exerc. Metab.* **2015**, *25*, 110–118. [CrossRef] [PubMed]
18. Oppliger, R.A.; Steen, S.A.; Scott, J.R. Weight loss practices of college wrestlers. *Int. J. Sport Nutr. Exerc. Metab.* **2003**, *13*, 29–46. [CrossRef] [PubMed]
19. Ebine, K.; Yoneda, I.; Hase, H. Physiological characteristics of exercise and findings of laboratory tests in Japanese elite judo athletes. *Med. Sport* **1991**, *65*, 73–79.
20. Little, N.G. Physical performance attributes of junior and senior women, juvenile, junior, and senior men judokas. *J. Sports Med. Phys. Fit.* **1991**, *31*, 510–520.
21. Franchini, E.; Huertas, J.R.; Sterkowicz, S.; Carratala, V.; Gutierrez-García, C.; Escobar-Molina, R. Anthropometrical profile of elite Spanish Judoka: Comparative analysis among ages. *Arch. Judo* **2011**, *7*, 239–245.
22. Bonitch, J.G.; Bonitch, J.; Padial, P.; Feriche, B. The effects os lactate concentration on de handgrip strength durin judo bouts. *J. Strength Cond. Assoc.* **2012**, *26*, 1863–1871. [CrossRef] [PubMed]
23. Boisseau, N.; Vera Perez, S.; Poortmans, J. Food and fluid Intake in adolescent female judo athletes before competition. *Pediatr. Exerc. Sci.* **2005**, *17*, 62–71.
24. Umeda, T.; Suzukawa, K.; Takahashi, I.; Yamamoto, Y.; Tanabe, M.; Kojima, A.; Katagiri, T.; Matsuzaka, M.; Totsuka, M.; Nakaji, S.; *et al.* Effects of intense exercise on the physiological and mental condition of female university judoists during a training camp. *J. Sports Sci.* **2008**, *26*, 897–904. [CrossRef] [PubMed]
25. Fukuda, D.H.; Stiut, J.R.; Kendall, K.L.; Smith, A.E.; Wray, M.E.; Hetrick, R.P. The effects of tournament preparation on anthropometric and sport-specific performance measures in youth judo athletes. *J. Strength Cond. Res.* **2013**, *27*, 331–339. [CrossRef] [PubMed]
26. Kubo, J.; Chishaki, T.; Nakamura, N.; Muramatsu, T.; Yamamoto, Y.; Ito, M.; Saitou, H.; Kukidome, T. Differences in fat-free mass and muscle thicknesses at various sites according to performance level among judo athletes. *J. Strength Cond. Res.* **2006**, *20*, 654–657. [CrossRef] [PubMed]
27. Krustulovic, S.; Zuvela, F.; Katic, R. Biomotor systems in elite junior judoists. *Coll. Antropol.* **2006**, *30*, 845–851.
28. Callister, R.; Callister, R.J.; Staron, R.S.; Fleck, S.J.; Tesch, P.; Dudley, G.A. Physiological characteristics of elite judo athletes. *Int. J. Sports Med.* **1991**, *12*, 196–203. [CrossRef] [PubMed]
29. Umeda, T.; Nakaji, S.; Shimoyama, T.; Kojima, A.; Yamamoto, Y.; Sugawara, K. Adverse effects of energy restriction on changes in immunoglobulins and complements during weight reduction in judoists. *J. Sports Med. Phys. Fit.* **2004**, *44*, 328–334.
30. Degoutte, F.; Jouanel, P.; Bègue, R.J.; Colombier, M.; Lac, G.; Pequignot, J.M.; Filaire, E. Food restriction, performance, biochemical, psychological, and endocrine changes in judo athletes. *Int. J. Sports Med.* **2006**, *27*, 9–18. [CrossRef] [PubMed]

31. Hernandez, R.; Torres-Luque, G.; Olmedilla, A. Relations among traning volumen, body weight, and profile of mood states for elite judoka during a competitive period. *Percept. Mot. Skills* **2009**, *109*, 870–880. [CrossRef] [PubMed]
32. Kim, S.H.; Kim, H.Y.; Kim, W.K.; Park, O.J. Nutritional status, iron-deficiency-related indices, and immunity of female athletes. *Nutrition* **2002**, *18*, 86–90. [CrossRef]
33. Torres-Luque, G.; Hernandez-Garcia, R.; Garatachea, N.; Nikolaidis, P.T. Anthropometric characteristics and neuromuscular function in young judo athletes by sex, age and weight category. *Sport Sci. Health* **2015**, *11*, 117–124. [CrossRef]
34. Kim, J.; Cho, H.C.; Jung, H.S.; Yoon, J.D. Influence of performance level on anaerobic power and body composition in elite male Judoists. *J. Strength Cond. Res.* **2011**, *25*, 1346–1354. [CrossRef] [PubMed]
35. Koral, J.; Dosseville, F. Combination of gradual and rapid weight loss: Effects on physical performance and psychological state of elite judo athletes. *J. Sports Sci.* **2009**, *27*, 115–120. [CrossRef] [PubMed]
36. Chaouachi, A.; Coutts, A.J.; Chamari, K.; Wong, P.; Chaouachi, M.; Chtara, M.; Amri, M. Effect of Ramadan intermittent fasting on aerobic and anaerobic performance and perception of fatigue in male elite judo athletes. *J. Strength Cond. Res.* **2009**, *23*, 2702–2709. [CrossRef] [PubMed]
37. El Abed, K.; Trabelsi, K.; Latiri, I.; Hakim, A.; Tabka, Z.; Zbidi, A. Effects of anaerobic exercise on the status of enzymatic antioxidants among Judo athletes during recovery level. *Sci. Sports* **2009**, *24*, 36–39. [CrossRef]
38. Souissi, N.; Chtourou, H.; Aloui, A.; Hammouda, O.; Dogui, M.; Chaouachi, A.; Chamari, K. Effects of time-of-day and partial sleep deprivation on short-term maximal performances of judo competitors. *J. Strength Cond. Res.* **2013**, *27*, 2473–2480. [CrossRef] [PubMed]
39. Iwai, K.; Okada, T.; Nakazato, K.; Fujimoto, H.; Yamamoto, Y.; Nakajima, H. Sport-specific characteristics of trunk muscles in collegiate wrestlers and judokas. *J. Strength Cond. Res.* **2008**, *22*, 350–358. [CrossRef] [PubMed]
40. Papacosta, E.; Gleeson, M.; Nassis, G.P. Salivary hormones, IgA, and performance during intense training and tapering in judo athletes. *J. Strength Cond. Res.* **2013**, *27*, 2569–2580. [CrossRef] [PubMed]
41. Saraiva, A.R.; Reis, V.M.; Costa, P.B.; Bentes, C.M.; Costae Silva, G.V.; Novaes, J.S. Chronic Effects of different resistance training exercise orders on flexibility in elite judo athletes. *J. Hum. Kinet.* **2014**, *40*, 129–137. [CrossRef] [PubMed]
42. Detanico, D.; Pupo, J.D.; Franchini, E.; Dos Santos, S.G. Effects of successive judo matches on fatigue and muscle damage markers. *J. Strength Cond. Res.* **2015**, *29*, 1010–1016. [CrossRef] [PubMed]
43. Bonitch-Góngora, J.G.; Bonitch-Domínguez, J.G.; Padial, P.; Feriche, B. The effect of lactate concentration on the handgrip strength during judo bouts. *J. Strength Cond. Res.* **2012**, *26*, 1863–1871. [CrossRef] [PubMed]
44. Sterkowicz-Przybycień, K.; Almansba, R. Sexual dimorphism of anthropometrical measurements in judoists vs untrained subject. *Sci. Sports* **2011**, *26*, 316–323. [CrossRef]
45. Ache Dias, J.; Wentz, M.; Külkamp, W.; Mattos, D.; Goethel, M.; Borges Júnior, N. Is the handgrip strength performance better in judokas than in non-judokas? *Sci. Sports* **2012**, *27*, e9–e14. [CrossRef]
46. Cottin, F.; Papelier, Y.; Durbin, F.; Maupu, P.; Escourrou, P. Heart rate comparative study by spectral analysis between two exercises: Ergocycle vs judo randori. *Sci. Sports* **2001**, *16*, 295–305. [CrossRef]
47. Morales, J.; Álamo, J.M.; García-Masso, X.; Buscà, B.; López, J.L.; Serra-Año, P.; González, L.M. Use of heart rate variability in monitoring stress and recovery in judo athletes. *J. Strength Cond. Res.* **2014**, *28*, 1896–1905. [CrossRef] [PubMed]
48. Silva, A.M.; Fields, D.A.; Heymsfield, S.B.; Sardinha, L.B. Body composition and power changes in elite judo athletes. *Int. J. Sports Med.* **2010**, *31*, 737–741. [CrossRef] [PubMed]
49. Silva, A.M.; Fields, D.A.; Heymsfield, S.B.; Sardinha, L.B. Relationship between changes in total-body water and fluid distribution with maximal forearm strength in elite judo athletes. *J. Strength Cond. Res.* **2011**, *25*, 2488–2495. [CrossRef] [PubMed]
50. Gonçalves, E.M.; Matias, C.N.; Santos, D.A.; Sardinha, L.B.; Silva, A.M. Assessment of total body water and its compartments in elite judo athletes: Comparison of bioelectrical impedance spectroscopy with dilution techniques. *J. Sports Sci.* **2015**, *33*, 634–640. [PubMed]
51. Drid, P.; Casals, C.; Mekic, A.; Radjo, I.; Stojanovic, M.; Ostojic, S.M. Fitness and anthropometric profiles of international *vs.* national judo medalists in half-heavyweight category. *J. Strength Cond. Res.* **2015**, *29*, 2115–2121. [CrossRef] [PubMed]

52. Schwartz, J.; Takito, M.Y.; Del Vecchio, F.B.; Antonietti, L.S.; Franchini, E. Health-related physical fitness in martial arts and combat sports practitioners. *Sport Sci. Health* **2015**, *11*, 171–180. [CrossRef]
53. Franchini, E.; Branco, B.M.; Agostinho, M.F.; Calmet, M.; Candau, R. Influence of linear and undulating strength periodization on physical fitness, physiological, and performance responses to simulated judo matches. *J. Strength Cond. Res.* **2015**, *29*, 358–367. [CrossRef] [PubMed]
54. Aziz, A.; Tan, B.; Teh, K.C. Physiological responses during matches and profile of elite pencak silat exponents. *J. Sport Sci. Med.* **2002**, *1*, 147–155.
55. Degoutte, F.; Jouanel, P.; Filaire, E. Energy demands during a judo match and recovery. *Br. J. Sports Med.* **2003**, *37*, 245–249. [CrossRef] [PubMed]
56. Franchini, E.; Artioli, G.G.; Brito, C.J. Judo Combat: Time-motion analysis and physiology. *Int. J. Perform. Anal. Sport* **2013**, *13*, 624–641.
57. Bonitch, J.; Ramirez, J.; Femia, P.; Feriche, B.; Padial, P. Validating the relation between heart rate and perceived exertion in a judo competition. *Med. Dello Sport* **2005**, *58*, 23–28.
58. Hernandez, R.; Torres-Luque, G.; Villaverde, C. Physiological requirements of judo combat. *Int. Sportmed. J.* **2009**, *10*, 145–151.
59. Arruza, J.; Alzate, R.; Valencia, J. Esfuerzo percibido y frecuencia cardiaca de la intensidad de los esfuerzos en el entrenamiento de judo. *Rev. Psicol. Deporte* **1996**, *9–10*, 29–40.
60. Serrano, M.A.; Salvador, A.; Gonzalez Bono, E.; Sanchis, C.; Suay, F. Relationships between recall of perceived exertion and blood lactate concentration in a judo competition. *Percept. Mot. Skills* **2001**, *92*, 1139–1148. [CrossRef] [PubMed]
61. Franchini, E.; Takito, M.; Kiss, M.A.P.D.M.; Strerkowicz, S. Physical fitness and anthropometrical differences between elite and non-elite judo players. *Biol. Sport* **2005**, *22*, 79–93.
62. Bonitch-Dominguez, J.; Bonitch Gongora, J., Padial, P.; Feriche, B. Changes in peak leg power induced by successive judo bouts and their relationship to lactate production. *J. Sports Sci.* **2010**, *28*, 1527–1534. [CrossRef] [PubMed]
63. Malczewska, J.; Stupnicki, R.; Blach, W.; Turek-Lepa, E. The effects of physical exercise on the concentrations of ferritin and transferrin receptor in plasma of male judoists. *Int. J. Sports Med.* **2004**, *25*, 516–521. [CrossRef] [PubMed]
64. Ostojic, S.M.; Ahmetovic, Z. Weekly training volume and hematological status in female top-level athletes of different sports. *J. Sports Med. Phys. Fit.* **2008**, *48*, 398–403.
65. Su, Y.C.; Lin, C.J.; Chen, K.T.; Lee, S.M.; Lin, J.S.; Tsai, C.C.; Chou, Y.; Lin, J.G. Effects of huangqi jianzhong tang on hematological and biochemical parameters in judo athletes. *Acta Pharmacol. Sin.* **2001**, *22*, 1154–1158. [PubMed]
66. Chinda, D.; Umeda, T.; Shimoyama, T.; Kojima, A.; Tanabe, M.; Nakaji, S.; Sugawara, K. The acute response of neutrophil function to a bout of judo training. *Luminescence* **2003**, *18*, 278–282. [CrossRef] [PubMed]
67. Filaire, E.; Maso, F.; Degoutte, F.; Jouanel, P.; Lac, G. Food restriction, performance, Psychological state and lipid values in judo atlethes. *Int. J. Sports Med.* **2001**, *22*, 454–459. [CrossRef] [PubMed]
68. Suay, F.; Salvador, A.; González, E.; Sanchis, C.; Simón, V.M.; Montoro, J.B. Testosterona y evaluacion de la conducta agresiva en jovenes judokas. *Rev. Psicol. Deporte* **1996**, *5*, 79–93.
69. Filaire, E.; Sagnol, M.; Ferrand, C.; Maso, F.; Lac, G. Psychophysiological stress in judo athletes during competitions. *J. Sports Med. Phys. Fit.* **2001**, *41*, 263–268.
70. Salvador, A.; Suay, F.; González-Bono, E.; Serrano, M.A. Anticipatory cortisol, testosterone and psychological responses to judo competition in young men. *Psychoneuroendocrinology* **2003**, *28*, 364–375. [CrossRef]
71. Obminski, Z. Pre and post star hormone levels in blood as an indicator of psychological load with junior competitors. *Pol. J. Sport Tour.* **2009**, *16*, 158–165.
72. Salvador, A.; Suay, F.; Martinez-Sanchis, S.; Simon, V.M.; Brain, P.F. Correlating testosterone and fighting in male participants in judo contests. *Physiol. Behav.* **1999**, *68*, 205–209. [CrossRef]

6

Vertical Jumping Tests *versus* Wingate Anaerobic Test in Female Volleyball Players: The Role of Age

Pantelis Theodoros Nikolaidis [1,2,*], Jose Afonso [3,†], Vicente Javier Clemente-Suarez [4,†], Jose Rafael Padilla Alvarado [5,†], Tarak Driss [6,†], Beat Knechtle [7,†] and Gema Torres-Luque [8,†]

1. Department of Physical and Cultural Education, Hellenic Army Academy, Athens 16673, Greece
2. Exercise Physiology Laboratory, Nikaia 18450, Greece
3. Faculty of Sport, University of Porto, Porto 4200-450, Portugal; jafonsovolei@hotmail.com
4. Department of Sport Science, European University of Madrid, Madrid 28670, Spain; vctxente@yahoo.es
5. Department of Physical Education, Universidad de Los Llanos Occedentales Ezequiel Zamora, Barinitas 7001, Venezuela; joserafael.pa@gmail.com
6. UFR STAPS, CeRSM (EA 2931), Université Paris Ouest Nanterre La Défense, Nanterre 92000, France; tarak.driss@u-paris10.fr
7. Instutute of Primary Care, University of Zurich, Zurich CH-8006, Switzerland; beat.knechtle@hispeed.ch
8. Area of Corporal Express, Faculty of Humanities and Science Education, University of Jaen, Jaen 3109, Spain; gtluque@ujaen.es

* Correspondence: pademil@hotmail.com

† These authors contributed equally to this work.

Academic Editor: Eling Douwe de Bruin

Abstract: Single and continuous vertical jumping tests, as well as the Wingate anaerobic test (WAnT), are commonly used to assess the short-term muscle power of female volleyball players; however, the relationship among these tests has not been studied adequately. Thus, the aim of the present study was to examine the relationship of single and continuous vertical jumps with the WAnT in female volleyball players. Seventy adolescent (age 16.0 ± 1.0 years, body mass 62.5 ± 7.1 kg, height 170.4 ± 6.1 cm, body fat 24.2% ± 4.3%) and 108 adult female volleyball players (age 24.8 ± 5.2 years, body mass 66.5 ± 8.7 kg, height 173.2 ± 7.4 cm, body fat 22.0% ± 5.1%) performed the squat jump (SJ), countermovement jump (CMJ), Abalakov jump (AJ), 30 s Bosco test and WAnT (peak power, P_{peak}; mean power, P_{mean}). Mean power in the Bosco test was correlated (low to large magnitude) with P_{mean} of the WAnT ($r = 0.27$, $p = 0.030$ in adolescents *versus* $r = 0.56$, $p < 0.001$ in adults). SJ, CMJ and AJ also correlated with P_{peak} ($0.28 \leqslant r \leqslant 0.46$ in adolescents *versus* $0.58 \leqslant r \leqslant 0.61$ in adults) and with P_{mean} ($0.43 \leqslant r \leqslant 0.51$ *versus* $0.67 \leqslant r \leqslant 0.71$, respectively) of the WAnT ($p < 0.05$). In summary, the impact of the Bosco test and WAnT on muscle power varied, especially in the younger age group. Single jumping tests had larger correlations with WAnT in adults than in adolescent volleyball players. These findings should be taken into account by volleyball coaches and fitness trainers during the assessment of short-term muscle power of their athletes.

Keywords: age groups; anaerobic power; exercise mode; performance analysis; physiological evaluation; short-term power; team sport

1. Introduction

Volleyball is an intermittent high intensity team sport, where a combination of physical characteristics and aerobic and anaerobic capacity is necessary in order to perform a sequence of well-coordinated, high demand activities [1]. While a minimal level of aerobic capacity is necessary to cope with the demands of training and the game, maximal effort during short periods of time (e.g., jumping, hitting the ball) usually determines the outcome of a game [2]. Therefore, volleyball players should posses adequate short-term muscle power to compete at a high level [3,4]. Short-term muscle power is usually assessed using cycling—e.g., the 30 s Wingate anaerobic test, (WAnT) and jumping tests including single jumps such as the squat (SJ), countermovement (CMJ) and Abalakov jump (AJ), and continuous jumps such as the 30 s Bosco test—within a laboratory setting [5,6].

Although both jumping and cycling tests have been used extensively to assess short-term power in volleyball players, very few studies have been conducted to evaluate the relationship among these tests [7–10]. A study on young basketball players had shown large correlations between CMJ and two indices of the WAnT (peak power, P_{peak}, and mean power, P_{mean}) [7]. More recently, research on male volleyball players found a large correlation between P_{mean} of the WAnT with P_{mean} of the Bosco test [8], whereas large to very large correlations were observed among SJ, CMJ, P_{peak} and P_{mean} of the WAnT in young track-and-field athletes [9]. The sample size in the abovementioned studies was between 9 and 24.

The abovementioned studies have enhanced our understanding of the relationship of jumping tests with the WAnT; however, none of them has addressed the effect of chronological age on this relationship. The knowledge of the relationship between cycling and jumping tests would contribute to an optimal measurement and evaluation of short-term muscle power [11,12], which would be of great practical value for volleyball coaches and fitness trainers. Moreover, understanding the effect of chronological age on this relationship might help volleyball professionals to use these tests according to age. Additionally, sex-related physiological differences in performance and in game demands have been identified in volleyball [13,14], thereby rendering generalization of studies on male samples to female samples a risky venture. Therefore, the aim of the present study was to examine the relationship between jumping tests of short-term muscle power and the WAnT in a wide range of chronological ages of female volleyball players.

2. Methods

2.1. Participants

A cross-sectional design was used to examine the relationship of single and continuous jumping tests with the WAnT in female volleyball. To accomplish this aim, 178 female volleyball players (<18 years, $n = 70$; ⩾18 years, $n = 108$) from teams in the region of Athens were measured in the context of their yearly routine physical fitness assessment (Table 1). Testing procedures were carried out on September 2014 during the preparative period of seasons 2014–2015, respectively. The participants were familiar with testing procedures, because the fitness battery was routinely administered to these teams in the past, *i.e.*, all participants have performed the particular fitness battery at least one time previously. They visited the laboratory where they were examined for anthropometric characteristics, single and continuous jumping tests and the WAnT under standard environmental conditions (temperature 22–24 °C and humidity 50%–54%). The study was carried out according to the ethical standards of Declaration of Helsinki of the World Medical Association in 1964 as it was modified in 2013 and approved by the local institutional review board. Informed consent was given by all players or their guardians (in the case of underage participants).

Table 1. Anthropometric characteristics of volleyball players according to age group.

Variable	Total (n = 178)	<18 Years (n = 70)	>18 Years (n = 108)	Mean Difference (95% CI)
Age (years)	21.1 ± 5.9	16.0 ± 1.0	24.8 ± 5.2 †	−8.8 (−10.1; −7.6), d = −2.4
Body mass (kg)	64.9 ± 8.4	62.5 ± 7.1	66.5 ± 8.8 *	−3.9 (−6.4; −1.5), d = −0.5
Height (cm)	172.1 ± 7.0	170.4 ± 6.1	173.2 ± 7.4 *	−2.8 (−4.9; −0.7), d = −0.4
BMI ($kg \cdot m^{-2}$)	21.9 ± 2.2	21.5 ± 1.9	22.1 ± 2.4	−0.6 (−1.3; 0.1), d = −0.3
BF (%)	22.9 ± 4.9	24.2 ± 4.3	22.0 ± 5.1 *	2.2 (0.8; 3.7), d = 0.5

BMI = body mass index, BF = body fat percentage, CI = confidence intervals, d = effect size Cohen's d; * and † significant difference at $p < 0.01$ and $p < 0.001$, respectively.

2.2. Protocols and Equipments

2.2.1. Anthropometry

We used an electronic body mass scale (HD-351 Tanita, Arlington Heights, IL, USA) and a portable stadiometer (SECA, Leicester, UK) to measure body mass in the nearest 0.1 kg and stature in the nearest 1 mm with participants being barefoot and in minimal clothing, respectively. These measurements were used to calculate body mass index (BMI) as the quotient of body mass (kg) to stature squared (m^2). Body fat percentage (BF) was calculated from the sum of 10 skinfolds [15], which were taken with a skinfold caliper (Harpenden, West Sussex, UK). Chronological age for each participant was calculated using a table of decimals of year [16].

2.2.2. Single Jumping Tests and Bosco Test

The participants performed two trials for each jumping exercise (squat jump (SJ), countermovement jump without arm-swing (CMJ) and with arm-swing (Abalakov jump, AJ)) and the best result was recorded [17]. Height of each jump was estimated using the Opto-jump (Microgate Engineering, Bolzano, Italy) and was expressed in cm. The coefficient of variation of these single jumps has been reported previously as ~2%–3%, respectively [18,19]. The validity of the Opto-jump has been tested against force plate and has been shown to be very high (intraclass correlation coefficient (0.997–0.998)); however, the Opto-jump consistently provided ~1 cm higher score than force plate [20]. This discrepancy should be attributed to the fact that the participant did not assume the same body configuration during takeoff and landing [21]. The reliability of this system has been examined previously using intraclass correlation coefficient and coefficient of variation which indicated excellent reliability (~0.985 and ~2.7%, respectively) [20]. The Opto-jump system calculates jump height from jump's flight time [21]. The Bosco test was conducted on the same equipment as the abovementioned jump tests. The participants were instructed to jump as high as possible for 30 s, while trying to retain short ground contact times [22]. They were also requested to keep their hands on their waist throughout the test. The mean power during the 30 s test was expressed in $W \cdot kg^{-1}$.

2.2.3. Wingate Anaerobic Test

The WAnT was performed on a cycle ergometer (Ergomedics 874, Monark, Sweden) [23]. This ergometer was modified with an extra photocell, placed on the floor exactly under the lowest position of right pedal, which was connected to a PC so each revolution was recorded in order to calculate the main indices of the test. Briefly, participants were asked to pedal as fast as possible for 30 s against a braking force that was determined by the product of body mass in kg by 0.075. Peak power (P_{peak}) was estimated as the average power over a 5 s period with the highest performance, which occurs usually in the first 5 s of the test. Mean power (P_{mean}) was calculated as the average power during the 30 s period. Both P_{peak} and P_{mean} were expressed in W and $W \cdot kg^{-1}$. Fatigue index (FI) was calculated as $FI = 100 \times (P_{peak}$—minimal power$)/P_{peak}$, where minimal power was the lowest power output over a 5 s period, occurring usually towards the end of the test. The coefficient of variation of power indices has shown ~1%–2% [19].

2.3. Statistical Analysis

Statistical analyses were performed using IBM SPSS v.20.0 (SPSS, Chicago, IL, USA). Data were expressed as mean and standard deviations of the mean (SD). An independent t-test examined differences between adolescent and adult participants. Mean difference together with 95% confidence intervals (CI) was calculated. To interpret the effect size for statistical differences in the t-test we used Cohen's d classified as $d \leqslant 0.2$, trivial; $0.2 < d \leqslant 0.6$, small; $0.6 < d \leqslant 1.2$, moderate; $1.2 < d \leqslant 2.0$, large; and $d > 2.0$, very large [24]. Pearson correlation coefficient r examined the relationships among jumping tests and the WAnT. To interpret the magnitude of correlations the following criteria were adopted: $r \leqslant 0.1$, trivial; $0.1 < r \leqslant 0.3$, small; $0.3 < r \leqslant 0.5$, moderate; $0.5 < r \leqslant 0.7$, large; $0.7 < r \leqslant 0.9$, very large; and $r > 0.9$, almost perfect [25]. The level of significance was set at $\alpha = 0.05$.

3. Results

The anthropometric characteristics of participants can be found in Table 1. Differences among age groups were shown for all variables, except BMI which approached but did not quite achieve statistical significance ($p = 0.075$). The younger age group was lighter and shorter with higher BF than the older groups ($p < 0.05$). These differences had a small magnitude.

The results of the jumping tests and WAnT can be found in Table 2. The age groups differed for all single jump tests (SJ, CMJ and AJ) and all indices of the WAnT (absolute and relative P_{peak} and P_{mean}) ($p < 0.05$), except FI. In these tests, adults scored higher than adolescent volleyball players. These differences were of moderate magnitude for SJ, absolute P_{peak} and P_{mean}, and small for CMJ, AJ, relative P_{peak} and P_{mean}.

Table 2. Short-term muscle power of volleyball players according to age group.

Variable	Total (n = 178)	<18 Years (n = 70)	>18 Years (n = 108)	Mean Difference (95% CI)
SJ (cm)	23.6 ± 4.1	22.1 ± 3.1	24.6 ± 4.4 ‡	−2.5 (−4.0; −1.1), d = −0.7
CMJ (cm)	25.2 ± 4.4	24.0 ± 2.9	25.9 ± 5.1 *	−1.9 (−3.5; −0.3), d = −0.5
AJ (cm)	30.5 ± 4.9	29.4 ± 4.5	31.1 ± 5.1 *	−1.7 (−3.2; 0.3), d = −0.4
Bosco (W·kg^{-1})	25.8 ± 5.0	25.4 ± 4.6	26.0 ± 5.3	−0.6 (−2.2; 0.9), d = −0.1
P_{peak} (W)	574 ± 88	537 ± 75	598 ± 88 ‡	61 (−86; −36), d = −0.7
P_{peak} (W·kg^{-1})	8.90 ± 0.95	8.63 ± 0.85	9.07 ± 0.97 †	−0.45 (−0.73; −0.16), d = −0.5
P_{mean} (W)	423 ± 66	393 ± 52	444 ± 66 ‡	−51 (−70; −33), d = −0.9
P_{mean} (W·kg^{-1})	6.57 ± 0.81	6.33 ± 0.72	6.73 ± 0.82 ‡	−0.40 (−0.64; −0.16), d = −0.5
FI (%)	45.5 ± 7.5	45.7 ± 7.7	45.4 ± 7.5	0.4 (−2.0; 2.7), d < 0.1

SJ = squat jump, CMJ = countermovement jump, Abalakov = jump, P_{peak} = peak power, P_{mean} = mean power, FI = fatigue index during the Wingate anaerobic test (WAnT). The symbols *, † and ‡ denoted significance at $p < 0.05$, $p < 0.01$ and $p < 0.001$, respectively.

Mean power in the Bosco test was correlated (low to large magnitude) with relative P_{mean} in the WAnT (Table 3, Figure 1). SJ, CMJ and AJ were also correlated with P_{peak} ($0.28 \leqslant r \leqslant 0.46$ in adolescents *versus* $0.58 \leqslant r \leqslant 0.61$ in adults) and with P_{mean} ($0.43 \leqslant r \leqslant 0.51$ *versus* $0.67 \leqslant r \leqslant 0.71$, respectively) of the WAnT ($p < 0.05$).

Table 3. Correlations among cycling and jumping tests of short-term muscle power in volleyball players.

Variable	SJ			CMJ			AJ			Bosco Test		
	<18 Years	>18 Years	Total	<18 Years	>18 Years	Total	<18 Years	>18 Years	Total	<18 Years	>18 Years	Total
P_{peak} (W)	0.14	0.26 *	0.32 ‡	<0.01	0.25 *	0.26 ‡	0.17	0.16	0.22 †	0.04	0.05	0.06
P_{peak} (W·kg^{-1})	0.33 *	0.61 ‡	0.58 ‡	0.28	0.58 ‡	0.54 ‡	0.46 ‡	0.59	0.56 ‡	0.08	0.46 ‡	0.33 ‡
P_{mean} (W)	0.28	0.41 ‡	0.45 ‡	0.15	0.39 †	0.39 ‡	0.26 *	0.28 †	0.32 ‡	0.21	0.14	0.18 *
P_{mean} (W·kg^{-1})	0.48 †	0.71 ‡	0.67 ‡	0.43 †	0.67 ‡	0.62 ‡	0.51 ‡	0.65 ‡	0.62 ‡	0.27 *	0.54 ‡	0.45 ‡
FI (%)	−0.23	0.02	−0.03	−0.23	0.02	−0.03	−0.06	0.05	0.01	−0.23	−0.01	−0.10

P_{peak} = peak power, P_{mean} = mean power, FI = fatigue index during the Wingate anaerobic test (WAnT), SJ = squat jump, CMJ = countermovement jump, AJ = Abalakov jump. The symbols *, † and ‡ denoted significance at $p < 0.05$, $p < 0.01$ and $p < 0.001$, respectively.

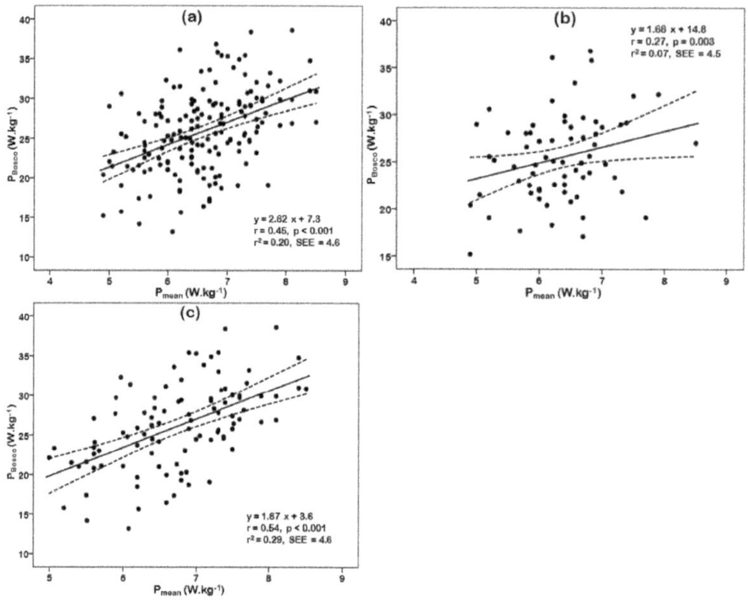

Figure 1. Relationship between mean power in the Wingate anaerobic test and mean power in the Bosco test in the total sample (**a**), adolescents (**b**), and adults (**c**). X axis represents mean power (W$\cdot$ kg^{-1}) in Wingate anaerobic test; y axis represents mean power (W$\cdot$ kg^{-1}) in Bosco test; SEE = standard error of estimate.

4. Discussion

The main findings of the present study were that (a) mean power in the Bosco test was correlated (low to large magnitude) with P_{mean} in the WAnT; (b) single jumps (SJ, CMJ and AJ) were correlated with P_{peak} and with P_{mean} of the WAnT; and (c) an age effect on the relationship between performance in jumping and cycling tests was observed (correlations of larger magnitude were found in adult rather than in adolescent volleyball players).

Although one would expect to observe a similar performance in the Bosco test and the WAnT, because both tests lasted the same time and required maximal effort, the findings confirmed this hypothesis only partially (*i.e.*, just in the case of adults). The magnitude of their correlation varied from small (adolescents) to large (adults), but even in the case of adults (Figure 1c), a large portion of variance (~71%) in performance in the Bosco test could not be accounted for by variance in performance in the WAnT. The differences in this correlation between adolescent and adult groups might be related to the athletes' experience in the realization of these tests. Although the participants were not asked about the exact number of times they previously participated in the fitness battery, according to their higher athletic experience, it was assumed that the adult volleyball players have performed both tests on more occasions than the adolescents. On the contrary, the lower correlation in the adolescents might be due to them having less expertise in the coordination of their arms (e.g., in AJ) or in the eccentric phase of movement (e.g., in CMJ). An interpretation of this relationship between the Bosco test and the WAnT might be the different mode of exercise (jumping *versus* cycling), which recruited different muscle groups, and the role of body mass (it moved against gravity in the former mode, whereas it was supported by the saddle in the latter mode).

The lower correlation between the Bosco test and the WAnT in the adolescent volleyball players compared to their older counterparts indicated a lower ability to "translate" anaerobic power as measured in the cycling test into a continuous jumping performance for the former group. This variation might result from the effect of a long-term training process, including practice in jumping during training and game-play in the latter group, which allowed them to perform continuous jumping more efficiently. Similarly, SJ, CMJ and AJ correlated with P_{peak} and with P_{mean} of the WAnT with higher magnitude in the adult compared to the adolescent volleyball players. Furthermore, it was likely that the lower correlations in the adolescent participants might be due to the choice of the braking force during the WAnT [26–29].

Even if the findings of the present study suggested that the 30 s Bosco test should not be used interchangeably with the WAnT, especially in adolescent volleyball players, this did not imply that the latter test was not suitable for monitoring volleyball players. The WAnT has been used extensively to evaluate anaerobic profile in this sport [8,30–32]. On the other hand, jumping tests provided additional information about sport-specific qualities, such as the stretch-shortening cycle or the use of the arm-swing.

5. Conclusions

In summary, the impact of the Bosco test and the WAnT on muscle power varied, especially in the younger age group. Single vertical jumping tests had larger correlations with WAnT in adult rather than in adolescent volleyball players. These findings should be taken into account by volleyball coaches and fitness trainers during the assessment of short-term muscle power of their athletes.

Acknowledgments: We thank all the volleyball players of the teams participating to this study for their collaboration.

Conflicts of Interest: The authors declare no conflict of interest.

References

1. Gabbett, T.; Georgieff, B. Physiological and anthropometric characteristics of Australian junior national, state, and novice volleyball players. *J. Strength Cond. Res.* **2007**, *21*, 902–908. [PubMed]
2. Grgantov, Z.; Milić, M.; Katić, R. Identification of explosive power factors as predictors of player quality in young female volleyball players. *Coll. Antropol.* **2013**, *37*, 61–68. [PubMed]
3. Nikolaidis, P.T.; Afonso, J.; Busko, K. Differences in anthropometry, somatotype, body composition and physiological characteristics of female volleyball players by competition level. *Sport Sci. Health* **2015**, *11*, 29–35. [CrossRef]
4. Nikolaidis, P.T.; Ziv, G.; Arnon, M.; Lidor, R. Physical characteristics and physiological attributes of female volleyball players-the need for individual data. *J. Strength Cond. Res.* **2012**, *26*, 2547–2557. [CrossRef] [PubMed]
5. Álvarez-Herms, J.; Julià-Sánchez, S.; Corbi, F.; Pagès, T.; Viscor, G. Anaerobic performance after endurance strength training in hypobaric environment. *Sci. Sports* **2014**, *29*, 311–318. [CrossRef]
6. Nikolaidis, P.T.; Afonso, J.; Buśko, K.; Ingebrigtsen, J.; Chtourou, H.; Martin, J.J. Positional differences of physical traits and physiological characteristics in female volleyball players—The role of age. *Kinesiology* **2015**, *47*, 75–81.
7. Hoffman, J.R.; Epstein, S.; Einbinder, M.; Weinstein, Y. A comparison between the Wingate anaerobic power test to both vertical jump and line drill tests in basketball players. *J. Strength Cond. Res.* **2000**, *14*, 261–264.
8. Dal Pupo, J.; Gheller, R.G.; Dias, J.A.; Rodacki, A.L.F.; Moro, A.R.P.; Santos, S.G. Reliability and validity of the 30-s continuous jump test for anaerobic fitness evaluation. *J. Sci. Med. Sport* **2014**, *17*, 650–655. [CrossRef] [PubMed]
9. Çakir-Atabek, H. Relationship between anaerobic power, vertical jump and aerobic performance in adolescent track and field athletes. *J. Phys. Educ. Sport* **2014**, *14*, 643–648.
10. Driss, T.; Vandewalle, H.; Monod, H. Maximal power and force-velocity relationships during cycling and cranking exercises in volleyball players: Correlation with the vertical jump test. *J. Sports Med. Phys. Fit.* **1998**, *38*, 286–293.
11. Vandewalle, H.; Peres, G.; Heller, J.; Panel, J.; Monod, H. Force-velocity relationship and maximal power on a cycle ergometer—Correlation with the height of a vertical jump. *Eur. J. Appl. Physiol. Occup. Physiol.* **1987**, *56*, 650–656. [CrossRef] [PubMed]

12. Rouis, M.; Attiogbé, E.; Vandewalle, H.; Jaafar, H.; Noakes, T.D.; Driss, T. Relationship between vertical jump and maximal power output of legs and arms: Effects of ethnicity and sport. *Scand. J. Med. Sci. Sports* **2015**, *25*, e197–e207. [CrossRef] [PubMed]
13. João, P.V.; Leite, N.; Mesquita, I.; Sampaio, J. Sex differences in discriminative power of volleyball game-related statistics. *Percept. Mot. Skills* **2010**, *111*, 893–900. [CrossRef] [PubMed]
14. Costa, G.; Afonso, J.; Brant, E.; Mesquita, I. Differences in game patterns between male and female youth volleyball. *Kinesiology* **2012**, *44*, 60–66.
15. Parizkova, J. Lean body mass and depot fat during autogenesis in humans. In *Nutrition, Physical Fitness and Health: International Series on Sport Sciences*; Parizkova, J., Rogozkin, V., Eds.; University Park Press: Baltimore, MD, USA, 1978.
16. Ross, W.D.; Marfell-Jones, M.J. Kinanthropometry. In *Physiological Testing of the High-Performance Athlete*; MacDougall, J.D., Wenger, H.A., Green, H.J., Eds.; Human Kinetics: Champaign, IL, USA, 1991.
17. Aragon-Vargas, L.F. Evaluation of four vertical jump tests: Methodology, reliability, validity, and accuracy. *Meas. Phys. Educ. Exerc. Sci.* **2000**, *4*, 215–228. [CrossRef]
18. Markovic, G.; Dizdar, D.; Jukic, I.; Cardinale, M. Reliability and factorial validiry of squat and countermovement jump tests. *J. Strength Cond. Res.* **2004**, *18*, 551–555. [PubMed]
19. Hopkins, W.G.; Schabort, E.J.; Hawley, J.A. Reliability of power in physical performance tests. *Sports Med.* **2001**, *31*, 211–234. [CrossRef] [PubMed]
20. Glatthorn, J.F.; Gouge, S.; Nussbaumer, S.; Stauffacher, S.; Impellizzeri, F.M.; Maffiueletti, N.A. Validity and reliability of Uptojump photoelectric cells for estimating vertical jump height. *J. Strength Cond. Res.* **2011**, *25*, 556–560. [CrossRef] [PubMed]
21. Linthorne, N.P. Analysis of standing vertical jumps using a force platform. *Am. J. Phys.* **2001**, *69*, 1198–1204. [CrossRef]
22. Sands, W.A.; McNeal, J.R.; Ochi, M.T.; Urbanek, T.L.; Jemni, M.; Stone, M.H. Comparison of the Wingate and Bosco anaerobic tests. *J. Strength Cond. Res.* **2004**, *18*, 810–815. [PubMed]
23. Driss, T.; Vandewalle, H. The measurement of maximal (anaerobic) power output on a cycle ergometer: A critical review. *BioMed Res. Int.* **2013**, *2013*. [CrossRef] [PubMed]
24. Cohen, J. *Statistical Power Analysis for the Behavioral Sciences*; Lawrence Erlbaum Associates: Hillsdale, NJ, USA, 1988.
25. Hopkins, W.G.; Marshall, S.W.; Batterham, A.M.; Hanin, J. Progressive statistics for studies in sports medicine and exercise science. *Med. Sci. Sports Exerc.* **2009**, *41*, 3–13. [CrossRef] [PubMed]
26. Doré, E.; Bedu, M.; França, N.M.; Diallo, O.; Duché, P.; van Praagh, E. Testing peak cycling performance: Effects of braking force during growth. *Med. Sci. Sports Exerc.* **2000**, *32*, 493–498. [PubMed]
27. Jaafar, H.; Rouis, M.; Coudrat, L.; Attiogbé, E.; Vandewalle, H.; Driss, T. Effects of load on Wingate test performances and reliability. *J. Strength Cond. Res.* **2014**, *28*, 3462–3468. [CrossRef] [PubMed]
28. Jaafar, H.; Rouis, M.; Attiogbé, E.; Vandewalle, H.; Driss, T. A Comparative study between the Wingate and Force-Velocity anaerobic cycling tests: Effect of physical fitness. *Int. J. Sports Physiol. Perform.* **2016**, *11*, 48–54. [CrossRef] [PubMed]
29. Doré, E.; Diallo, O.; França, N.M.; Bedu, M.; van Praagh, E. Dimensional changes cannot account for all differences in short-term cycling power during growth. *Int. J. Sports Med.* **2000**, *21*, 360–365. [CrossRef] [PubMed]
30. Eliakim, A.; Portal, S.; Zadik, Z.; Meckel, Y.; Nemet, D. Training reduces catabolic and inflammatory response to a single practice in female volleyball players. *J. Strength Cond. Res.* **2013**, *27*, 3110–3115. [CrossRef] [PubMed]
31. Nikolaidis, P.T. Body mass index and body fat percentage are associated with decreased physical fitness in adolescent and adult female volleyball players. *J. Res. Med. Sci.* **2013**, *18*, 22–26. [PubMed]
32. Fernández-Campos, C.; Dengo, A.L.; Moncada-Jiménez, J. Acute consumption of an energy drink does not improve physical performance of female volleyball players. *Int. J. Sport Nutr. Exerc. Metab.* **2015**, *25*, 271–277. [CrossRef] [PubMed]

7

Effects of Intermittent Neck Cooling During Repeated Bouts of High-Intensity Exercise

Andrew J. Galpin [1,*], James R. Bagley [2], Blake Whitcomb [1], Leonard D. Wiersma [1], Jakob Rosengarten [1], Jared W. Coburn [1] and Daniel A. Judelson [1]

[1] Center for Sport Performance, Department of Kinesiology, California State University, Fullerton, CA 92834, USA; blake.whitcomb@gmail.com (B.W.); lwiersma@fullerton.edu (L.D.W.); jakoblpc@googlemail.com (J.R.); jcoburn@fullerton.edu (J.W.C.); dan.judelson@nike.com (D.A.J.)

[2] Department of Kinesiology, San Francisco State University, San Francisco, CA 94132, USA; jrbagley@sfsu.edu

* Correspondence: agalpin@fullerton.edu

Academic Editor: Eling de Bruin

Abstract: The purpose of this investigation was to determine the influence of intermittent neck cooling during exercise bouts designed to mimic combat sport competitions. Participants ($n = 13$, age = 25.3 ± 5.0 year height = 176.9 ± 7.5 cm, mass = 79.3 ± 9.0 kg, body fat = 11.8% ± 3.1%) performed three trials on a cycle ergometer. Each trial consisted of two, 5-min high-intensity exercise (HEX) intervals (HEX1 and HEX2—20 s at 50% peak power, followed by 15 s of rest), and a time to exhaustion (TTE) test. One-minute rest intervals were given between each round (RI1 and RI2), during which researchers treated the participant's posterior neck with either (1) wet-ice (ICE); (2) menthol spray (SPRAY); or (3) no treatment (CON). Neck (T_{NECK}) and chest (T_{CHEST}) skin temperatures were significantly lower following RI1 with ICE (vs. SPRAY). Thermal sensation decreased with ICE compared to CON following RI1, RI2, TTE, and a 2-min recovery. Rating of perceived exertion was also lower with ICE following HEX2 (vs. CON) and after RI2 (vs. SPRAY). Treatment did not influence TTE (68.9 ± 18.9s). The ability of intermittent ICE to attenuate neck and chest skin temperature rises during the initial HEX stages likely explains why participants felt cooler and less exerted during equivalent HEX bouts. These data suggest intermittent ICE improves perceptual stress during short, repeated bouts of vigorous exercise.

Keywords: mixed martial arts; recovery; combat sports; endurance; performance; ice

---

1. Introduction

The scientific community has recently drawn interest in the complex physiological demands of combat sports (e.g., wrestling, boxing, judo) [1]. Their energetic requirements and activity patterns differ from steady-state sports such as cycling or running whereby they require alternating bouts of maximal exertion (usually 5–15 s) and active rest (usually 5–40 s), repeated for 2–6 min, per round, with most competitions requiring 3–10 rounds [1–4]. Causes of fatigue during these activities, or similar forms of high-intensity exercise (HEX), are multifaceted as various physiological, and perceptual inputs interact to control both physical capacity and the desire to perform it [5–7]. Specifically, a combination of body temperature and the conscious perception of thermal distress [8], thermal sensation (TS), and the rating of perceived exertion (RPE) [9] combine to determine exercise workload/performance [5–7,10].

Reducing skin temperature in thermally sensitive areas (face, hands, specific exercising muscles, or a combination of these) may reduce TS, thermal discomfort, and RPE, which improves exercise performance and perception [7,10,11]. Applying cooling agents (e.g., ice packs) to these locations before or during the rest intervals (RI) of HEX (i.e., "intermittent cooling") has been shown to increase exercise power output [12] and time to fatigue [10,13,14]. Unfortunately, cooling these areas is not practical for combat sports due to the number of muscles involved, the equipment, and sport rules [9]. Coaches typically circumvent this problem by placing an ice bag on the back of an athlete's necks between rounds. Neck cooling typically enhances performance during low- [15–17] and moderate-intensity exercise (⩽70% VO_2max) [16,17]. However, little is known about its effectiveness during HEX.

A growing collection of parallel research strongly supports thermal perception as a thermoregulatory controller [7,8,18]. Thus, researchers are now also investigating the effects of perceived (i.e., non-thermal) cooling on thermoregulation and performance [5–7,18], particularly when applied to the neck. The early indications suggest that non-thermal cooling (usually menthol sprays) does not alter core and skin temperatures, skin blood flow, or skin sweat rate [5], but does promote positive changes in TS and RPE.

Taken together, while the literature supports a relationship between body cooling and exercise performance, it is still unclear (1) if intermittent neck cooling during HEX alters performance, TS, or the perception of difficulty, and (2) if these alterations are a result of actual physical cooling, or simply the perception of cooling. Therefore, the purpose of this study was to investigate physiological and perceptual effects of intermittent neck cooling during the rest periods of repeated HEX bouts designed to mimic combat sport competition energetic demands.

2. Materials and Method

2.1. Study Design

Participants reported to the laboratory on four separate occasions (each separated by ⩾48 and ⩽168 h), which included one familiarization and three experimental trials (Figure 1). Each trial consisted of repeated bouts of HEX cycling. During the rest intervals (RI) between acute HEX bouts, participants had (A) a wet-ice bag (ICE) [19], (B) a menthol spray (SPRAY), or (C) nothing (CON) placed on their cervical spine. This was designed to mimic a typical 3-round combat sport event (i.e., 3 × 5-min rounds, with 1-min rest between rounds). Only one treatment (ICE, SPRAY, or CON) was used per experimental trial, and the order was randomized.

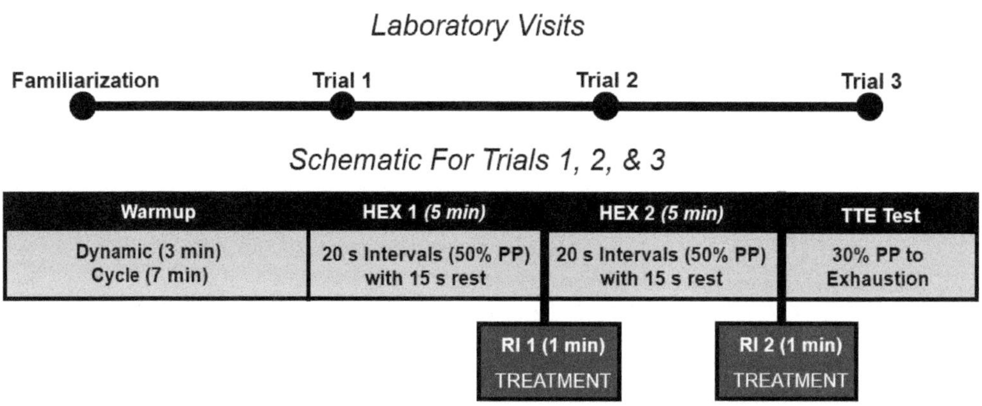

Figure 1. Laboratory visits timeline and schematic showing repeated high-intensity exercise bouts. For each visit, the TREATMENT included either ICE (wet ice), SPRAY (menthol spray), or CON (control, no treatment). Abbreviations: HEX: high-intensity bout of exercise; PP: peak power; RI: rest interval; TTE: time to exhaustion.

2.2. Experimental Controls

All trials took place in the Exercise Physiology Laboratory (maintained at 25.0 ± 1.0 °C, 53.0% ± 1.0% relative humidity) with the same technicians, at the same time of the day (within participant). Participants were asked to not exercise the 24 h before each trial, but were encouraged to maintain their normal training routine throughout the duration of the study. Participants were instructed to consume a diet similar to their first trial for all subsequent trials. To verify consistency, hydration and food logs were recorded 24 h prior to each trial. Participants were further instructed to consume 500 mL of water the night before and 500 mL in the morning before the start of the trial. Height, mass, and body fat percentage (via bioelectrical impedance analysis) was recorded prior to each trial. To minimize confounding influences of motivation, participants were given no feedback on their performance, nor did they receive verbal (or any other) encouragement at any point of the study.

2.3. Participants

Physically active males ($n = 13$, age = 25.3 ± 5.0 year, height = 176.9 ± 7.5 cm, mass = 79.3 ± 9.0 kg, body fat = 11.8% ± 3.1%) without previous experience with neck cooling were recruited for this investigation. In order to participate, volunteers were required to have performed repeated HEX bouts (which we defined as repeated bouts of ⩾90% maximal perceived exertion and/or heart rate) ⩾3 times per week for at least six weeks prior to testing, and to have been free of any current joint, musculoskeletal, or neuromuscular injuries. Prior to participation, volunteers signed an informed consent form and filled out a physical activity questionnaire previously approved by the California State University, Fullerton Institutional Review Board.

2.4. Familiarization and Experimental Trials

Before every trial (familiarization and three experimental), participants performed a 10-min warm-up consisting of 3 min (total) of knee hugs, toe touches, lunges, power skips, and side shuffles, and 7 min of cycling at 50 Watts (self-selected cadence). For the familiarization trial, participants followed the warm-up with a 10-s Wingate test (to measure peak power (PP)), rested for 10 min, and then completed the full experimental trial (including scale reading practice and wearing of the metabolic cart headgear or mouthpiece). For the experimental trials, 1 min of rest was given between the end of the warm-up and beginning of the HEX.

Each experimental trial was performed on a cycle ergometer (Ergomedic 839E, Monark Exercise AB, Sweden) and consisted of two, 5-min HEX bouts (20 s maximal cadence cycling, plus 15 s passive rest) at 50% PP, plus a single bout to exhaustion (TTE) at 30% PP. Pilot work suggested 50% PP allowed participants to reach maximal effort within a 20-s interval, while still being physically capable of completing the full protocol. The work-to-rest ratio of 20:15 s was chosen because it is a standard protocol used among HEX practitioners, and it also represents the typical activity pattern observed during combat sport competitions [3]. Exhaustion during the TTE was defined as the participant's inability to pedal ⩾60 revolutions per min for more than 5 consecutive seconds. Pilot data also suggested 30% PP would allow most participants to reach exhaustion between 1–5 min, which is the length of most combat sport rounds.

A 1-min passive RI separated all three bouts of exercise (the two HEX and the one TTE). During the RI, participants remained on the bike but were not allowed to cycle, as combat sport athletes typically sit passively on a stool during competition RI. However, during the RI between HEX round 1 (HEX1) and HEX round 2 (HEX2), and between HEX2 and TTE, the posterior neck was treated with either ICE, SPRAY, or CON. The treatment (ICE, SPRAY, or CON) was consistent within each trial, but the order of each trial was randomized (e.g., Participant 1 received SPRAY Day 1; CON, Day 2; ICE, Day 3, while Participant 2 received CON, Day 1; ICE, Day 2; SPRAY, Day 3).

For ICE, participants had a researcher hold an ice bag (Mueller Sport Medicine, Inc., Prairie Du Sac, Wisconsin) filled with 1 quart of ice (immediately from freezer) and 600 mL of room temperature water on the back of the neck (in direct contact with only the skin) [19]. This method mimics the cooling technique frequently used in combat sport competitions. SPRAY was achieved by having a researcher apply 2–4 mL of a commercially available 8% menthol spray (Stopain: DRJ Group, Inc., Hazelton, Pennsylvania) directly on the participant's neck at the beginning of RI1 and RI2. The spray was wiped off the neck with a towel immediately following RI1 and RI2 to prevent potential residual influences on subsequent exercise bouts (i.e., HEX2 and TTE) [7]. Participants were not informed of the reason for including the SPRAY treatment. Participants received no treatment during either RI1 or RI2 during the CON trial.

2.5. Skin Temperature

Skin temperature was recorded every second from the beginning of the cycling warm-up until the end of recovery. Four calibrated surface thermistors (DS1922L-F5# Thermochron, Ibutton, Whitewater, Wisconsin) were secured in place with surgical tape to the neck (T_{NECK}), the right side of the pectoralis major (T_{CHEST}), the upper arm (T_{ARM}), and the quadriceps (T_{LEG}). Data were reported at the same time points as TS and RPE. Core temperature was not reported, as similar cooling research indicated that it would not be influenced by our treatments [7,17,18].

2.6. Expired Gas and Heart Rate

Expired gases were collected with a metabolic cart (Parvo Medics 2400, Sandy, Utah) throughout every trial (i.e., cycling warm-up through recovery). A chest monitor (Polar FS1, Lake Success, New York) was used to record heart rate (HR) through the same period. Expired gas and HR data were recorded every 15 s from the beginning of the cycling warm-up until the end of recovery.

2.7. Perceptual Measures

TS and rating of RPE were measured by having participants point to visual scales (1) immediately (<2 s) following HEX1/start of RI1, (2) immediately following RI1/the start of HEX2, (3) immediately following HEX2/start of RI2, (4) immediately following RI2/the start of TTE, (5) immediately following TTE, and (6) 2 min after the end of TTE (recovery). TS was rated with a 9-point scale, ranging from 0 (unbearably cold) to 8 (unbearably hot), with 4 as comfortable (neutral). RPE was measured on the 15-grade Borg scale ranging from 6 (no exertion) to 20 (maximal exertion).

2.8. Statistical Analysis

All statistical analyses were performed on IBM SPSS Statistics 20.0. Alpha was set at $p < 0.05$. TTE was analyzed using a 3×1 (treatment $\times$ time) repeated measures ANOVA. A 3×6 (treatment $\times$ time) factorial ANOVA was used to analyze TS, RPE, skin temperature, VO_2, RER, VE, and HR. Where appropriate, LSD post hoc test comparisons were used. Standardized effect size (Cohen's d; *d*) analyses were used in interpreting the magnitude of differences between treatments. An effect size was classified as trivial (<0.20), small (0.20–0.49), moderate (0.50–0.79), or large (>0.80) as expressed by dividing the mean difference by the between-participant SD. All data are presented as mean $\pm$ SD.

3. Results

3.1. Skin Temperature

The condition x time interaction was not significant for any skin temperature. Significant ($p < 0.05$) main effects existed for time (T_{NECK}: F = 10.77, T_{CHEST}: F = 11.16, T_{ARM}: 49.32, T_{LEG}: F = 7.58) and condition (T_{NECK}: F = 4.24, T_{CHEST}: 3.41, T_{ARM}: 3.45). Pairwise comparisons revealed the following. T_{NECK} following RI1 was significantly lower during ICE than SPRAY ($p < 0.05$) (Figure 2). T_{CHEST} was significantly lower during ICE than SPRAY ($p < 0.05$) and tended to be lower than CON ($p = 0.08$, $d = 0.48$) following RI1 (Figure 2). T_{CHEST} was significantly lower ($p < 0.05$) during ICE than both SPRAY and CON both immediately following HEX2, and after RI2. T_{ARM} tended to be lower during ICE compared to CON and SPRAY, both immediately following HEX2 ($p = 0.07$; $d = 0.59$, $p = 0.08$; $d = 0.63$, respectively) and after RI2 ($p = 0.08$; $d = 0.44$, $p = 0.08$; $d = 0.80$, respectively). T_{LEG} did not change at any time point, for any condition.

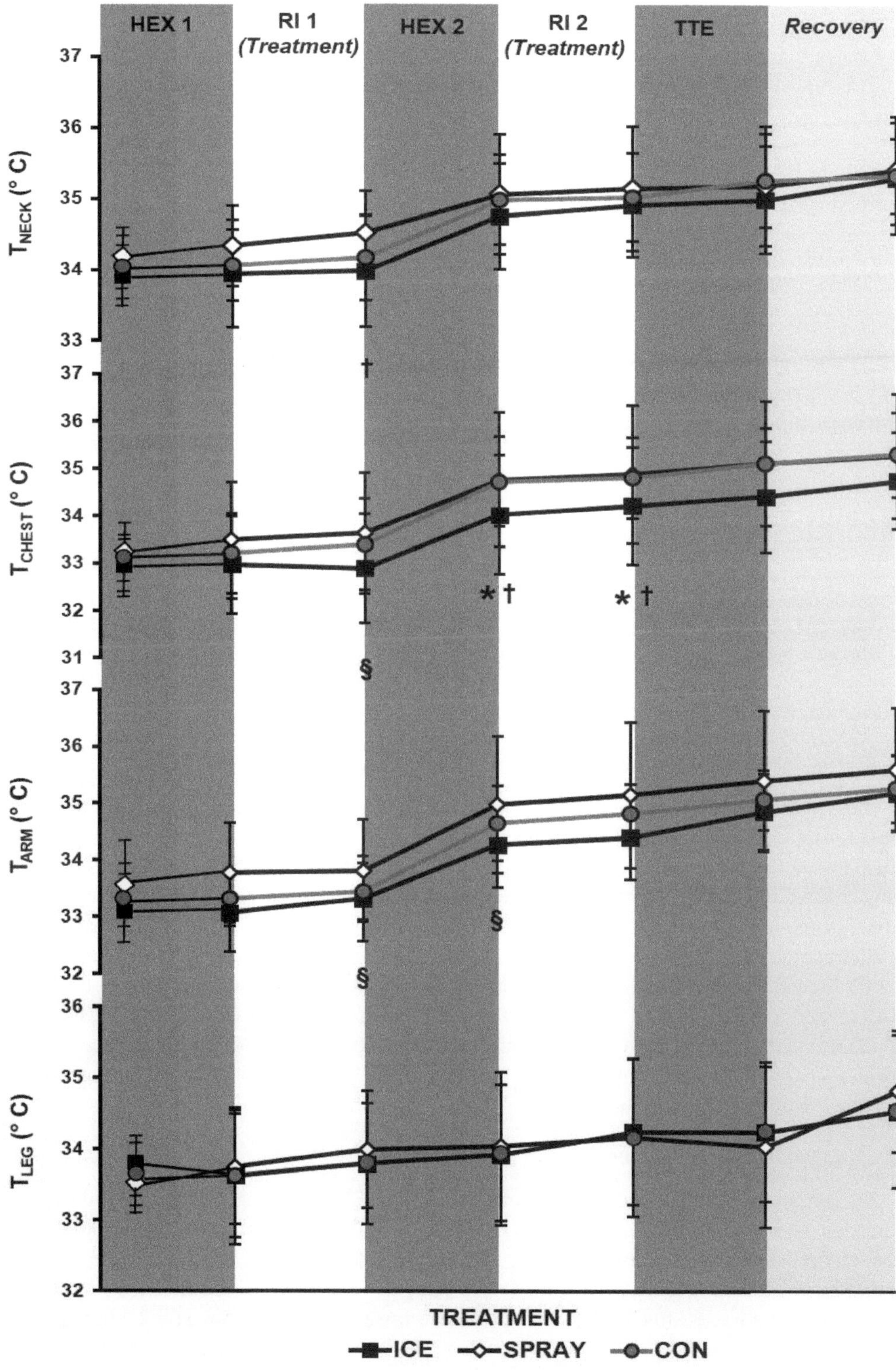

Figure 2. Skin temperatures (T_{NECK}, neck; T_{CHEST}, chest) during exercise bouts (HEX: high-intensity exercise interval; TTE: time-to-exhaustion) with intermittent rest intervals (RI) and neck cooling treatments (ICE: "wet ice" bag; SPRAY: non-thermal cool spray; or CON: control). Significance among treatments: * ICE vs. CON ($p < 0.05$), § ICE vs. CON (*trend*; $p \leqslant 0.08$), † ICE vs. SPRAY ($p < 0.05$). Mean ± SD.

3.2. Expired Gas and Heart Rate

No significant differences existed among treatments at any time point in metabolic and cardiovascular variables. Thus, data were collapsed between treatments and reported across time (Table 1).

Table 1. The cardiovascular and metabolic variables collapsed between treatments and displayed across time.

Variable	HEX 1	HEX 2	TTE
RER_{AVE}	1.00 ± 0.5	0.97 ± 0.03	1.01 ± 0.04
RER_{PEAK}	1.12 ± 0.07	1.22 ± 0.09 *	1.13 ± 0.07
VE_{AVE} ($L \cdot min^{-1}$)	67.6 ± 12.8	80.3 ± 16.1 *	75.1 ± 17.0 ¥
VE_{PEAK} ($L \cdot min^{-1}$)	89.8 ± 17.5	90.9 ± 18.1	89.9 ± 19.1
HR_{AVE} (bpm)	147.7 ± 17.7	163.6 ± 14.0*	157.3 ± 15.7
HR_{PEAK} (bpm)	169.7 ± 11.2	175.7± 10.6 §	173.3 ± 11.4
VO_{2AVE} ($mL \cdot kg^{-1} \cdot min^{-1}$)	35.5 ± 5.9	39.0 ± 6.3	32.6 ± 6.5
VO_{2PEAK} ($mL \cdot kg^{-1} \cdot min^{-1}$)	45.1 ± 6.1	44.8 ± 7.5	41.7 ± 8.2

Data are reported as mean ± SD. * signifies $p < 0.05$ compared to HEX 1 and TTE, § signifies $p < 0.05$ compared to HEX 1, ¥ signifies $p = 0.07$ compared to HEX 2.

3.3. Perceptual Measures

3.3.1. Thermal Sensation

The condition x time interaction was significant (F = 2.717, $p = 0.034$). A significant main effect existed for time (F = 19.46, $p = 0.001$) and condition (F = 4.22, $p = 0.029$). Pairwise analysis showed participants felt significantly cooler during ICE than CON ($p = 0.02$) and tended to feel cooler than during SPRAY ($p = 0.10$). Analysis of the simple main effects showed TS was the same among treatments immediately after HEX1 and HEX2. However, following RI1 and RI2 (i.e., after treatment administration), TS decreased (i.e., participants felt significantly cooler) with ICE compared to CON ($p < 0.05$; Figure 3) and tended to decrease with ICE compared to SPRAY after RI1 ($p = 0.10$; $d = 0.35$). SPRAY tended to have a similar cooling affect as ICE following RI2 when compared to CON ($p = 0.07$, $d = 0.67$). Immediately following TTE, TS significantly ($p < 0.05$) decreased during ICE compared to CON and tended to decrease compared to SPRAY ($p = 0.09$; $d = 0.58$). This continued through recovery as ICE was significantly lower than CON ($p < 0.05$).

3.3.2. Rating of Perceived Exertion (RPE)

The condition x time interaction was not significant ($p = 0.519$). A significant main effect existed for time (F = 44.808, $p < 0.000$) and condition (F = 6.26, $p = 0.040$). Pairwise analysis showed participants felt significantly less exerted during ICE than CON ($p = 0.018$). Analysis of simple main effects showed RPE was the same among treatments immediately after HEX1 (Figure 3). Additionally, no differences existed among treatments after RI1. However, RPE was lower in ICE following HEX2 when compared to CON ($p < 0.05$) and tended to be lower when compared to SPRAY ($p = 0.10$; $d = 0.38$). RPE was also lower with ICE compared to SPRAY and tended to be lower compared to CON ($p = 0.08$; $d = 0.41$) after RI2. RPE was not different between treatments immediately following TTE but tended to be lower in ICE during recovery compared to SPRAY ($p = 0.10$; $d = 0.40$) and CON ($p = 0.12$; $d = 0.37$).

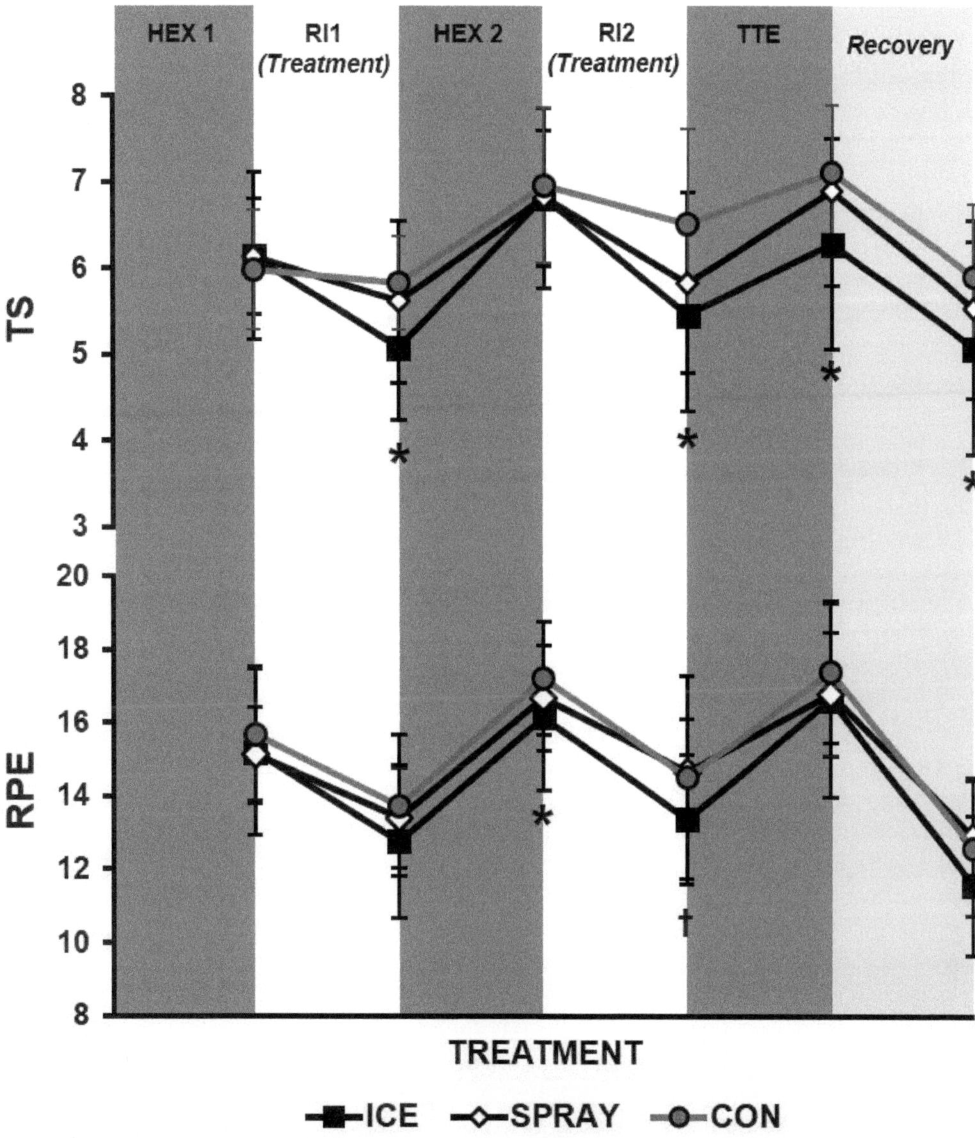

Figure 3. Perceptual responses to repeated exercise bouts (HEX: high-intensity exercise interval; TTE: time-to-exhaustion) with intermittent rest intervals (RI) and neck cooling treatments (ICE: "wet ice" bag; SPRAY: non-thermal cool spray; or CON: control). TS: thermal sensation; RPE: rating of perceived exertion. Significance among treatments: * ICE vs. CON ($p < 0.05$), † ICE vs. SPRAY ($p < 0.05$). Mean ± SD.

3.4. Time To Exhaustion

Treatment did not influence TTE (ICE = 66.5 ± 16.6, SPRAY = 74.0 ± 23.7, CON = 65.9 ± 16.6 s).

4. Discussion

Our findings provide new insight into the relationship between neck cooling, physiological and perceived fatigue, skin temperature, and actual performance during repeated, high-intensity exercise intervals. These data show that holding an ice bag on the back of the neck for one minute between rounds of HEX attenuates the rise in skin temperature and, as a result, makes participants feel cooler and, at times, less exerted, but does not alter cardiovascular or metabolic function. Thus, intermittent neck cooling may function as an effective, practical, and legal cooling option for combat sport athletes (or others who participate in repeated HEX for sport or recreation) to utilize during competition and training.

Temperature, Perception, and Performance

Temperature, perception, and actual exercise performance significantly influence each other [20]. In fact, Mündel [4] suggested the temperature of a skin surface area $\leqslant$10% of the body may significantly effect hormonal and perceptual responses to exercise [9]. The attenuated rise in neck, chest, and arm skin temperature seen here with ICE did not correspond with a reduced rise in heart rate (or altered metabolic function) as proposed by others [20]. However, the ability of ICE to cool the skin is similar to previous research [21] and likely explains our improvements in TS [13]. This reduction in TS allowed participants to enter subsequent exercise bouts feeling cooler. Interestingly, while the effect of the first application of ICE on TS was eliminated by the next round of exercise (i.e., post HEX2 TS was not different between treatments), its effects on RPE persisted (i.e., post HEX2 RPE was significantly lower in ICE). This continued through RI2, suggesting that participants both (1) completed the standardized exercise bout (HEX2) and (2) went into the third bout of exercise (TTE) feeling less exerted and cooler, even though several cardiovascular and metabolic markers (RER_{PEAK}, VE_{AVE}, HR_{AVE}, and HR_{PEAK}) indicated HEX2 was more physiologically challenging than HEX1. They also felt cooler after a matched workload (TTE) and 2 min into recovery. Additionally, lower pre-exercise TS corresponded with lower post-exercise RPE (when compared to a standardized work bout—HEX2). Unfortunately, our study design eliminated the ability to determine if the reduced post-RI2 RPE was a function of ICE (1) aiding recovery from HEX1; (2) pre-cooling the neck in preparation for HEX2; (3) or both. Research from others suggests intermittent cooling of other body parts reduces RPE [22], but we are the first to show such changes with intermittent neck cooling.

The ability of ICE to attenuate the rise in skin temperature diminished as the exercise session extended. This means changes in skin temperature either (1) did not fully explain the continual decrease in TS or RPE; or, more likely, (2) caused a continued perception of cooling, even when actual cooling was not occurring. Actual temperature changes are not required to alter thermoregulatory responses or to improve performance [7]. We chose to globally account for both actual and perceived cooling by including a treatment group that received an over-the-counter spray (SPRAY) containing menthol, a substance that interacts with cold receptors in sensory neurons [6] and alters exercise performance [5,23]. Recent evidence suggests an L-menthol spray with a concentration of 0.2% lowers TS [23]. Our data show a limited effectiveness of SPRAY, which is probably a result of differences in exercise protocols (i.e., our repeated HEX vs. 40 min of steady-state) [5,23], or our use of an 8% commercially available product. None of our participants reported skin irritation or discomfort from SPRAY, as has been reported in some previous studies. Thus, it was unlikely to explain our findings.

Changes in physical and perceptual markers during intermittent [13,14] or pre-cooling [20] of the actual exercising muscle, face and palm, and/or neck usually correspond with improvements in endurance and time trial performance [24]. The inability of ICE to influence leg temperature and subsequently improve TTE in our study is most likely explained by a combination of (a) the location and (b) a short duration (1 min) of cooling, and the (c) high-intensity and (d) short duration (~1 min) of TTE. Cooling the legs directly would obviously maximize the influence on skin temperature and likely improve TTE performance [14]. However, this strategy is unrealistic for combat sport athletes or during any exercise bout that uses multiple muscle groups. As opposed to previous research, which typically use >5 min [24–26] or even leaves the cooling device on the neck during the actual exercise [17], our cooling period was limited to 1 min. This distinction is important as the amount of cooling time significantly alters its effectiveness [27]. Our time was chosen as it reflects the timeframe of combat sports, and excessive cooling may actually harm repeated sprint performance [26].

Cooling is typically effective for exercise tasks performed at 40–70% VO_2max that last ~20–60 min [14,17], but not always [15]. We are the first to examine intermittent neck cooling at normal room temperature at this high of exercise intensity. Drust et al. (2005) showed that performance during a 40-min high-intensity, intermittent cycling protocol (15 s on, 15 s off) was worse when performed in a hot room compared to a normal temperature room [28]. Moreover, the effects of intermittent cooling during high-intensity exercise may be enhanced when in hot environments. Individual perception of recovery, independent of physiological measures [27], relates to subsequent sprint performance [29]. Therefore, the fact that our reduced TS persisted through HEX2 suggests that RPE and performance might have actually improved if a standardized HEX was performed instead of the short TTE (TTE required maximal effort, eliminating our ability to compare the effects of ICE during RI2 on post-TTE RPE), or had additional rounds of HEX been performed. The combination of short duration, high RPE, and reduced cardiovascular or metabolic demand (which was significantly greater in HEX2, but not TTE, compared to HEX1) suggest that failure during TTE was a muscle, not cardiovascular issue. The apparent delayed improvements in perception caused by reduced skin temperature means intermittent cooling might enhance performance in exercise tasks lasting longer than were tested here.

In concert with previous literature, our data suggest ICE might be effective for combat sports or other activities that require repeated, high-intensity exercise intervals that last more than two rounds and result in high physiological and perceived fatigue ratings [2]. ICE could also help long-term training motivation as how one (athlete or non-athlete) feels during exercise predicts future exercise intentions and behavior [30], which is probably why RPE is regarded as a highly effective tool for monitoring combat sport training [31]. The specific mechanisms explaining our findings are unknown. Several postulates exist (e.g., altered sensory perception, pain reduction, Gate Control Theory, and Central Fatigue Theory) and have been reviewed elsewhere [14].

Not measuring core temperature during our study was a limitation. However, extensive research on humans exercising at normal environmental temperatures supports our position [7,17,18]. Specifically, one study showed neck icing does not significantly alter core temperature more than simple passive rest [32]. Improvements in exercise performance have even been noted with cooling when core temperature did not change [25] or even increased [33]. Moreover, core temperature changes slower than skin temperature, making skin the more likely primary thermal signal [18]. We also acknowledge that our exercise task was atypical for exercise physiology research and would be considered novel to most participants. This left us potentially susceptible to a familiarity effect during visits 3 and 4. With this in mind, we specifically utilized participants with a history of frequent, high-intensity exercise intervals. We also analyzed and confirmed that no depended variables were altered by visit order ($p > 0.4$).

5. Conclusions

Small durations (i.e., 2 min total) of intermittent wet-ice neck cooling (i.e., an ice bag) partially attenuated the rise in skin temperature during repeated bouts of high-intensity exercise. This made participants feel cooler and less exerted (at times) over the course of 12–15 min (total) of exercise. However, time to exhaustion during a ~1 min cycling protocol was not altered. The benefits of neck cooling may be limited for activities primarily limited by power or muscular endurance. However, it may benefit combat sport athletes or other individuals during exercise of more than two, 5-min HEX rounds. Practitioners may incorporate intermittent neck cooling as an effective, practical, and legal cooling option for combat sport athletes. Future research should focus on physiological and performance outcomes during actual competition.

Acknowledgments: The research team would like to thank all the participants for their hard work and effort in this exhausting task.

Author Contributions: Andrew J. Galpin, James R. Bagley, Blake Whitcomb, Leonard D. Wiersma, Jared W. Coburn, and Daniel A. Judelson conceived and designed the experiment; Andrew J. Galpin, Blake Whitcomb, and Jakob Rosengarten performed the experiments; Andrew J. Galpin, James R. Bagley,

Blake Whitcomb, Jakob Rosengarten, and Daniel A. Judelson analyzed the data; Andrew J. Galpin, James R. Bagley, Blake Whitcomb, Leonard D. Wiersma, Jakob Rosengarten, Jared W. Coburn, and Daniel A. Judelson wrote the paper.

Conflicts of Interest: The authors declare no conflict of interest.

References

1. Davis, P.; Benson, P.R.; Pitty, J.D.; Connorton, A.J.; Waldock, R. The activity profile of elite male amateur boxing. *Int. J. Sports Physiol. Perform.* **2015**, *10*, 53–57. [CrossRef] [PubMed]
2. Chaabene, H.; Mkaouer, B.; Franchini, E.; Souissi, N.; Selmi, M.A.; Nagra, Y.; Chamari, K. Physiological responses and performance analysis difference between official and simulated karate combat conditions. *Asian J. Sports Med.* **2014**, *5*, 21–29. [CrossRef] [PubMed]
3. Del Vecchio, F.B.; Hirata, S.M.; Franchini, E. A review of time-motion analysis and combat development in mixed martial arts matches at regional level tournaments. *Percept. Mot. Skills* **2011**, *112*, 639–648. [CrossRef] [PubMed]
4. Mundel, T.; Bunn, S.J.; Hooper, P.L.; Jones, D.A. The effects of face cooling during hyperthermic exercise in man: Evidence for an integrated thermal, neuroendocrine and behavioural response. *Exp. Physiol.* **2007**, *92*, 187–195. [CrossRef] [PubMed]
5. Gillis, D.J.; House, J.R.; Tipton, M.J. The influence of menthol on thermoregulation and perception during exercise in warm, humid conditions. *Eur. J. Appl. Physiol.* **2010**, *110*, 609–618. [CrossRef] [PubMed]
6. Kozyreva, T.V.; Tkachenko, E.I.A. Effect of menthol on human temperature sensitivity. *Fiziol. Cheloveka* **2008**, *34*, 99–103. [CrossRef] [PubMed]
7. Schlader, Z.J.; Simmons, S.E.; Stannard, S.R.; Mündel, T. Skin temperature as a thermal controller of exercise intensity. *Eur. J. Appl. Physiol.* **2011**, *111*, 1631–1639. [CrossRef] [PubMed]
8. Cheung, S.S. Interconnections between thermal perception and exercise capacity in the heat. *Scand. J. Med. Sci. Sports* **2010**, *20* (Suppl. 3), 53–59. [CrossRef] [PubMed]
9. Radomski, M.W.; Cross, M.; Buguet, A. Exercise-induced hyperthermia and hormonal responses to exercise. *Can. J. Physiol. Pharmacol.* **1998**, *76*, 547–552. [CrossRef] [PubMed]
10. Verducci, F.M. Interval cryotherapy decreases fatigue during repeated weight lifting. *J. Athl. Train.* **2000**, *35*, 422–426. [PubMed]
11. Armada-da-Silva, P.A.; Woods, J.; Jones, D.A. The effect of passive heating and face cooling on perceived exertion during exercise in the heat. *Eur. J. Appl. Physiol.* **2004**, *91*, 563–571. [CrossRef] [PubMed]
12. Dixon, P.G.; Kraemer, W.J.; Volek, J.S.; Howard, R.L.; Gomez, A.L.; Comstock, B.A.; Dunn-Lewis, C.; Fragala, M.S.; Hooper, D.R.; Hakkinen, K.; et al. The impact of cold-water immersion on power production in the vertical jump and the benefits of a dynamic exercise warm-up. *J. Strength Cond. Res.* **2010**, *24*, 3313–3317. [CrossRef] [PubMed]
13. Grahn, D.A.; Cao, V.H.; Nguyen, C.M.; Liu, M.T.; Heller, H.C. Work volume and strength training responses to resistive exercise improve with periodic heat extraction from the palm. *J. Strength Cond. Res.* **2012**, *26*, 2558–2569. [CrossRef] [PubMed]
14. Kwon, Y.S.; Robergs, R.A.; Schneider, S.M. Effect of local cooling on short-term, intense exercise. *J. Strength Cond. Res.* **2013**, *27*, 2046–2054. [CrossRef] [PubMed]
15. Bulbulian, R.; Shapiro, R.; Murphy, M.; Levenhagen, D. Effectiveness of a commercial head-neck cooling device. *J. Strength Cond. Res.* **1999**, *13*, 198–205. [CrossRef]
16. Tyler, C.J.; Sunderland, C.; Cheung, S.S. The effect of cooling prior to and during exercise on exercise performance and capacity in the heat: A meta-analysis. *Br. J. Sports Med.* **2015**, *49*, 7–13. [CrossRef] [PubMed]
17. Tyler, C.J.; Wild, P.; Sunderland, C. Practical neck cooling and time-trial running performance in a hot environment. *Eur. J. Appl. Physiol.* **2010**, *110*, 1063–1074. [CrossRef] [PubMed]
18. Schlader, Z.J.; Prange, H.D.; Mickleborough, T.D.; Stager, J.M. Characteristics of the control of human thermoregulatory behavior. *Physiol. Behav.* **2009**, *98*, 557–562. [CrossRef] [PubMed]
19. Dykstra, J.H.; Hill, H.M.; Miller, M.G.; Cheatham, C.C.; Michael, T.J.; Baker, R.J. Comparisons of cubed ice, crushed ice, and wetted ice on intramuscular and surface temperature changes. *J. Athl. Train.* **2009**, *44*, 136–141. [CrossRef] [PubMed]

20. Wegmann, M.; Faude, O.; Poppendieck, W.; Hecksteden, A.; Frohlich, M.; Meyer, T. Pre-cooling and sports performance: A meta-analytical review. *Sports Med.* **2012**, *42*, 545–564. [CrossRef] [PubMed]
21. Siegel, R.; Laursen, P.B. Keeping your cool: Possible mechanisms for enhanced exercise performance in the heat with internal cooling methods. *Sports Med.* **2012**, *42*, 89–98. [CrossRef] [PubMed]
22. Bishop, S.H.; Herron, R.; Ryan, G.; Katica, C.; Bishop, P. The effect of intermittent arm and shoulder cooling on baseball pitching velocity. *J. Strength Cond. Res.* **2016**, *30*, 1027–1032. [CrossRef] [PubMed]
23. Gillis, D.J.; Weston, N.; House, J.R.; Tipton, M.J. Influence of repeated daily menthol exposure on human temperature regulation and perception. *Physiol. Behav.* **2015**, *139*, 511–518. [CrossRef] [PubMed]
24. Marsh, D.; Sleivert, G. Effect of precooling on high intensity cycling performance. *Br. J. Sports Med.* **1999**, *33*, 393–397. [CrossRef] [PubMed]
25. Duffield, R.; Dawson, B.; Bishop, D.; Fitzsimons, M.; Lawrence, S. Effect of wearing an ice cooling jacket on repeat sprint performance in warm/humid conditions. *Br. J. Sports Med.* **2003**, *37*, 164–169. [CrossRef] [PubMed]
26. Schniepp, J.; Campbell, T.S.; Powell, K.L.; Pincivero, D.M. The effects of cold-water immersion on power output and heart rate in elite cyclists. *J. Strength Cond. Res.* **2002**, *16*, 561–566. [CrossRef] [PubMed]
27. Minett, G.M.; Duffield, R. Is recovery driven by central or peripheral factors? A role for the brain in recovery following intermittent-sprint exercise. *Front. Physiol.* **2014**, *5*, 24. [CrossRef] [PubMed]
28. Drust, B.; Rasmussen, P.; Mohr, M.; Nielsen, B.; Nybo, L. Elevations in core and muscle temperature impairs repeated sprint performance. *Acta Physiol. Scand.* **2005**, *183*, 181–190. [CrossRef] [PubMed]
29. Cook, C.J.; Beaven, C.M. Individual perception of recovery is related to subsequent sprint performance. *Br. J. Sports Med.* **2013**, *47*, 705–709. [CrossRef] [PubMed]
30. Ekkekakis, P. Let them roam free? Physiological and psychological evidence for the potential of self-selected exercise intensity in public health. *Sports Med.* **2009**, *39*, 857–888. [CrossRef] [PubMed]
31. Padulo, J.; Chaabene, H.; Tabben, M.; Haddad, M.; Gevat, C.; Vando, S.; Maurino, L.; Chaouachi, A.; Chamari, K. The construct validity of session rpe during an intensive camp in young male karate athletes. *Muscles Ligaments Tendons J.* **2014**, *4*, 121–126. [CrossRef] [PubMed]
32. Yang, Z.; Svetlana, N.; P, K.C.; B, C.A.; Catalina, C.; Gytis, B.; Jesper, S.; A, B.P. Effect of half time cooling on thermoregulatory responses and soccer-specific performance tests. *Monten. J. Sports Sci. Med.* **2014**, *3*, 17–22.
33. Uckert, S.; Joch, W. Effects of warm-up and precooling on endurance performance in the heat. *Br. J. Sports Med.* **2007**, *41*, 380–384. [CrossRef] [PubMed]

8

Lateral Squats Significantly Decrease Sprint Time in Collegiate Baseball Athletes

Jason B. White [1,†], Trevor P. Dorian [2,†] and Margaret T. Jones [1,*]

[1] Health and Human Performance, George Mason University, Manassas, VA 20110, USA; jwhite35@gmu.edu
[2] Exercise Science and Sport Studies, Springfield College, Springfield, MA 01109, USA
* Correspondence: mjones15@gmu.edu
† These authors contributed equally to this work.

Academic Editor: Lee E. Brown

Abstract: The purpose was to examine the effect of prior performance of dumbbell lateral squats (DBLS) on an agility movement-into-a-sprint (AMS) test. Twelve collegiate, resistance-trained, baseball athletes participated in three sessions separated by three days. Session One consisted of AMS baseline test, DBLS 5-RM test, and experimental protocol familiarization. Subjects were randomly assigned the protocol order for Sessions Two and Three, which consisted of warm up followed by 1-min sitting (no-DBLS) or performing the DBLS for 1 × 5 repetitions @ 5RM for each leg. Four minutes of slow recovery walking preceded the AMS test, which consisted of leading off a base and waiting for a visual stimulus. In reaction to stimulus, subjects exerted maximal effort while moving to the right by either pivoting or drop stepping and sprinting for 10 yards (yd). In Session Three, subjects switched protocols (DBLS, no-DBLS). Foot contact time (FCT), stride frequency (SF), stride length (SL), and 10-yd sprint time were measured. There were no differences between conditions for FCT, SF, or SL. Differences existed between DBLS (1.85 $\pm$ 0.09 s) and no-DBLS (1.89 $\pm$ 0.10 s) for AMS (p = 0.03). Results from the current study support the use of DBLS for performance enhancement prior to performing the AMS test.

Keywords: agility; complex training; lower body strength; postactivation potentiation; speed

---

1. Introduction

The importance of lower body muscular power to performance in sporting activities is well documented [1–3] Therefore, training techniques designed to improve lower body power are of interest, and methods such as plyometrics and complex training are commonly employed [4–6]. These training methods utilize exercises similar to the movements of sporting activity in order to provide sport specific enhancements and improve power development.

The response of skeletal muscle to specific stimuli is a function of the prior contraction history [7]. Complex training, a method that involves performing a moderate to heavy resistance exercise as a conditioning contraction followed by a lighter-resistance ballistic activity, has been shown to elicit greater lower body power production in subsequent explosive movements [8,9]. An example of complex training is performing a squat as the heavy strength exercise, followed by explosive vertical jumps. Acute performance enhancement found in power movements following a conditioning contraction exercise, such as a heavily loaded resistance exercise or maximal voluntary contractions (MVC), is likely due to post-activation potentiation (PAP) [10–14], which is defined as an increase in muscle function following a preload stimulus [7]. The application of complex training to elicit PAP, both acutely and in training programs, has long been thought to improve lower body power [4,15–17]. Both PAP and neuromuscular fatigue are stimulated by the same factors [18] and can occur simultaneously [19], but the greatest motor performance occurs with minimal neuromuscular fatigue [7]. It may be for this reason that the numerous studies that have examined complex training and PAP have pursued acute identification of the optimal load or the timing after loading where peak power production occurs. Previous research with resistance-trained athletes indicates that the optimal load for complex training may be achieved using MVCs [11] or 60%–85% 1-RM [20] and 3 to 8 min rest between the heavy strength exercise and the ensuing explosive movement [20,21]. However, the effect of complex training on PAP has been shown to vary with the individual's training status, exercise intensity, exercise volume, and length of rest period between the strength exercise and the explosive activity [20,22]. Further, it has been suggested that the interplay between a subject's individual characteristics and the protocol design (e.g., strength and power exercise selection) may have an important effect on the extent of potentiation elicited [23].

Strength is critical to developing force rapidly and is integral to the baseball skills of batting, throwing, and running [24], and agility movements (e.g., drop step, pivot, shuffle) are important when reacting to a stimulus (e.g., fielding, leading off of a base). Previous methodology to induce PAP has utilized dynamic movements, such as squat [13], bench press [25], Olympic lifts [26], loaded drop jumps [27], as well as isometric MVC [11,28]. Little research exists to indicate how PAP induced by lateral movements acutely impacts lower body power development. Further, because most studies have used the squat and vertical jump as the conditioning contraction exercise and ensuing explosive movement, respectively, little is known about the impact of loaded lateral strength exercises on explosive movement and power production. Yet, sports such as baseball, basketball, hockey, and football require as much as 50%–90% agility movements in a lateral direction [29]. Additionally, little research has been completed analyzing methods to improve the first stride in a frontal plane following a stationary athletic position. Therefore, the purpose of the current study was to examine the acute impact of dumbbell lateral squat (DBLS) exercise on an agility movement-into-a-sprint (AMS) test in collegiate baseball players.

2. Material and Methods

2.1. Subjects

Twelve ($n = 12$) National Collegiate Athletic Association (NCAA) Division-III resistance-trained baseball position players volunteered to participate in the current study. All subjects were proficient weight lifters and had $\geqslant$ 1 year of formal strength and conditioning training experience. All subjects were medically cleared for intercollegiate athletic participation, had the risks and benefits explained to them beforehand, signed an institutionally approved consent form to participate, and completed a medical history form. The Institutional Review Board for Human Subjects approved all procedures. Exclusion criteria consisted of severe musculoskeletal injuries of the lower body or spinal injuries within 6 months before the start of the study. The subjects were instructed to refrain from lower body exercise for 72 h before each testing session. Also, they were asked to consume an identical diet for the 24 h before each testing session. Testing sessions were conducted during the off-season training period. All subjects in the current study were members of the same baseball team, and were familiar with the DBLS exercise and the AMS test from their participation in the same collegiate strength and conditioning off-season program. Physical characteristics are included in Table 1.

Table 1. Physical characteristics of baseball athletes.

Physical Characteristic	Mean	*SD*
Age (y)	19.9	1.2
Training experience (y)	3.2	2.1
Height (cm)	175.9	6.6
Body mass (kg)	79.9	10.9
5-RM DBLS (kg)	18.2	4.9

$n = 12$. Year (y); Centimeter (cm); Kilogram (kg); Standard deviation (*SD*).

2.2. Experimental Design

The purpose of the current study was to investigate the acute effect of DBLS exercise on an agility movement into a 10 yd sprint. A within-subject randomized crossover design was used as subjects completed the AMS test following DBLS exercise and a control condition (no-DBLS) without DBLS exercise. In both the DBLS and no-DBLS conditions, four minutes of slow recovery walking preceded the AMS test.

2.3. Procedures

2.3.1. Session One: 5-RM DBLS Testing and Protocol Familiarization

Session One consisted of completing the informed consent and medical history forms, familiarization with the 10-min supervised standardized warm-up (*i.e.*, five minutes of stationary cycling at 70–80 RPM with a 0.5-kg load and five min of dynamic flexibility exercises), application of reflective markers, baseline AMS test, and 5-RM DBLS test. Prior to testing and familiarization, subjects' height and body mass were determined to the nearest 0.1 cm and 0.1 kg, respectively, using a stadiometer (Tanita; Arlington Heights, IL, USA) and self-calibrating digital scale (Tanita; Arlington Heights, IL, USA) with subjects in sock feet.

2.3.2. Sessions Two and Three: Experimental Protocol

Seventy-two hours after Session One, subjects returned to the laboratory at the same time of day on two separate occasions, each separated by seventy-two hours, to perform two randomly ordered experimental trials (DBLS, no-DBLS). Athletes were randomly assigned to the DBLS or no-DBLS protocol. In Session Three, which took place 72 h later, the subjects switched protocols. On the day of each experimental trial, subjects arrived having refrained from lower body resistive exercise since the previous experimental trial. After a supervised, standardized, 10-min warm-up identical to that performed prior to testing during session one, subjects performed DBLS exercise of 1×5 repetitions @ 5-RM for each leg or sat quietly for 1 min, depending upon their assigned protocol. The DBLS exercise was performed according to the methods described for the 5-RM test. However, both legs were trained. After the left knee flexed to meet the proper squat depth five consecutive times, the right leg followed. Following four minutes of slow recovery walking subjects performed the AMS test.

2.3.3. 5-RM DBLS Test

Lateral squat [30] strength was assessed for the right leg with a 5-RM test using dumbbells. Briefly, subjects completed a 10-min whole body warm up followed by supervised warm up sets for the DBLS test. While performing the DBLS, the athlete assumed a stance approximately twice that of shoulder width (Figure 1). Each subject's foot placement was measured and recorded. The pelvis was tilted posteriorly and the subject performed a downward squatting motion until the anterior thigh was parallel to the floor. When the subject reached parallel squat depth, a sound was emitted from the safety squat beeper (Bigger, Faster, Stronger, Inc., Salt Lake City, UT, USA), which had been placed anteriorly on the thigh of the right leg [24]. The beeper location was noted for each subject and repeated for subsequent experimental sessions. In the down position of the DBLS, both heels remained in contact with the floor. The down position was held for one second. Upon completion of the down position, the subject rose to the upward position with full extension in the hips and knees, while keeping the feet in contact with ground. Dumbbells were rested upon the anterior deltoids of the subject in a front squat hold position. A timed rest of three minutes was taken before each maximal effort set. Weight was increased based upon the performance of the previous attempt, and the subject continued to perform sets of five repetitions until failure or until it was determined that he could no longer perform the DBLS safely with proper form. After two failures, testing was stopped, and the best lift for 5-RM was recorded.

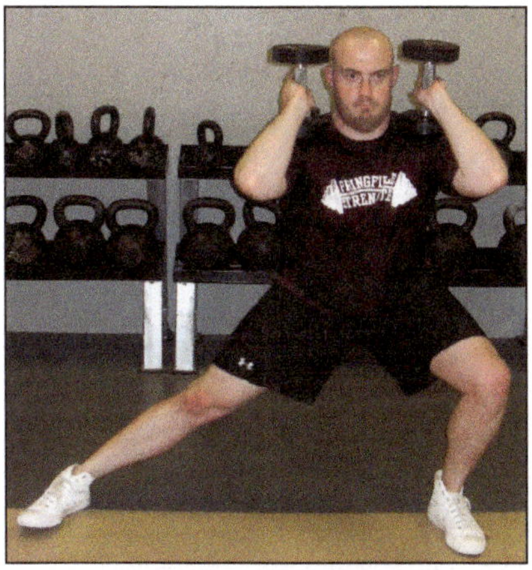

Figure 1. Mid-range of the DBLS exercise.

2.3.4. AMS Test

The AMS test was conducted in the laboratory following the DBLS or no-DBLS exercise. All subjects performed a 4-min slow walking recovery [21] prior to the start of the AMS test. The AMS consisted of performing a 10-yd sprint from a base runner's stance for the starting position. Ten reflective markers were applied to the body: left and right anterior superior iliac spine, center of the left and right patella, left and right mid-thigh, distal anterior portion of the left and right tibia, medial malleolus on the right leg, and lateral malleolus on the left leg. Individual anatomical locations of marker placements were located and marked on each subject with semi-permanent ink to enable reproducibility for subsequent measures. Athletes were required to wear compression shorts to clarify movement of the lower extremities for the video analysis. Prior to the initiation of the agility movement, the subject was stationary and had a stance slightly wider than shoulder width, with slight flexion in the knees and hips. Body weight was distributed evenly on the balls of the feet, and both feet were parallel with the sagittal plane. Each subject's foot placement was measured and recorded. The direction of movement was to the right of the subject in the frontal plane, which is identical to stealing a base in baseball; consequently, athletes were well versed in the movement. The initial movement began upon reaction to a visual stimulus, which was a light emitting diode. The subject exerted maximal effort while moving to the right by either pivoting both feet or drop stepping with the right foot in order to place the feet in a position similar to that of a linear sprint during initial acceleration. The subject maximally sprinted for 10 yd. Each athlete's choice of a pivot or drop step was noted by the researcher and repeated during subsequent testing sessions.

In AMS testing Sessions Two and Three, the foot contact time (FCT) and stride length (SL) for the Stride 1 and Stride 2, and stride frequency (SF) for Segment 1 and Segment 2 were recorded by a video camera (50 fps, JVC GR-DVL9800 Mini, JVC USA, Wayne, NJ), which was placed perpendicular to the sagittal plane of the subject and 10 yd from the running lane. Markers were placed at 0, 5, and 10 yd on the blank wall that was parallel to the running lane. The same trained researcher analyzed all recordings using two-dimensional video analysis software (Dartfish 5.0 Connect, Fribourg, Switzerland). Timing sensors with single beamed infrared photocells (Brower Timing Systems, Salt Lake City, UT, USA) were placed to capture the time at the 5 and 10 yd locations.

Test-retest reliability for the AMS was determined from data collected during baseline AMS tests in session one and the subsequent no-DBLS condition, which was either Session Two or Three depending upon the random order assignment of each subject's no-DBLS condition.

Foot contact time (FCT). The FCT time was defined as the time that each foot was in contact with the ground following initial lower body movement. The initial movement pattern varied based upon how the athletes were taught to steal a base (*i.e.*, drop step *vs.* pivot). Approximately half of the athletes drop stepped with the right foot prior to pivoting and striding with the left. Only FCT prior to a stride was recorded in order to maintain consistency among measures. Athletes repeated their chosen initial movement (*i.e.*, drop step, pivot) for both DBLS and no-DBLS conditions.

Stride frequency (SF). For comparison of SF or number of strides per section of distance, the AMS test was divided into two segments: 0–5 (Segment 1) and 6–10 yd (Segment 2). Using video analysis, SF for each segment was determined from the total number of strides taken during the total time taken to cover Segment 1 and to cover Segment 2.

Stride length (SL). Stride length for Stride 1 and Stride 2 were determined from video analysis and recorded in inches for both experimental sessions. Stride 1 was defined as the distance covered between first two successive ground contacts by the left foot. Stride 2 was defined as the distance covered between next two successive ground contacts by the right foot.

2.4. Statistical Analyses

Normality of data was assessed by the Kolmogorov-Smirnov test of normality, which determined all primary outcome measures of interest to be normally distributed. Foot contact (FCT), stride frequency (SF), and stride length (SL) were analyzed with 2 (condition: DBLS, no-DBLS) × 2 [time (FCT), distance (SL), number (SF)] repeated measures analysis of variance (ANOVA). The AMS test was analyzed by a 2 (condition) × 3 (segment 1, segment 2, total time) repeated measures ANOVA. Bonferroni's pairwise post hoc analyses examined differences across condition and within testing periods. Effect sizes were calculated and a modified classification system (trivial, 0.0–0.2; small, 0.2–0.6; moderate, 0.6–1.2; large, 1.2–2.0; very large, >2.0; extremely large, >4.0) was used [31]. Test-retest reliability was determined through the intra-class correlation coefficient (ICC). Statistical procedures were conducted using the Statistical Package for the Social Sciences (IBM SPSS Statistics 20.0, IBM Corporation, Armonk, NY, USA). The alpha level was set at $p < 0.05$.

3. Results

There was no significant interaction between the DBLS and no-DBLS conditions for FCT ($p = 0.70$), SF ($p = 0.28$), or SL ($p = 0.79$) (Table 2). Significant differences were found for FCT (ES = 5.3, $p = 0.0001$) and SL (ES = 1.2, $p = 0.0004$) between Stride 1 and Stride 2. The SF for Segment 2 (6–10 yard) was significantly (ES = 2.2, $p < 0.0002$) less than for Segment 1 (0–5 yard). A significant difference existed between conditions for the AMS test for Segment 1 time (ES = 0.61, $p = 0.01$, DBLS: 1.11 ± 0.06 s; no-DBLS: 1.15 ± 0.07 s), and total time (ES = 0.42, $p = 0.03$, DBLS: 1.85 ± 0.09 s; no-DBLS: 1.89 ± 0.10 s) (Figure 2). There was no significant difference ($p = 0.414$) in overall AMS time between session one (1.90 ± 0.09 s) and the no-DBLS condition (1.89 ± 0.10 s), and the ICC of 0.98 between the two testing sessions was considered strong.

Table 2. Foot contact, stride frequency, and stride length for DBLS and no-DBLS conditions.

Measure	DBLS Condition M ± *SD*	no-DBLS Condition M ± *SD*
Foot Contact Time (FCT) (s):		
Stride 1	0.39 ± 0.05	0.38 ± 0.04
Stride 2	0.64 ± 0.04 *	0.63 ± 0.06 *
Stride Frequency (SF):		
0–5 yd (Segment 1)	3.75 ± 0.45	3.75 ± 0.45
6–10 yd (Segment 2)	2.92 ± 0.29 #	2.67 ± 0.49 #
Stride Length (SL) (in):		
Stride 1	46.52 ± 3.97	46.19 ± 5.75
Stride 2	52.23 ± 5.36 *	51.54 ± 7.11 *

* Significant difference ($p < 0.001$) between Stride 1 and Stride 2; # significant difference ($p < 0.001$) between 0 and 5 yd (Segment 1) and 6 and 10 yd (Segment 2); $n = 12$, yd (yard), s (second), in (inch).

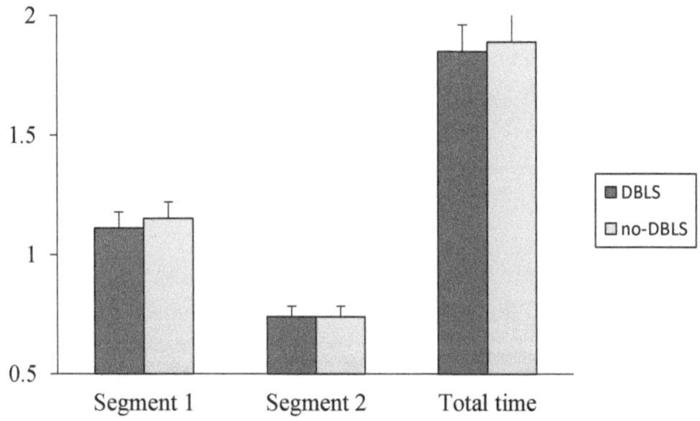

Figure 2. AMS test time (s) for DBLS and no-DBLS conditions. # significant difference ($p < 0.05$) between total LMS time for DBLS and no-DBLS conditions; * significant difference ($p < 0.05$) between Segment 1 (0–5 yd) and Segment 2 (6–10 yd).

4. Discussion

This is the first study to examine whether or not an acute bout of DBLS exercise would enhance agility movement and the subsequent sprint in resistance-trained, collegiate baseball athletes. It was hypothesized that measures of FCT, SF, SL, and AMS time would improve as a result of acute lower body resistive exercise. The overall findings supported a positive effect on the use of resistive exercise on AMS time; however, no difference was found for FCT, SF, or SL across the DBLS and no-DBLS conditions. To our knowledge, no study to date has reported on the effect of complex training on an agility movement-into-a-sprint, FCT, SF, or SL in baseball athletes, yet, baseball is a sport that requires a large percentage of agility movements in a lateral direction [29]. The performance measure (AMS test) in the current study was comparable to the baseball specific movement of stealing a base [32]. It required reaction to a visual stimulus, quick change of direction, and a short burst sprint, all of which are regularly used movement patterns in baseball [33].

The mechanisms responsible for eliciting PAP and the optimal conditions for performance enhancement from complex training have not been clearly defined. The utilization of dynamic strength movements for a conditioning exercise to induce PAP during plyometric exercise has yielded mixed results [10,14,23,34–36]. Previous research has demonstrated improved sprint times following single joint and isometric strength exercise [37]. However, the effect of dynamic strength exercise on sprint time is equivocal and varies by individual and rest time [21,22]. Further, the exercise selection and intensity of the conditioning contraction can impact subsequent power production [20]. Complex training has resulted in improved 10-m shuttle run time [38], 10-m [22], 40-m [13], and 100-m [39] sprint times. In contrast, other research has shown no effect on 10-m [13], 30-m [24] and 40-m [26] sprint times.

In the current study, complex training did not elicit a PAP response for the FCT, which was defined as the time that each foot was in contact with the ground following initial lower body movement until the foot completed the stride. The contact time for Stride 1 was significantly lower than Stride 2, irrespective of DBLS or no-DBLS condition. This was likely due to the required movement direction to the right, which was similar to that necessary when stealing a base. As a result, the left foot always completed Stride 1, and the right foot stayed in contact with the ground for a longer period of time. Varying differences in the agility movement patterns (drop step, pivot) were existent, but not the focus of the current study.

Complex training did not elicit a PAP response for the SF. In both conditions the SF for Segment 1 was significantly greater than Segment 2, which is likely a result of the short explosive strides required during the initial acceleration of Segment 1 *versus* the longer strides of Segment 2 as the athlete increased his running speed [40].

The primary purpose of examining SL was to determine change in SL due to PAP; however, the condition (DBLS, no-DBLS) had no effect on SL in the current study. Irrespective of condition, Stride 2 was significantly greater than Stride 1, and this finding was likely due to the specific mechanical tendencies of the movement pattern. The initial agility movement that was performed prior to sprinting was identical to that of a baseball player attempting to steal a base; therefore, the subject was required to move to his right in the frontal plane following a stationary athletic position. After visual examination of the digital recordings of running mechanics it was clear that an initial stride of the subject with the left foot was needed in order to rotate the hips and shoulders to the right and rapidly move the center of gravity so that the momentum of the subject was correctly oriented toward the target. The pivoting limited the initial stride of the left foot. The subject could then make a significantly greater second stride with the left foot because he was facing in the direction of the sprinting destination.

Regardless of condition (DBLS, no-DBLS) the AMS test time for Segment 2 (6–10 yd) was significantly lower than Segment 1 (0–5 yd), which is likely a result of the athlete beginning the AMS test from a stationary athletic stance position. After accelerating through the 5 yd sensor and completing Segment 1, the athlete had created enough momentum to propel himself through Segment 2 and the final 10 yd sensor at a faster speed.

While FCT, SL, and SF, did not differ between DBLS and no-DBLS conditions, AMS Segment 1 and total time were significantly lower (0.04 s) for the DBLS condition than the no-DBLS condition; therefore, the resistive exercise may have induced PAP, which enhanced the sprint time. Segment 1 was 3.6% faster and the total AMS time was 2.2% faster when the AMS was preceded by DBLS. Although the effect size was small, milliseconds can determine whether or not a base runner is safe or out, therefore, such a magnitude of improvement might have noteworthy ramifications during competition. In the current study, the DBLS exercise was followed by a 4-min rest period during which the subjects completed a slow recovery walk prior to performing the AMS test. In previous research reporting a significant PAP effect during sprinting distances of 10-m [22], 30-m [38], 40-m [13], and 100-m [39], the dynamic resistance exercise selection and intensity have varied for the conditioning contraction, but the most effective rest periods have consistently been $\geqslant$ 4 min. The design of the current study was unique because it examined the effects of PAP on a ballistic agility movement that led into a sprint. The use of resistance-trained baseball athletes who were familiar with the AMS test and the DBLS in conjunction with the standardization of all warm-up procedures may have also been contributing factors in the positive results of the current study.

We acknowledge some study limitations. First, although all subjects in the current study were resistance-trained collegiate baseball position players, the sample size of twelve was small. A larger sample size may have resulted in other differences between the DBLS and no-DBLS conditions. It has been demonstrated that results from studies examining PAP in relation to performance on field tests are equivocal, in part due to the varied individual response to complex training methods [20,22,26]. Second, a higher grade of video analysis software may have allowed for better discrimination in measures of FCT, SL, and SF.

It is well known that responses to a PAP protocol may vary depending upon the individual's training background and strength level [14,23,34,36,39]. Future research that examines the effects of dynamic strength movements on varied sprint distances, repeated sprint measures, and the establishment of how long the PAP effect remains are warranted. The investigation of efficiency of various agility movement patterns (e.g., drop step, pivot) for directional change would also be of interest. Further, the effect of implementing such complex training methods between innings during game play would be of interest to the baseball practitioner.

5. Conclusions

Results from the current study are applicable to sport and training. Successful skill execution in baseball often requires the development of power over a short period of time. Effective use of PAP (movement specific conditioning exercise, proper rest time) in the form of complex training can enable an individual to train at a greater intensity, therefore, attaining superior gains in power production. Program implementation of complex training, which pairs DB lateral squats with short sprints, may provide an adequate training stimulus for enhancing agility movements and, thereby, improve base running.

Acknowledgments: The authors would like to thank the athletic trainers, coaches, and student-athletes from the intercollegiate baseball program, for their contribution to the study.

Author Contributions: All authors were involved in study design, data collection, data interpretation, and manuscript writing.

Conflicts of Interest: The authors declare no conflict of interest.

References

1. Baker, D.; Nance, S. The relation between strength and power in professional rugby league players. *J. Strength Cond. Res.* **1999**, *13*, 224–229. [CrossRef]
2. Hawley, J.A.; Williams, M.M.; Vickovic, M.M.; Handcock, P.J. Muscle power predicts freestyle swimming performance. *Br. J. Sport Med.* **1992**, *26*, 151–155. [CrossRef]
3. Silvestre, R.; West, C.; Maresh, C.M.; Kraemer, W.J. Body composition and physical performance in men's soccer: A study of a national collegiate athletic association division I team. *J. Strength Cond. Res.* **2007**, *20*, 177–183. [CrossRef] [PubMed]
4. Bauer, T.; Thayer, R.E.; Baras, G. Comparison of training modalities for power development in the lower extremity. *J. Strength Cond. Res.* **1990**, *4*, 115–121. [CrossRef]
5. Dodd, D.J.; Alvar, B.A. Analysis of acute explosive training modalities to improve lower-body power in baseball players. *J. Strength Cond. Res.* **2007**, *21*, 1177–1182. [CrossRef] [PubMed]
6. Potteiger, J.A.; Lockwood, R.H.; Haub, M.D.; Dolezal, B.A.; Almuzaini, K.S.; Schroeder, J.M.; Zebas, C.J. Muscle power and fiber characteristics following 8 weeks of plyometric training. *J. Strength Cond. Res.* **1999**, *13*, 275–279. [CrossRef]
7. Hodgson, M.; Docherty, D.; Robbins, D. Post-activation potentiation underlying physiology and implications for motor performance. *Sports Med.* **2005**, *35*, 585–595. [CrossRef] [PubMed]
8. Chiu, L.Z.; Fry, A.C.; Weiss, L.W.; Schilling, B.K.; Brown, L.E.; Smith, S.L. Postactivation potentiation response in athletic and recreationally trained individuals. *J. Strength Cond. Res.* **2003**, *17*, 671–677. [CrossRef] [PubMed]
9. Tillin, M.N.A.; Bishop, D. Factors modulating post-activation potentiation and its effect on performance of subsequent explosive activities. *Sports Med.* **2009**, *39*, 147–166. [CrossRef] [PubMed]
10. Baker, D. Acute effect of alternating heavy and light resistance on power output during upper-body complex power training. *J. Strength Cond. Res.* **2003**, *17*, 493–497. [CrossRef] [PubMed]
11. Gullich, A.; Schmidtbleicher, D. MVC-induced short-term potentiation of explosive force. *New Stud. Athlet.* **1996**, *11*, 67–81.
12. Hamada, T.; Sale, D.G.; Macdougall, J.D.; Tarnopolsky, M.A. Postactivation potentiation, fiber type, and twitch contraction time in human knee extensor muscles. *J. Appl. Physiol.* **2000**, *88*, 2131–2144. [PubMed]
13. McBride, J.; Nimphius, S.; Erickson, T.M. The acute effects of heavy-load squats and loaded countermovement jumps on sprint performance. *J. Strength Cond. Res.* **2005**, *19*, 893–897. [CrossRef] [PubMed]
14. Young, W.B.; Jenner, A.; Griffiths, K. Acute enhancement of power performance from heavy load squats. *J. Strength Cond. Res.* **1998**, *12*, 82–84. [CrossRef]
15. Adams, K.; O'Shea, J.P.; O'Shea, K.L.; Climstein, M. The effect of six weeks of squat, plyometric and squat-plyometric training on power production. *J. Strength Cond. Res.* **1992**, *6*, 36–41. [CrossRef]
16. Ebben, W.P.; Watts, P.B. A review of combined weight training and plyometric training modes: Complex training. *Strength Cond. J.* **1998**, *20*, 18–27. [CrossRef]
17. Verkhoshansky, Y.; Tetyan, V. Speed-strength preparation of future champions. *Legk. Athlet.* **1973**, *2*, 12–13.
18. Rassier, D.; Herzog, W. The effects of training on fatigue and twitch potentiation in human skeletal muscle. *Eur. J. Sport Sci.* **2001**, *1*, 177–192. [CrossRef]
19. Rassier, D.E.; MacIntosh, B.R. Coexistence of potentiation and fatigue in skeletal muscle. *Braz. J. Med. Biol. Res.* **2000**, *30*, 499–508. [CrossRef]

20. Wilson, J.M.; Duncan, N.M.; Marin, P.J.; Brown, L.E.; Loenneke, J.P.; Wilson, S.M.C.; Jo, E.; Lowery, R.P.; Ugrinowitsch, C. Meta-analysis of postactivation potentiation and power: Effects of conditioning activity, volume, gender, rest periods, and training status. *J. Strength Cond. Res.* **2013**, *27*, 854–859. [CrossRef] [PubMed]
21. Comyns, T.M.; Harrison, A.J.; Hennessy, L.K.; Jensen, R.L. The optimal complex training rest interval for athletes from anaerobic sports. *J. Strength Cond. Res.* **2006**, *20*, 471–476. [CrossRef] [PubMed]
22. Bevan, H.R.; Cunningham, D.J.; Tooley, E.P.; Owen, N.J.; Cook, C.J.; Kilduff, L.P. Influence of postactivation potentiation on sprinting performance in professional rugby players. *J. Strength Cond. Res.* **2010**, *24*, 701–705. [CrossRef] [PubMed]
23. Suchomel, T.J.; Lamont, H.S.; Moir, G.L. Understanding vertical jump potentiation: A deterministic model. *Sports Med.* **2015**. [CrossRef] [PubMed]
24. Jones, M.T. Effect of compensatory acceleration training in combination with accommodating resistance on upper body strength in collegiate athletes. *Open Access J. Sports Med.* **2014**, *5*, 183–189. [CrossRef] [PubMed]
25. Hrysomallis, D.; Kidgell, D. Effect of heavy dynamic resistive exercise on acute upper-body power. *J. Strength Cond. Res.* **2001**, *15*, 426–430. [CrossRef] [PubMed]
26. Guggenheimer, J.D.; Dickin, D.C.; Reyes, G.F.; Dolny, D.G. The effects of specific preconditioning activities on acute sprint performance. *J. Strength Cond. Res.* **2009**, *23*, 1135–1139. [CrossRef] [PubMed]
27. Lima, J.B.; Marin, D.P.; Barquilha, G.; Da Silva, L.O.; Puggina, E.F.; Pithon-Curi, T.C.; Hirabarai, S.M. Acute effects of drop jump potentiation protocol on sprint and counter movement vertical jump performance. *Hum. Mov. Sci.* **2011**, *12*, 324–330.
28. Lim, J.H.; Kong, P.W. Effects of isometric and dynamic postactivation potentiation protocols on maximal sprint performance. *J. Strength Cond. Res.* **2013**, *27*, 2730–2736. [CrossRef] [PubMed]
29. MacClean, C.R. Sport-specific and lateral conditioning. *Scholast. Coach* **1993**, 14–17.
30. Hedrick, A. Using free weights to improve lateral movement performance. *Strength Cond. J.* **1999**, *21*, 21–25. [CrossRef]
31. Hopkins, W.; Marshall, S.; Batterham, A.; Hanin, J. Progressive statistics for studies in sports medicine and exercise science. *Med. Sci. Sports Exerc.* **2009**, *41*, 3–12. [CrossRef] [PubMed]
32. Caliendo, P. *Youth Baseball Drills*, 1st ed.; Human Kinetics: Champaign, IL, USA, 2014; pp. 134–151.
33. Priest, J.W.; Jones, J.N.; Conger, B.; Marble, D.K. Performance measures of NCAA baseball tryouts obtained from the new 60-yd run-shuttle. *J. Strength Cond. Res.* **2011**, *25*, 2872–2878. [CrossRef] [PubMed]
34. Duthie, G.M.; Young, W.B.; Aitken, D.A. The acute effects of heavy loads on jump squat performance: An evaluation of the complex and contrast methods of power development. *J. Strength Cond. Res.* **2002**, *16*, 530–538. [CrossRef] [PubMed]
35. Gourgoulis, V.; Aggeloussis, N.; Kasimatis, P.; Mavromatis, G.; Garas, A. Effect of a submaximal half-squats warm-up program on vertical jumping ability. *J. Strength Cond. Res.* **2003**, *17*, 342–344. [CrossRef] [PubMed]
36. Rixon, K.P.; Lamont, H.S.; Bemben, M.G. Influence of type of muscle contraction, gender, and lifting experience on postactivation potentiation performance. *J. Strength Cond. Res.* **2007**, *21*, 500–505. [CrossRef] [PubMed]
37. Sale, D.G. Postactivation potentiation: Role in human performance. *Exerc. Sport Sci. Rev.* **2002**, *30*, 138–143. [CrossRef] [PubMed]
38. Okuno, N.M.; Tricoli, V.; Silva, S.B.C.; Bertuzzi, R.; Moreira, A.; Kiss, M.A.P.D.M. Postactivation potentiation on repeated-sprint ability in elite handball players. *J. Strength Cond. Res.* **2013**, *27*, 662–668. [CrossRef] [PubMed]
39. Linder, E.E.; Prins, J.H.; Murata, N.M.; Derenne, C.; Morgan, C.F.; Solomon, J.R. Effects of preload 4 repetition maximum on 100-m sprint times in collegiate women. *J. Strength Cond. Res.* **2010**, *24*, 1184–1190. [CrossRef] [PubMed]
40. Plisk, S. Speed, agility and speed-endurance development. In *Essentials of Strength Training and Conditioning*, 3rd ed.; Baechle, T.R., Earle, R.W., Eds.; Human Kinetics: Champaign, IL, USA, 2008; pp. 457–485.

9

The Effects of a Multi-Ingredient Performance Supplement on Hormonal Profiles and Body Composition in Male College Athletes

Matthew H. Sharp [1,*], Kevin A. Shields [2,†], Jacob T. Rauch [2,†], Ryan P. Lowery [1,†], Shane E. Durkee [3,†], Gabriel J. Wilson [3,†] and Eduardo O. De Souza [2,†]

1 Applied Science and Performance Institute, Tampa, FL 33607, USA; ryanplowery@gmail.com
2 Department of Health Sciences and Human Performance, The University of Tampa, Tampa, FL 33606, USA; kevinshields31@gmail.com (K.A.S.); jacobrauch1@gmail.com (J.T.R.); edesouza@ut.edu (E.O.D.S.)
3 Maximum Human Performance, West Caldwell, NJ 07006, USA; sdurkee@maxperformance.com (S.E.D.); gwilson@maxperformance.com (G.J.W.)
* Correspondence: msharp2113@gmail.com
† These authors contributed equally to this work.

Academic Editor: Beat Knechtle

Abstract: Periods of intense training can elicit an acute decline in performance and body composition associated with weakened hormone profiles. This study investigated the effects of a multi-ingredient performance supplement (MIPS) on body composition and hormone levels in college athletes following a six-week training protocol. Twenty male college athletes were equally assigned to MIPS and placebo (PLA) groups for supplementation (three pills, twice daily) in conjunction with resistance training and specialized sports training (e.g., nine total sessions/week) for six weeks. Dual Energy X-ray Absorptiometry determined body composition at weeks 0 and 6. Serum samples collected at weeks 0 and 6 determined free testosterone (FT), total testosterone (TT), IGF-1 and total estrogen (TE) levels. PLA experienced a significant decline in lean body mass (LBM) (−1.5 kg; $p < 0.05$) whereas the MIPS sustained LBM. The MIPS increased TT 21.9% (541.5 ± 48.7 to 639.1 ± 31.7) and increased FT 15.2% (13.28 ± 1.1 to 15.45 ± 1.3 ng/dL) ($p < 0.05$). Conversely, PLA decreased TT 7.9% (554.5 ± 43.3 to 497.2 ± 39.1 ng/dL), decreased FT 17.4% (13.41 ± 1.8 to 11.23 ± 2.55 ng/dL), and decreased FT:E 12.06% ($p < 0.05$). These findings suggest the MIPS can prevent decrements in LBM and anabolic hormone profiles during intense training periods.

Keywords: lean body mass; resistance training; testosterone; herbal ingredients

---

1. Introduction

Testosterone is an anabolic, androgenic steroid hormone, which, like other steroid hormones, is derived from cholesterol. In addition, higher testosterone levels have been demonstrated to contribute to increased muscle growth and activation of the nervous system, resulting in enhanced power and strength, mood, libido, and several other benefits [1]. On the other hand, the current literature suggests that as little as a 10% decline in testosterone concentration can significantly reduce gains in strength and muscle hypertrophy [2]. Interestingly, there are conflicting results regarding the anabolic role of testosterone in strength training-induced adaptations [3,4] while other studies have demonstrated positive association of testosterone response on functional performance and body composition [5,6].

Despite the aforementioned conflicts, a growing interest in herbal ingredients to increase testosterone levels among athletic populations remains. However, with treatment or supplementation with multi-ingredient performance supplements (MIPS) that contain multiple herbal ingredients (*i.e.*, fenugreek and tribulus terrestris) said to improve the testosterone profile, there is concern with the excess production of endogenous testosterone metabolites such as estrogen and dihydrotestosterone (DHT). These metabolites can cause side effects and also operate in a negative feedback loop by inhibiting the body's natural production of luteinizing hormone and testosterone [7].

To date, no research exists to examine the interaction of MIPS on hormone levels, body composition and blood and urine clinical markers in college athletes. Therefore, the first purpose of this study was to examine the efficacy of a MIPS combined with regular training on lean body mass and hormonal profiles in collegiate athletes. In addition, research shows that imbalances in training load and recovery may impair hormonal levels. For instance, there is a significant negative linear correlation (*i.e.*, $r = -0.60$, $p < 0.01$) between overtraining and salivary testosterone concentration [8]. Studies have also found a linear, negative relationship between increased training volume in endurance athletes and testosterone levels [9]. These findings suggest that athletes are at risk of suffering declines in anabolic hormone levels and performance during a competitive season in which high levels of fatigue brought on by high physical demands are likely prevalent. Therefore, the second purpose of this study was to investigate the effects of a MIPS on hormone levels during high levels of specialized sports training combined with resistance training.

2. Materials and Methods

2.1. Experimental Design

This study utilized a randomized, double-blind, placebo-controlled parallel design to test the effects of a multi-ingredient sports supplement (MHP's T-BOMB 3XTREME Maximum Human Performance, LLC, 165 Clinton Road, West Caldwell, NJ 07006) (Supplementary Table S1) on hormone profiles and body composition in college athletes during season. Baseline testing prior to supplementation included assessments of body composition via Dual-Energy X-ray Absorptiometry (DEXA), hormone, serum and blood clinical profiles by venipuncture techniques and urine samples for analysis. Following baseline testing, subjects were stratified according to body composition and age and then randomly assigned the placebo (PLA) or MIPS such that baseline values for these parameters were not statistically different. Subjects performed a high frequency training cycle which consisted of four resistance training sessions and five specialized sports training sessions each week for six weeks. All workout sessions were supervised by trained personnel. During the study, both groups consumed three pills with the breakfast meal and three pills post-workout, or with dinner on non-training days. Subjects were retested post-supplementation (week 6) in a manner identical to baseline testing.

2.2. Subjects

Twenty college male athletes aged 21 ± 2 years who had a minimum of three years of experience in resistance training volunteered for this study. Subjects could not participate if they were currently taking any medications including anti-inflammatory agents, any performance-enhancing supplements, if they smoked, or if they had any respiratory or metabolic disorders. In an effort to control post-workout nutrition, all participants were supplementing with one serving (1 g CHO, 0 g Fat, 25 g PRO) of whey protein isolate after resistance training. This was considered in their macronutrient profile. Each participant signed an informed consent approved by the Institutional Review Board before participating in the study. The baseline characteristics for each group are provided in Table 1.

2.3. Dietary Records

Subjects were required to perform a three-day dietary recall including two weekdays and one weekend day, while none of the three days used were in succession of one another during weeks 0 and 6. The dietary recalls were assessed using a free mobile app (MyFitnessPal, Inc, San Francisco, CA, USA) to determine the average daily macronutrient intake of carbohydrate (CHO), fat, and protein (PRO) to the nearest gram. Each subject recorded their dietary logs at the necessary times for 100% compliance.

Table 1. Physical baseline characteristics of participants.

Characteristic	PLA (n = 10)	MIPS (n = 10)
Age (years)	21 ± 0	21 ± 2
LBM (kg)	69.58 ± 1.75	70.13 ± 2.01
FM (kg)	14.40 ± 1.12	13.58 ± 1.00
TM (kg)	83.98 ± 2.16	83.71 ± 1.87
BF%	17.0 ± 1.1	16.2 ± 1.1

The baseline characteristics expressed as mean ± standard error for both groups are shown in Table 1. There were no between-group difference for any variable at week 0 of the study ($p > 0.05$). LBM = Lean Body Mass; FM = Fat Mass; TM = Total Mass; BF % = Body Fat Percent; kg = kilograms.

2.4. Training

The resistance training program was designed to train all major muscle groups centered on compound movements for the upper and lower body. Subjects trained on Monday, Tuesday, Thursday, and Friday of each week. Table 2 contains the specifics of exercise selection, sets, repetitions and rest periods. Monday and Tuesday consisted of hypertrophy training while Thursday and Friday was strength. Training loads were progressively increased by 2%–5% for a given exercise if the subject could lift the target repetitions with proper technique prior to muscular failure. In the event in which target repetitions could not be lifted, the load was decreased by 5%–10% until the repetition scheme was reached. Additionally, all subjects participated in specialized sports training sessions (3–4 h) on days Monday through Friday. In conjunction with resistance training and specialized sports training, all subjects trained, on average, nine times per week. All training sessions were supervised to ensure proper technique, maximal effort and intensity.

Table 2. Resistance training protocol.

Day 1 and 3				Day 2 and 4			
Exercise	Sets	Reps	Rest	Exercise	Sets	Reps	Rest
Banded BB Back Squat	5	3	3 min	Banded BB Deadlift	4	2	3 min
DB Hip Bridge	3	10	1–2 min	(1) Supinated Pull-Up	3	5	1–2 min
(1) BB Bent Row	3	6	1–2 min	(2) DB Romanian Deadlift	3	5	
(2) BB Lateral Lunge	3	6		(3) Cable Row	3	12	
(1) Neutral Grip DB Press	3	6	1–2 min	(1) BB Split Squat	2	6	1–2 min
(2) Cable Paloff Press	3	10		(2) Unilateral DB Row	2	6	
BB Reverse Lunge	2	8	1–2 min	(1) DB Lateral Step-Up (2) DB Cuban Press	2	6	1–2 min

BB = barbell; DB = dumbbell. Numbered exercises indicate that the movements were performed subsequently without rest, then rested after performing the final numbered movement.

2.5. Body Composition

A whole body DEXA (Hologic, Bedford, MA, USA) scan was utilized to measure body composition. Lean body mass (LBM) and fat mass (FM) were determined for the total body with the subject laying in a supine position with the knee extended and instructed not to move for the entire duration of the scan (~10 min). Results from each scan were uploaded and accessed on a computer directly connected to the DEXA device. All DEXA scans were conducted from baseline and after completion of the study following a 10 h overnight fast. The coefficient of variation (CV) for body composition assessment was 1.5%.

2.6. Blood Collection

All blood samples were collected at baseline and at the end of week 6 via venipuncture by a trained phlebotomist. All samples were collected after a 10 h overnight fast at the same time range

(0700–1000 h). After coagulation, blood was centrifuged at 1500 *g* for 15 min at 4 °C. Serum was aliquoted and stored at −80 °C for further analysis.

2.7. Statistical Analysis

Normality was confirmed by visual inspection of box plots and Shapiro Wilk test. A two-way ANOVA for repeated measures was performed for each dependent variable, assuming supplementation (PLA and MIPS) and time (pre and post) as fixed factors (GraphPad Prism 6, La Jolla, CA, USA). Whenever a significant F-value was obtained, a *post-hoc* test with Bonferroni's adjustment was used for multiple comparison purposes. The significance level was set at $p < 0.05$. Results are expressed as mean ± standard error.

3. Results

3.1. Dietary Analysis

There were no significant differences between groups in total caloric or macronutrient intake of carbohydrate (CHO), fat, or protein (PRO) over the course of the three-day dietary recall at week 0 or week 6 (Table 3; $p > 0.05$).

Table 3. Three-day dietary recalls for PLA and MIPS groups at weeks 0 and 6.

Dietary Variable	PLA		MIPS	
	Week 0	Week 6	Week 0	Week 6
CHO (g/kg)	4.3 ± 0.5	4.3 ± 0.4	4.3 ± 0.4	4.4 ± 0.4
Fat (g/kg)	1.0 ± 0.1	1.0 ± 0.1	0.9 ± 0.1	1.0 ± 0.1
PRO (g/kg)	1.9 ± 0.1	2.0 ± 0.1	2.0 ± 0.2	2.1 ± 0.2
Total kcals	2832 ± 40	2857 ± 60	2818 ± 41	2925 ± 58

No significant differences were observed between groups for total calories or macronutrient intakes ($p > 0.05$).

3.2. Body Composition

There were no significant differences for TM and FM after six weeks for PLA and MIPS groups ($p > 0.05$). There was a significant group × time interaction for LBM in which the PLA group experienced a decline in LBM (−1.5 kg) ($p < 0.05$) after six weeks (Figure 1).

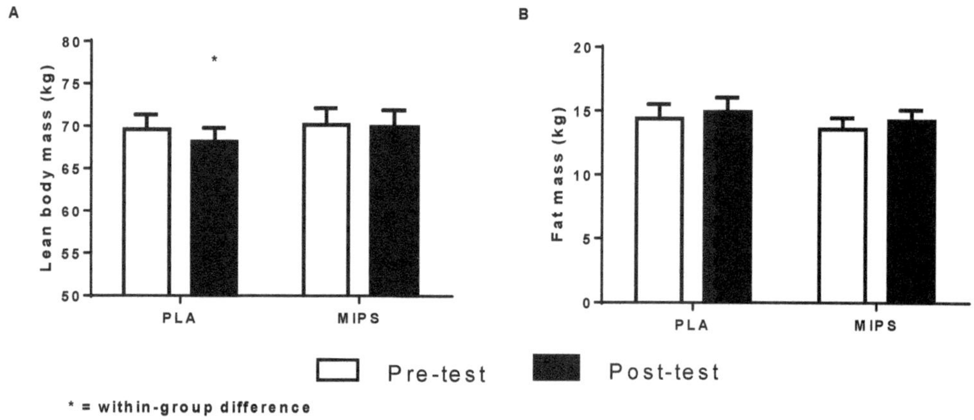

Figure 1. Body composition. (**A**) Group pre- and post-test lean body mass values; (**B**) Group pre- and post-testing fat mass values.

3.3. Hormone Profiles

There was a significant group × time interaction ($p < 0.0007$) favoring an increase in total testosterone for the MIPS group. In addition, the pairwise comparison revealed between-group differences at week 6 (MIPS: 21.9% *vs.* PLA: −7.9%; $p < 0.03$). Likewise, there was a significant group × time interaction ($p < 0.0006$) in which MIPS increased free testosterone 15.2% ($p < 0.01$) and the PLA group decreased −17.4% ($p < 0.01$) (Figure 2). The pairwise comparison did not reveal a between-group difference ($p > 0.05$). Results for total and free testosterone to estrogen ratios (TT:E and FT:E) are presented in Figure 3A and 3B, respectively. No significant between-groups differences were detected prior to the experimental period ($p > 0.05$). There was a significant group × time interaction for TT:E ($p < 0.006$) (Figure 3). Pairwise comparisons revealed that only the MIPS group significantly increased TT:E 11.71% ($p < 0.05$), whereas PLA tended to have declined in TT:E by −8.41% ($p = 0.072$). Likewise, there was a significant group × time interaction for FT:E ($p < 0.003$) in which the pairwise comparisons revealed that the MIPS group increased 10.51% ($p < 0.05$), whereas the PLA significantly decreased −12.06% ($p < 0.03$).

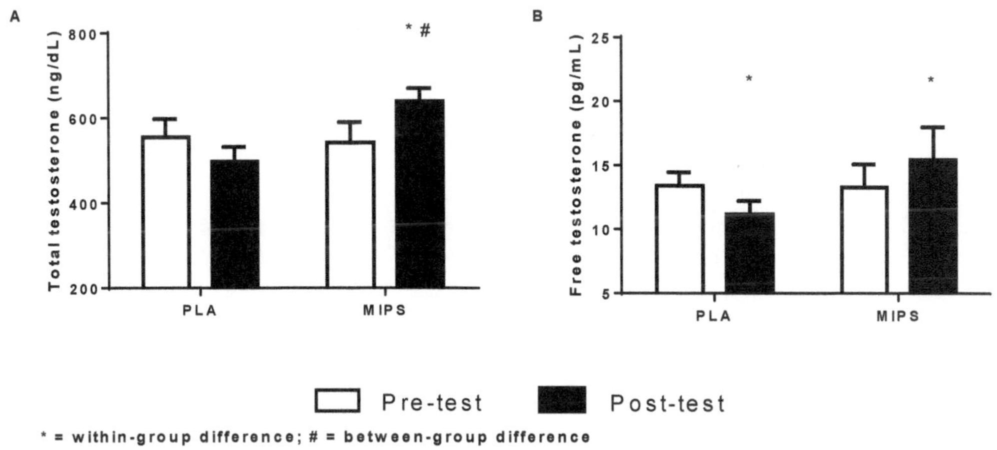

Figure 2. Measures of Plasma Total & Free Testosterone. (**A**) Group pre- and post-test total testosterone levels; (**B**) Group pre- and post-testing free testosterone levels.

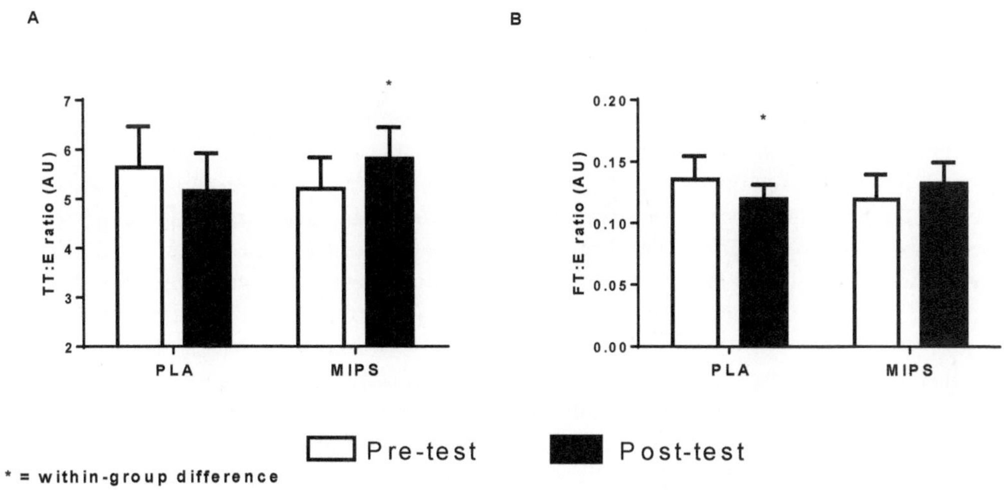

Figure 3. Total Testosterone to Estrogen (TT:E) & Free Testosterone to Estrogen (FT:E) Ratios, (**A**) Group pre- and post-testing TT:E values; (**B**) Group pre- and post-testing FT:E values.

3.4. Clinical Safety Data

There were no group × time interactions or main effects ($p > 0.05$) observed in any whole blood, serum or urinary clinical safety markers tested (Supplementary Tables S2–S4).

4. Discussion

The current study's purpose was two-fold: (I) to examine the efficacy of a MIPS on lean body mass and hormonal profiles in college athletes during the season; and (II) to investigate the effects of a MIPS on hormone levels during high levels of specialized sports training combined with resistance training. The main finding of the current study was that MIPS staved off the declines seen in LBM and testosterone during high intensity training. These findings have broad implications for athletes seeking to optimize testosterone levels and maintain LBM during training seasons.

Athletes often undergo periods of rigorous training in order to compete or prepare for competitions. It is important to mention that athletes in this trial trained, on average, nine times per week throughout the duration of the study, combining both resistance training and specialized sports training. Furthermore, only the PLA group demonstrated significant declines in total and free testosterone as well as LBM. However, the MIPS group sustained LBM associated with positive changes in hormonal profile. This beneficial effect observed in the MIPS group could be associated with the fact that the MIPS used in this study contains multiple ingredients which may have contributed to elevated total and free testosterone as observed in Figure 2A,B. For instance, key ingredients contained in the MIPS have been shown to improve free and total testosterone. Among them are herbal plant extracts fenugreek [10], tribulus and tongkat ali [11], as well as the minerals zinc and magnesium aspartate (ZMA) [12] (Supplementary Table S1). While the dose of these ingredients is proprietary, they approximate the clinical doses used in previous research which have shown that a range of 300–600 mg of fenugreek [10] as well as tribulus [13], 50 mg of zinc [14,15], and 30 mg of magnesium can support testosterone levels [16]. Ingredients in the MIPS such as stinging nettle leaf are known for increasing the amount of free (active) testosterone by binding the testosterone inhibitor sex hormone binding globulin (SHBG) [17]. In addition, the effects of ingredients in the investigated MIPS on LBM mass and hormone profiles are controversial. Some studies have demonstrated positive adaptations while other trials have not demonstrated any treatment effect on hormone profiles and LBM [11,12,17–26]. Moreover, some studies have demonstrated that testosterone might induce muscle growth in specific situations [27], but the post-exercise hormone responses are still not associated with a higher protein synthesis rate or muscle hypertrophy [28]. However, it is important to mention that the present study was the first to investigate the effects of MIPS in college athletes during an intense training phase (*i.e.*, nine sessions/week). Thus, our results suggest that athletic populations might have positive outcomes when supplementing with a MIPS that claims to improve hormone profiles. Furthermore, additional research is necessary to understand the mechanism for producing such outcomes.

Another important finding of the current study was that no significant elevation of plasma estrogen levels occurred in the MIPS group. It has been demonstrated that elevations in testosterone caused by drug therapy have caused deleterious side effects. Included among these side effects are increased estrogen and DHT as well as a decline in natural testosterone production [7]. In this study, the MIPS significantly increased testosterone with no change in estrogen levels. The ability of the MIPS to attenuate a rise in estrogen may be due to multiple ingredients including chrysin [29], DIM (diindolymethane) [26] and stinging nettle leaf [17]. These extracts have been demonstrated to attenuate the activity of aromatase and also compete for estrogen at its receptor binding site.

Finally, there were no adverse side effects reported from the participants and no significant changes in hemodynamic measures and in clinical chemistry markers measured in whole blood, serum, or urine, suggesting that the MIPS at the investigated dosages for a period of six weeks appears safe (Supplementary Tables S2–S4).

5. Conclusions

The collective results of this research indicate that a MIPS used in the current study results in positive hormonal profiles while sustaining lean body mass in college athletes after six weeks of training with a high frequency (nine sessions/week) protocol compared to a visually identical, volume-matched placebo. Therefore, our findings suggest that athletes and resistance-trained individuals may avoid lean body mass loss during high intensity training cycles by supplementing with MIPS formulas. In addition, further studies are needed to elucidate the athletic performance–related effects and the mechanisms of action of MIPS in sustaining lean mass in trained populations, as this manuscript lacks any performance data. Moreover, these results should be further examined to discover if MIPS can be used to help other populations which seek to sustain or improve lean body mass during catabolic conditions combined with resistance training. The effects of the MIPS in female athletes also warrants further examination. It is important to note that catabolic conditions (e.g., LBM decrements) should be avoided by monitoring an athlete's recovery and decreasing physical stress in order to optimize on-field performance.

Acknowledgments: Maximum Human Performance, LLC, 165 Clinton Road, West Caldwell, NJ 07006 provided the supplement for this study. No other remuneration was provided.

Author Contributions: Ryan P. Lowery conceived and designed the experiment; Matthew H. Sharp, Kevin A. Shields, Ryan P. Lowery and Jacob T. Rauch performed the experiment; Eduardo O. De Souza and Matthew H. Sharp analyzed the data; Matthew H. Sharp, Shane E. Durkee, Gabriel J. Wilson and Eduardo O. De Souza were involved in writing the manuscript.

Conflicts of Interest: Matthew H. Sharp, Kevin A. Shields, Jacob T. Rauch, Ryan P. Lowery and Eduardo O. De Souza declare no conflicts of interest. These authors were in charge of designing and performing the study, as well as manuscript preparation. Shane E. Durkee and Gabriel J. Wilson work for Maximum Human Performance who sell the MIPS tested in this study. They were involved in writing the manuscript, but had no involvement in performing the study.

References

1. Herbst, K.L.; Bhasin, S. Testosterone action on skeletal muscle. *Curr. Opin. Clin. Nutr. Metab. Care* **2004**, *7*, 271–277. [CrossRef] [PubMed]
2. Alen, M.; Rahkila, P. Anabolic-androgenic steroid effects on endocrinology and lipid metabolism in athletes. *Sports Med.* **1988**, *6*, 327–332. [CrossRef] [PubMed]
3. Phillips, S.M. Strength and hypertrophy with resistance training: Chasing a hormonal ghost. *Eur. J. Appl. Physiol.* **2012**, *112*, 1981–1983. [CrossRef] [PubMed]
4. West, D.W.; Phillips, S.M. Anabolic processes in human skeletal muscle: Restoring the identities of growth hormone and testosterone. *Phys. Sportsmed.* **2010**, *38*, 97–104. [CrossRef] [PubMed]
5. Rønnestad, B.R.; Nygaard, H.; Raastad, T. Physiological elevation of endogenous hormones results in superior strength training adaptation. *Eur. J. Appl. Physiol.* **2011**, *111*, 2249–2259. [CrossRef] [PubMed]
6. Frx, A.C.; Kraemer, W.J.; Stone, M.H.; Koziris, L.P.; Thrush, J.T.; Fleck, S.J. Relationships between serum testosterone, cortisol, and weightlifting performance. *J. Strength Cond. Res.* **2000**, *14*, 338–343. [CrossRef]
7. Tilbrook, A.J.; Clarke, I.J. Negative feedback regulation of the secretion and actions of gonadotropin-releasing hormone in males. *Biol Reprod.* **2001**, *64*, 735–742. [CrossRef] [PubMed]
8. Maso, F.; Lac, G.; Filaire, E.; Michaux, O.; Robert, A. Salivary testosterone and cortisol in rugby players: Correlation with psychological overtraining items. *Br. J. Sports Med.* **2004**, *38*, 260–263. [CrossRef] [PubMed]
9. Hackney, A.C. Endurance exercise training and reproductive endocrine dysfunction in men: Alterations in the hypothalamic-pituitary-testicular axis. *Curr. Pharm. Des.* **2001**, *7*, 261–273. [CrossRef] [PubMed]
10. Wilborn, C.; Taylor, L.; Poole, C.; Foster, C.; Willoughby, D.; Kreider, R. Effects of a purported aromatase and 5 α-reductase inhibitor on hormone profiles in college-age men. *Int. J. Sport Nutr.* **2010**, *20*, 457–465.
11. Tambi, M.; Imran, M.; Henkel, R. Standardised water-soluble extract of eurycoma longifolia, tongkat ali, as testosterone booster for managing men with late-onset hypogonadism? *Andrologia* **2012**, *44*, 226–230. [CrossRef] [PubMed]

12. Brilla, L.; Conte, V. Effects of a novel zinc-magnesium formulation on hormones and strength. *J. Exerc. Physiol. Online* **2000**, *3*, 26–36.
13. Brown, G.A.; Vukovich, M.D.; Reifenrath, T.A.; Uhl, N.L.; Parsons, K.A.; Sharp, R.L.; King, D.S. Effects of anabolic precursors on serum testosterone concentrations and adaptations to resistance training in young men. *Int J. Sport Nutr Exerc. Metab.* **2000**, *10*, 340–359. [PubMed]
14. Neek, L.S.; Gaeini, A.A.; Choobineh, S. Effect of zinc and selenium supplementation on serum testosterone and plasma lactate in cyclist after an exhaustive exercise bout. *Biol. Trace Elem. Res.* **2011**, *144*, 454–462. [CrossRef] [PubMed]
15. Prasad, A.S.; Mantzoros, C.S.; Beck, F.W.; Hess, J.W.; Brewer, G.J. Zinc status and serum testosterone levels of healthy adults. *Nutrition* **1996**, *12*, 344–348. [CrossRef]
16. Cinar, V.; Polat, Y.; Baltaci, A.K.; Mogulkoc, R. Effects of magnesium supplementation on testosterone levels of athletes and sedentary subjects at rest and after exhaustion. *Biol. Trace Elem. Res.* **2011**, *140*, 18–23. [CrossRef] [PubMed]
17. Chrubasik, J.E.; Roufogalis, B.D.; Wagner, H.; Chrubasik, S. A comprehensive review on the stinging nettle effect and efficacy profiles. Part ii: Urticae radix. *Phytomedicine* **2007**, *14*, 568–579. [CrossRef] [PubMed]
18. Poole, C.; Bushey, B.; Foster, C.; Campbell, B.; Willoughby, D.; Kreider, R.; Taylor, L.; Wilborn, C. The effects of a commercially available botanical supplement on strength, body composition, power output, and hormonal profiles in resistance-trained males. *J. Int. Soc. Sports Nutr.* **2010**, *7*, 34. [CrossRef] [PubMed]
19. Rogerson, S.; Riches, C.J.; Jennings, C.; Weatherby, R.P.; Meir, R.A.; Marshall-Gradisnik, S.M. The effect of five weeks of tribulus terrestris supplementation on muscle strength and body composition during preseason training in elite rugby league players. *J. Strength Cond. Res.* **2007**, *21*, 348–353. [CrossRef] [PubMed]
20. Safarinejad, M.R. Urtica dioica for treatment of benign prostatic hyperplasia: A prospective, randomized, double-blind, placebo-controlled, crossover study. *J. Herb. Pharmacother.* **2005**, *5*, 1–11. [CrossRef] [PubMed]
21. Gambelunghe, C.; Rossi, R.; Sommavilla, M.; Ferranti, C.; Rossi, R.; Ciculi, C.; Gizzi, S.; Micheletti, A.; Rufini, S. Effects of chrysin on urinary testosterone levels in human males. *J. Med. Food* **2003**, *6*, 387–390. [CrossRef] [PubMed]
22. Wilborn, C.D.; Kerksick, C.M.; Campbell, B.I.; Taylor, L.W.; Marcello, B.M.; Rasmussen, C.J.; Greenwood, M.C.; Almada, A.; Kreider, R.B. Effects of zinc magnesium aspartate (ZMA) supplementation on training adaptations and markers of anabolism and catabolism. *J. Int. Soc. Sports Nutr.* **2004**, *1*, 12–20. [CrossRef] [PubMed]
23. Talbott, S.M.; Talbott, J.A.; George, A.; Pugh, M. Effect of tongkat ali on stress hormones and psychological mood state in moderately stressed. *J. Int. Soc. Sports Nutr.* **2013**, *10*, 28. [CrossRef] [PubMed]
24. Sareena, H.; Ashril, Y. The ergogenic effects of eurycoma longifolia jack: A pilot study. Joint conference of basem and bases. *Br. J. Sports Med.* **2003**, *37*, 464–470.
25. Suzuki, M.; Ito, Y.; Fujino, T.; Abe, M.; Umegaki, K.; Onoue, S.; Noguchi, H.; Yamada, S. Pharmacological effects of saw palmetto extract in the lower urinary tract. *Acta Pharmacol. Sin.* **2009**, *30*, 271–281. [CrossRef] [PubMed]
26. Jellinck, P.H.; Gekforkert, P.; Riddick, D.S.; Okey, A.B.; Michnovicz, J.J.; Bradlow, H.L. Ah receptor binding properties of indole carbinols and induction of hepatic estradiol hydroxylation. *Biochem. Pharmacol.* **1993**, *45*, 1129–1136. [CrossRef]
27. Bhasin, S.; Storer, T.W.; Berman, N.; Callegari, C.; Clevenger, B.; Phillips, J.; Bunnell, T.J.; Tricker, R.; Shirazi, A.; Casaburi, R. The effects of supraphysiologic doses of testosterone on muscle size and strength in normal men. *N. Engl. J. Med.* **1996**, *335*, 1–7. [CrossRef] [PubMed]
28. West, D.W.; Kujbida, G.W.; Moore, D.R.; Atherton, P.; Burd, N.A.; Padzik, J.P.; de Lisio, M.; Tang, J.E.; Parise, G.; Rennie, M.J. Resistance exercise-induced increases in putative anabolic hormones do not enhance muscle protein synthesis or intracellular signalling in young men. *J. Physiol.* **2009**, *587*, 5239–5247. [CrossRef] [PubMed]
29. Collins, B.M.; McLachlan, J.A.; Arnold, S.F. The estrogenic and antiestrogenic activities of phytochemicals with the human estrogen receptor expressed in yeast. *Steroids* **1997**, *62*, 365–372. [CrossRef]

10

Analysis of Physiological, Technical, and Tactical Analysis during a Friendly Football Match of Elite U19

Juan Ignacio Ortega [1], Carlos Evangelio [1], Filipe Manuel Clemente [2,3], Fernando Manuel Lourenço Martins [3,4] and Sixto González-Víllora [1,*]

[1] Physical Education Department, University of Castilla-La Mancha, Edificio Fray Luis de León, 16071 Cuenca, Spain; naichzzz@gmail.com (J.I.O); carletes_92@hotmail.com (C.E)
[2] Instituto Politécnico de Viana do Castelo, Escola Superior de Desporto e Lazer, Complexo Desportivo e Lazer Comendador Rui Solheiro—Monte de Prado, 4960-320 Melgaço, Portugal; filipe.clemente5@gmail.com
[3] Instituto de Telecomunicações, Delegação da Covilhã, Instituto Superior Técnico—Torre Norte —Piso 10, Av. Rovisco Pais, 1, 1049-001 Lisboa, Portugal; fmlmartins@ubi.pt
[4] Instituto Politécnico de Coimbra, Escola Superior de Educação, Departamento de Educação, IIA, RoboCorp, ASSERT, Rua Dom João III, 3030-329 Coimbra, Portugal
* Correspondence: sixto.gonzalez@uclm.es

Academic Editor: Eling Douwe de Bruin

Abstract: The main objective was to analyze a friendly match of youth elite soccer players identifying the variance of tactical and physiological response parameters during the game. In addition, detecting the impact of both halves on player performance. For the purposes of this study twenty-two U19 players were analyzed playing 11v11. Activity profile, heart rate (HR and HRmax), grouped in five different zones were analyzed via Bluetooth technology, technical performance was analyzed by the Team Sport Assessment Procedure (TSAP), and tactical performance was measured by Social Network Analysis. A comparison of heart rate responses showed significant main effects in the halves ($p = 0.001$; $\eta_p^2 = 0.623$). A comparison between tactical position and technical performance had significant main effects ($p = 0.001$; $\eta_p^2 = 0.390$). Tactical position showed statistically significant effects on tactical prominence ($p = 0.002$; $\eta_p^2 = 0.296$). Therefore, fatigue is a component distinguished in technical/tactical parameters, such as volume of play and efficiency index. Results suggest that fatigue effects may constrain technical performance and, for that reason, the use of instruments to monitor the fatigue effect during matches may be suggested.

Keywords: performance analysis; match analysis; network analysis; soccer; adjacency matrices

---

1. Introduction

The game of football requires a great dynamic and movements that depend on the ball location, teammates, and opponents' behaviors [1,2]. The movements made by players constrains the physiological and physical demands; thus, team dynamics should be analyzed in association with the personal demands [3]. Despite this, the analysis has been performed not considering the dynamic of the game. Match analysis (about the patterns of play) and performance analysis (based on internal and external load) have been working alone without an association.

Research conducted on soccer have been found that heart rate (HR) responses varies between 80% and 90% of HRmax and ~75% of VO_{2max} [4,5]. These values are in line with the lactate threshold, thus prominently varying between oxidative and glycolytic systems [6]. These acute responses depend from the time-motion profile of the players. Commonly, 10–12 km per game are covered by players during a full match [7]. During the match, 1000 to 1400 short activities changing every 4–6 s are made [8]. Moreover, technical activity and performance may also influence the individual impact of the game in a player [9]. Thus, time-motion analysis and acute physiological responses confirms the variability of demands that occurs during the match.

Nevertheless, the time-motion profile is constrained by the specificity of a team's dynamics and decisions made during the emergence of the game [10,11]. Some observational methods have characterized the team dynamics by using some mathematical algorithms and observational methods [12,13]. In the specific case of teammates' interactions, network analysis based on graph theory have been used [14,15]. Results have showed that midfielders and external defenders are the prominent players in the building of passing sequences [16]. On the other hand, during attacking transition and counter-attack, forwards assume a great prominence [17]. Thus, the phases of the game and the tactic specificity of the team contribute to the individual participation of each player during the match.

Despite of this isolated analysis to acute physiological responses and collective organization, no study has analyzed both at the same time, as far we know. However, such analysis is extremely important to identify the impact of the style of play in the physiological demands. This information will help optimize the training methodology and specificity.

For that reason, the aim of this study is to analyze a full match of youth elite soccer players and identify the variance of physiological and collective organization parameters during the game. It also aims to identify the impact of halves on the performance.

2. Methods

2.1. Participants

Twenty-two elite youth soccer players (age 19.85 ± 1.2 years old; height 178.91 ± 4.5 cm; body mass 71.56 ± 6.1 kg; competitive playing experience 9.23 ± 1.8 years) from two squads of a Spanish National Youth Premier League soccer club (highest state competition) volunteered to participate in this study. Eleven players from each squad were selected to participate in the study and were free of illness and injury at the time of testing. A minimum of five years of experience in elite youth soccer and the regular four weekly training sessions were the criteria to include the players in this study. All participants signed informed consent forms outlining commitment, benefits, potential risks, and the study's procedures in line with the ethical standards of Declaration of Helsinki for the study in humans. The study also complied with ethical standards of the University of Castilla-la Mancha.

2.2. Procedures of Heart Rate Monitoring

An initial session was used to assess fitness levels and familiarize participants with all testing procedures. Participants completed the Yo-Yo Intermittent Recovery Test level 1 by using soccer boots in an official turf field during which HRmax was determined [18]. The HR data was recorded via Bluetooth technology (Polar Team App, Polar Electro Oy, Pakkalankuja, Finland) in all training sessions. The HR results were grouped into five different zones of % HRmax: zone 1 [Z1] (50–60 % HRmax), zone 2 [Z2] (60–70 % HRmax), zone 3 [Z3] (70–80 % HRmax), zone 4 [Z4] (80–90 % HRmax), and zone 5 [Z5] (⩾90 % HRmax). After the preliminary testing protocol, the 11v11 game was promoted in an official turf field during two halves of 30 min with 15 min of rest. A smaller period of time (30 min and not the regular 45) was used based on the temperature of 25 °C recorded during the match.

2.3. Assesment of Technical Performance

The technical performance it was analyzed following the Team Sport Assessment Procedure (TSAP) protocol [19,20]. This instrument allowed to identify the following observational indicators [20]: (CB) Conquered Ball represents the moment in which the player intercepts the ball from the opponent; (RB) Received Balls represent the moment in which the player receives the ball from a teammate;

(LB) Lost Ball represents the action of losing control of the ball; (NB) Neutral Ball represents a routine pass made without penetrating the opponent's region or does not allow moving forward; (P) Pass that allows displacing the ball into the opponent's defensive region; and (SS) Successful Shot on Goal, which represents the action of scoring or a shot that ensures to the team keeps possession of the ball. Using the indicators, it was possible to compute the following indices of technical performance: (i) volume of play ($Volume\ of\ Play\ (VP) = CB + RB$); (ii) attacks with ball ($Attacks\ with\ ball\ (AB) = P + SS$); (iii) efficiency index ($Efficiency\ Index\ (EI) = \frac{AB}{10+LB}$); and (iv) performance score ($Performance\ Score\ (PS) = \left(\frac{VP}{2}\right) + (EI \times 10)$).

The observational process was made after video collection by the same researcher with experience in match analysis. The reliability was tested by using a test-retest protocol (20-day interval) following by the Cohen's Kappa test [21]. After testing 15% of the full data, a Kappa value of 0.95 was observed, thus achieving a recommended value for this type of procedure [21].

2.4. Network Measurements

In our study it was analyzed the teammates' interaction during attacking moments based on a Social Network Analysis. This approach have been used in the last few years in order to identify the tendencies of interactions between teammates [22]. In our case only attacking interaction represented by passes between teammates it was analyzed. The protocol of observation followed previous studies in this field of analysis [23]. The following network metrics were computed in the SocNetV (version 1.9).

2.5. OutDegree

The OutDegree metric identifies the centrality level of a player in to pass the ball to their teammates. The following algorithm was used for the case of weighted digraphs (directed graphs), as a standard measure [24]; that is, the proportion of weights of the nodes that are adjacent to n_i.

$$C'^{w}_{(D-out)}(n_i) = \frac{k_i^{w-out}}{\sum_{i=1}^{n}\sum_{\substack{j=1 \\ j\neq i}}^{n} a_{ij}},$$

2.6. InDegree

The InDegree represents the centrality level of a player in the team. Specifically, it identifies the most recruited players to receive the ball. The following algorithm it was used in order to standardize the group size n [24]; that is, the proportion of weights of the nodes that are adjacent to n_i.

$$P'^{w}_{(D-in)}(n_i) = \frac{k_i^{w-in}}{\sum_{i=1}^{n}\sum_{\substack{j=1 \\ j\neq i}}^{n} a_{ij}},$$

2.7. Betweennees Centrality

Betweenness centrality measures the intermediate players between neighbors. The standard of betweenness centrality for weighted digraphs is calculated as [25]:

$$C'_b(n_k) = \frac{C_b(n_k)}{(n-1)(n-2)}$$

2.8. Statistical Procedures

The influences of tactical position and halves of match on the average % HRmax, % Time per HRmax Zone (% of total time), volume of play, efficiency index, performance score, % InDegree,

% OutDegree, and % Betweenness were analyzed using two-way MANOVA after validating normality and homogeneity assumptions. The assumption of normality for each univariate dependent variable was examined using Kolmogorov-Smirnov tests ($p > 0.05$). The assumption of the homogeneity of each group's variance/covariance matrix was examined with the Box's M Test. When the MANOVA detected significant statistical differences between the two factors, we proceeded to the two-way ANOVA for each dependent variable, followed by Tukey's HSD *post hoc* test [26]. When the two-way ANOVA showed an interaction between factors, it also generated a new variable that crossed the two factors (e.g., GK * 1st half; GK * 2nd half) for each dependent variable to identify statistical significance. Ultimately, the statistical procedures used were one-way ANOVA and Tukey HSD *post hoc*. If no interactions were detected in two-away ANOVA, a one-way ANOVA was used for each independent variable. All statistical analyses were performed using IBM SPSS Statistics (version 22) at a significance level of $p < 0.05$. The following scale was used to classify the effect size (partial eta square) of the test [27]: small, 0.2–0.49; moderate, 0.50–0.79; and large, 0.80–1.

3. Results

3.1. Heart Rate Analysis

The two-way MANOVA revealed that the halves ($p = 0.001$; $\eta_p^2 = 0.623$; moderate effect size) had significant main effects on the heart rate responses. No statistical differences were found between tactical positions ($p = 0.376$; $\eta_p^2 = 0.160$; small effect size). There was no significant interaction (Pillai's Trace = 0.572; F = 0.946; $p = 0.541$; $\eta_p^2 = 0.143$; small effect size) between tactical position and halves on heart rate responses.

In the case of % HRmax average, Z1, Z2, Z3, Z4, and Z5, a one-way ANOVA was performed on each independent variable because no interaction was found between factors. The statistical values resulted from the comparison between tactical positions can be observed in the following Table 1.

Table 1. One-way ANOVA values of halves in each tactical position in % HRmax average, Z1, Z2, Z3, Z4, and Z5.

Variable	Half	Position	M(SD)	F	p	η_p^2
% HRmax average	1st half	GK	–	1.325	0.299	0.228
		ED	69.00 (15.94)			
		CD	82.33 (7.57)			
		CMF	70.63 (17.85)			
		EMF	85.00 (4.90)			
		FW	67.00 (18.52)			
	2nd half	GK	–	1.427	0.265	0.241
		ED	79.75 (5.06)			
		CD	77.00 (3.61)			
		CMF	75.25 (6.90)			
		EMF	74.20 (6.57)			
		FW	69.00 (5.57)			
Z1	1st half	GK	–	0.936	0.465	0.172
		ED	7.50 (9.26)			
		CD	0.33 (0.58)			
		CMF	8.50 (12.87)			
		EMF	0.80 (1.79)			
		FW	9.67 (8.74)			
	2nd half	GK	–	0.706	0.598	0.136
		ED	4.25 (6.65)			
		CD	5.33 (6.11)			
		CMF	12.00 (10.85)			
		EMF	8.60 (7.16)			
		FW	9.00 (4.58)			

Table 1. *Cont.*

Variable	Half	Position	M(SD)	F	p	η_p^2
Z2	1st half	GK	–	0.385	0.816	0.079
		ED	7.75 (5.68)			
		CD	4.00 (4.58)			
		CMF	6.00 (5.83)			
		EMF	4.40 (3.65)			
		FW	7.33 (5.51)			
	2nd half	GK	–	1.368	0.284	0.233
		ED	14.75 (3.76)			
		CD	19.33 (4.34)			
		CMF	19.25 (2.66)			
		EMF	26.20 (3.36)			
		FW	19.33 (4.34)			
Z3	1st half	GK	–	0.496	0.739	0.099
		ED	19.25 (13.07)			
		CD	35.33 (26.84)			
		CMF	24.50 (17.91)			
		EMF	23.00 (14.83)			
		FW	31.00 (8.72)			
	2nd half	GK	–	2.747	0.061	0.379
		ED	30.00 (9.83)			
		CD	40.00 (8.19)			
		CMF	28.25 (10.89)			
		EMF	29.80 (9.26)			
		FW	47.33 (6.81)			
Z4	1st half	GK	–	1.821	0.169	0.288
		ED	29.25 (21.19)			
		CD	38.67 (11.72)			
		CMF	25.00 (12.86)			
		EMF	44.60 (8.47)			
		FW	37.00 (13.23)			
	2nd half	GK	–	0.683	0.613	0.132
		ED	33.00 (5.60)			
		CD	33.67 (15.14)			
		CMF	29.13 (11.17)			
		EMF	25.00 (11.25)			
		FW	23.67 (1.53)			
Z5	1st half	GK	–	0.303	0.872	0.063
		ED	11.25 (7.68)			
		CD	21.67 (37.53)			
		CMF	23.50 (26.75)			
		EMF	27.20 (26.34)			
		FW	15.00 (6.56)			
	2nd half	GK	–	1.799	0.173	0.286
		ED	18.00 (14.54)			
		CD	1.67 (2.08)			
		CMF	11.38 (10.72)			
		EMF	10.40 (9.99)			

Legend: % HRmax average, average of the % heart rate max achieved during the period of analysis; Z1, % of time in Zone 1 of heart rate intensity; Z2, % of time in Zone 2 of heart rate intensity; Z3, % of time in Zone 3 of heart rate intensity; Z4, % of time in Zone 4 of heart rate intensity; and Z5, % of time in Zone 5 of heart rate intensity.

One-way ANOVA was also carried out to compare the values between formats for the variables of % HRmax average, Z1, Z2, Z3, Z4, and Z5. The values can be verified in the following Table 2.

Table 2. One-way ANOVA values of tactical positions in each half in in % HRmax average, Z1, Z2, Z3, Z4, and Z5.

Variable	Position	Half	M(SD)	F	p	η_p^2
% HRmax average	GK	1st Half 2nd Half	– –	–	–	–
	ED	1st Half 2nd Half	69.00 (15.94) 79.75 (5.06)	1.653	0.246	0.216
	CD	1st Half 2nd Half	82.33 (7.57) 77.00 (3.61)	1.213	0.333	0.233
	CMF	1st Half 2nd Half	70.63 (17.85) 75.25 (6.90)	0.467	0.505	0.032
	EMF	1st Half 2nd Half	85.00 (4.90) [b] 74.20 (6.57) [a]	8.679	0.019	0.520
	FW	1st Half 2nd Half	67.00 (18.52) 69.00 (5.57)	0.032	0.867	0.008
Z1	GK	1st Half 2nd Half	– –	–	–	–
	ED	1st Half 2nd Half	7.50 (9.26) 4.25 (6.65)	0.325	0.589	0.051
	CD	1st Half 2nd Half	0.33 (0.58) 5.33 (6.11)	1.991	0.231	0.332
	CMF	1st Half 2nd Half	8.50 (12.87) 12.00 (10.85)	0.346	0.566	0.024
	EMF	1st Half 2nd Half	0.80 (1.79) [b] 8.60 (7.16) [a]	5.582	0.046	0.411
	FW	1st Half 2nd Half	9.67 (8.74) 9.00 (4.58)	0.014	0.912	0.003
Z2	GK	1st Half 2nd Half	– –	–	–	–
	ED	1st Half 2nd Half	7.75 (5.68) 14.75 (6.95)	2.435	0.170	0.289
	CD	1st Half 2nd Half	4.00 (4.58) [b] 19.33 (4.04) [a]	18.893	0.012	0.825
	CMF	1st Half 2nd Half	6.00 (5.83) [b] 19.25 (8.83) [a]	12.548	0.003	0.473
	EMF	1st Half 2nd Half	4.40 (3.65) [b] 26.20 (8.23) [a]	29.336	0.001	0.786
	FW	1st Half 2nd Half	7.33 (5.51) [b] 19.33 (3.51) [a]	10.125	0.033	0.717
Z3	GK	1st Half 2nd Half	– –	–	–	–
	ED	1st Half 2nd Half	19.25 (13.07) 30.00 (9.83)	1.727	0.237	0.224
	CD	1st Half 2nd Half	35.33 (26.84) 40.00 (8.19)	0.083	0.788	0.020
	CMF	1st Half 2nd Half	24.50 (17.91) 28.25 (10.89)	0.256	0.621	0.018
	EMF	1st Half 2nd Half	23.00 (14.83) 29.80 (9.26)	0.756	0.410	0.086
	FW	1st Half 2nd Half	31.00 (8.72) 47.33 (6.81)	6.542	0.063	0.621

Table 2. *Cont.*

Variable	Position	Half	M(SD)	F	p	η_p^2
Z4	GK	1st Half 2nd Half	– –	–	–	–
	ED	1st Half 2nd Half	29.25 (21.19) 33.00 (5.60)	0.117	0.744	0.019
	CD	1st Half 2nd Half	38.67 (11.72) 33.67 (15.14)	0.205	0.675	0.049
	CMF	1st Half 2nd Half	25.00 (12.86) 29.13 (11.17)	0.469	0.505	0.032
	EMF	1st Half 2nd Half	44.60 (8.47) [b] 25.00 (11.25) [a]	9.686	0.014	0.548
	FW	1st Half 2nd Half	37.00 (13.23) 23.67 (1.53)	3.008	0.158	0.429
Z5	GK	1st Half 2nd Half	– –	–	–	–
	ED	1st Half 2nd Half	11.25 (7.68) 18.00 (14.54)	0.674	0.443	0.101
	CD	1st Half 2nd Half	21.67 (37.53) 1.67 (2.08)	0.849	0.409	0.175
	CMF	1st Half 2nd Half	23.50 (26.75) 11.38 (10.72)	1.417	0.254	0.092
	EMF	1st Half 2nd Half	27.20 (26.34) 10.40 (9.99)	1.778	0.219	0.182
	FW	1st Half 2nd Half	15.00 (6.56) [b] 0.67 (1.15) [a]	13.902	0.020	0.777

Significantly different compared with GK [a]; ED [b] at $p < 0.05$. **Legend:** % HRmax average, average of the % heart rate max achieved during the period of analysis; Z1, % of time in Zone 1 of heart rate intensity; Z2, % of time in Zone 2 of heart rate intensity; Z3, % of time in Zone 3 of heart rate intensity; Z4, % of time in Zone 4 of heart rate intensity; and Z5, % of time in Zone 5 of heart rate intensity.

3.2. Technical Performance

The two-way MANOVA revealed that the tactical position ($p = 0.001$; $\eta_p^2 = 0.390$; small effect size) had significant main effects on the technical performance. No statistical differences were found between halves ($p = 0.173$; $\eta_p^2 = 0.107$; small effect size). There was no significant interaction (Pillai's Trace = 0.241; F = 0.878; $p = 0.558$; $\eta_p^2 = 0.121$; small effect size) between tactical position and halves on technical performance.

In the case of Volume of Play, Efficiency Index, and Performance Score, a one-way ANOVA was performed on each independent variable because no interaction was found between factors. The statistical values resulted from the comparison between tactical positions can be observed in the following Table 3.

Table 3. One-way ANOVA values of halves in each tactical position in Volume of Play, Efficiency Index, and Performance Score.

Variable	Half	Position	M(SD)	F	p	η_p^2
Volume of Play	1st half	GK ED CD CMF EMF FW	6.50 (2.12) [d] 14.25 (6.29) 18.25 (5.62) 24.00 (6.96) [a] 17.75 (6.24) 11.00 (1.41)	3.448	0.026	0.519
	2nd half	GK ED CD CMF EMF FW	7.50 (5.31) 10.75 (3.75) 11.75 (3.75) 13.67 (3.06) 11.75 (3.75) 11.50 (5.31)	0.221	0.948	0.065

Table 3. *Cont.*

Variable	Half	Position	M(SD)	F	p	η_p^2
Efficiency Index	1st half	GK	1.05 (0.96)	2.922	0.046	0.477
		ED	0.67 (0.36)			
		CD	1.01 (0.31)			
		CMF	0.71 (0.34)			
		EMF	0.24 (0.18)			
		FW	0.13 (0.09)			
	2nd half	GK	0.55 (0.63)	0.840	0.541	0.208
		ED	0.42 (0.27)			
		CD	0.69 (0.61)			
		CMF	0.48 (0.34)			
		EMF	0.20 (0.18)			
		FW	0.20 (0.15)			
Performance Score	1st half	GK	13.70 (10.70)	1.949	0.142	0.379
		ED	13.99 (6.74)			
		CD	19.25 (5.77)			
		CMF	19.10 (6.32)			
		EMF	11.30 (4.37)			
		FW	6.75 (1.18)			
	2nd half	GK	9.28 (8.09)	0.303	0.904	0.087
		ED	9.61 (6.04)			
		CD	12.79 (9.06)			
		CMF	11.59 (8.01)			
		EMF	7.83 (4.29)			
		FW	7.79 (0.41)			

Significantly different compared with GK [a]; CMF [d] at $p < 0.05$. **Legend:** % HRmax average, average of the % heart rate max achieved during the period of analysis; Z1, % of time in Zone 1 of heart rate intensity; Z2, % of time in Zone 2 of heart rate intensity; Z3, % of time in Zone 3 of heart rate intensity; Z4, % of time in Zone 4 of heart rate intensity; and Z5, % of time in Zone 5 of heart rate intensity.

The one-way ANOVA it was also carried out to compare the values between formats for the variables of Volume of Play, Efficiency Index, and Performance Score. The values can be verified in the following Table 4.

Table 4. One-way ANOVA values of tactical positions in each half in Volume of Play, Efficiency Index, and Performance Score.

Variable	Position	Half	M(SD)	F	p	η_p^2
Volume of Play	GK	1st Half	6.50 (2.12)	0.118	0.764	0.056
		2nd Half	7.50 (3.53)			
	ED	1st Half	14.25 (6.29)	0.530	0.494	0.081
		2nd Half	10.75 (7.27)			
	CD	1st Half	18.25 (5.62)	2.491	0.166	0.293
		2nd Half	11.75 (6.02)			
	CMF	1st Half	24.00 (6.96)	4.466	0.061	0.309
		2nd Half	13.67 (9.75)			
	EMF	1st Half	17.75 (6.24)	1.678	0.243	0.219
		2nd Half	11.75 (6.85)			
	FW	1st Half	11.00 (1.41)	0.077	0.808	0.037
		2nd Half	11.50 (2.12)			
Efficiency Index	GK	1st Half	1.05 (0.96)	0.365	0.607	0.154
		2nd Half	0.55 (0.63)			
	ED	1st Half	0.68 (0.36)	1.362	0.287	0.185
		2nd Half	0.42 (0.27)			
	CD	1st Half	1.01 (0.31)	0.871	0.387	0.127
		2nd Half	0.69 (0.61)			
	CMF	1st Half	0.71 (0.34)	1.468	0.254	0.128
		2nd Half	0.48 (0.34)			
	EMF	1st Half	0.24 (0.18)	0.139	0.722	0.023
		2nd Half	0.20 (0.18)			
	FW	1st Half	0.13 (0.09)	0.423	0.582	0.175
		2nd Half	0.20 (0.15)			

Table 4. *Cont.*

Variable	Position	Half	M(SD)	F	p	η_p^2
Performance Score	GK	1st Half 2nd Half	13.70 (10.70) 9.28 (8.09)	0.218	0.687	0.098
	ED	1st Half 2nd Half	13.99 (6.74) 9.61 (6.04)	0.938	0.370	0.135
	CD	1st Half 2nd Half	19.25 (5.80) 12.79 (9.06)	1.442	0.275	0.194
	CMF	1st Half 2nd Half	19.10 (6.32) 11.59 (8.01)	3.253	0.101	0.245
	EMF	1st Half 2nd Half	11.30 (4.37) 7.83 (4.29)	1.283	0.301	0.176
	FW	1st Half 2nd Half	6.75 (0.18) 7.79 (0.41)	10.911	0.081	0.845

Legend: % HRmax average, average of the % heart rate max achieved during the period of analysis; Z1, % of time in Zone 1 of heart rate intensity; Z2, % of time in Zone 2 of heart rate intensity; Z3, % of time in Zone 3 of heart rate intensity; Z4, % of time in Zone 4 of heart rate intensity; and Z5, % of time in Zone 5 of heart rate intensity.

3.3. Network Analysis

The two-way MANOVA revealed that the tactical position ($p = 0.002$; $\eta_p^2 = 0.296$; small effect size) had significant main effects on the tactical prominence. No statistical differences were found between halves ($p = 0.678$; $\eta_p^2 = 0.049$; small effect size). There was no significant interaction (Pillai's Trace = 0.207; F = 0.475; $p = 0.948$; $\eta_p^2 = 0.069$; small effect size) between tactical position and halves on network variables.

In the case of % InDegree, % OutDegree, and % Betweenness, a one-way ANOVA was performed on each independent variable because no interaction was found between factors. The statistical values resulted from the comparison between tactical positions can be observed in the following Table 5.

Table 5. One-way ANOVA values of halves in each tactical position in % InDegree, % OutDegree, and % Betweenness.

Variable	Half	Position	M(SD)	F	p	η_p^2
%InDegree	1st half	GK ED CD CMF EMF FW	0.00 (0.00) 9.46 (4.80) 10.18 (3.92) 11.81 (6.04) 8.80 (3.42) 7.69 (5.90)	1.908	0.149	0.374
	2nd half	GK ED CD CMF EMF FW	0.00 (0.00) 11.07 (7.88) 9.95 (3.43) 12.98 (5.10) 6.92 (1.20) 5.20 (0.09)	2.909	0.047	0.476
% OutDegree	1st half	GK ED CD CMF EMF FW	0.00 (0.00) [d] 7.63 (4.34) 9.75 (4.39) 12.38 (3.82) [a] 9.21 (4.72) 9.46 (2.21)	2.976	0.044	0.482
	2nd half	GK ED CD CMF EMF FW	0.00 (0.00) [d] 6.94 (1.30) [d] 8.24 (2.90) 14.58 (5.13) [a,b] 8.85 (2.92) 8.22 (0.47)	6.304	0.002	0.663

Table 5. *Cont.*

Variable	Half	Position	M(SD)	F	p	η_p^2
% Betweenness	1st half	GK	0.00 (0.00)	1.484	0.250	0.317
		ED	2.21 (1.83)			
		CD	3.46 (0.80)			
		CMF	5.39 (4.45)			
		EMF	4.39 (2.03)			
		FW	4.83 (1.42)			
	2nd half	GK	0.00 (0.00)	1.479	0.251	0.316
		ED	6.82 (10.21)			
		CD	5.45 (2.75)			
		CMF	11.73 (7.42)			
		EMF	4.73 (5.82)			
		FW	0.84 (0.39)			

Significantly different compared with GK [a]; ED [b]; CMF [d] at $p < 0.05$. **Legend:** % HRmax average, average of the % heart rate max achieved during the period of analysis; Z1, % of time in Zone 1 of heart rate intensity; Z2, % of time in Zone 2 of heart rate intensity; Z3, % of time in Zone 3 of heart rate intensity; Z4, % of time in Zone 4 of heart rate intensity; and Z5, % of time in Zone 5 of heart rate intensity.

One-way ANOVA was also carried out to compare the values between formats for the variables of network density, clustering coefficient, and total arcs. The values can be verified in the following Table 6.

Table 6. One-way ANOVA values of tactical positions in each half in % InDegree, % OutDegree, and % Betweenness.

Variable	Position	Half	M(SD)	F	p	η_p^2
% InDegree	GK	1st Half	0.00 (0.00)	0.001	0.999	0.001
		2nd Half	0.00 (0.00)			
	ED	1st Half	9.46 (4.80)	0.121	0.740	0.020
		2nd Half	11.07 (7.88)			
	CD	1st Half	10.18 (3.92)	0.008	0.932	0.001
		2nd Half	9.95 (3.43)			
	CMF	1st Half	11.81 (6.04)	0.131	0.725	0.013
		2nd Half	12.98 (5.10)			
	EMF	1st Half	8.80 (3.42)	1.076	0.340	0.152
		2nd Half	6.92 (1.20)			
	FW	1st Half	7.69 (5.90)	0.356	0.611	0.151
		2nd Half	5.20 (0.09)			
% OutDegree	GK	1st Half	0.00 (0.00)	0.001	0.999	0.001
		2nd Half	0.00 (0.00)			
	ED	1st Half	7.63 (4.34)	0.094	0.770	0.015
		2nd Half	6.94 (1.30)			
	CD	1st Half	9.75 (4.39)	0.331	0.586	0.052
		2nd Half	8.24 (2.90)			
	CMF	1st Half	12.38 (3.82)	0.709	0.420	0.066
		2nd Half	14.58 (5.13)			
	EMF	1st Half	9.21 (4.72)	0.018	0.899	0.003
		2nd Half	8.85 (2.92)			
	FW	1st Half	9.46 (2.21)	0.596	0.521	0.230
		2nd Half	8.22 (0.47)			

Table 6. *Cont.*

Variable	Position	Half	M(SD)	F	p	η_p^2
% Betweenness	GK	1st Half 2nd Half	0.00 (0.00) 0.00 (0.00)	0.001	0.999	0.001
	ED	1st Half 2nd Half	2.21 (1.83) 6.82 (10.21)	0.790	0.408	0.116
	CD	1st Half 2nd Half	3.46 (0.80) 5.45 (2.75)	1.938	0.213	0.244
	CMF	1st Half 2nd Half	5.39 (4.45) 11.73 (7.42)	3.214	0.103	0.243
	EMF	1st Half 2nd Half	4.39 (2.03) 4.73 (5.82)	0.012	0.916	0.002
	FW	1st Half 2nd Half	4.83 (1.42) 0.84 (0.39)	14.664	0.062	0.880

Legend: % HRmax average, average of the % heart rate max achieved during the period of analysis; Z1, % of time in Zone 1 of heart rate intensity; Z2, % of time in Zone 2 of heart rate intensity; Z3, % of time in Zone 3 of heart rate intensity; Z4, % of time in Zone 4 of heart rate intensity; and Z5, % of time in Zone 5 of heart rate intensity.

4. Discussion

The objective of this study was to analyze the influence of tactical positioning of the players in a friendly football match during two halves of 30 min. Moreover, heart rate response, technical analysis, and collective behavior were related with parameters.

Statistical differences in HR responses were found between halves. Descriptive statistics showed that external defenders, midfielders, and forwards increased HR values from the 1st to the 2nd half. Opposite effects were found in the remaining tactical positions. Generally, HR values, blood lactate concentrations and VO_2max decreases from the 1st to the 2nd half based on the decrease of carbohydrates and glycogen storage [8,28,29].

Moreover, when the fatigue increases in the 2nd half, the efficiency index decreases for all playing positions, except for the forward, who increases his volume of play to take advantage of the tiredness of the defenders. Thus, forwards covered more distance than defenders [30] when they can create chances of goal for the condition of play.

Consequently, the volume of play decreases for the tactical playing position, in the same way, than that of the efficiency index. This is due to the possession of the ball replacing the attack play in the 2nd half since fatigue does not allow effective vertical play due to reduced physical condition. The coordination, the muscle participation, agility, and the decision-making of the game are affected due to fatigue [4].

Moreover, the style of play decided by the coach has an influence on the volume of play. In this way, the team evaluated has a direct style of play for the attacking phases, and a pressuring of the ball for the defensive phases of the game, attending for the physiological, physical, and technical/tactical demands of the team [31]. For this reason, forwards increase their volume of play and efficiency index.

On the one hand, % InDegree between halves increase in positions without risk of losing the ball, like external defenders or central midfielders. Moreover, the Z5 of the % HR (Table 2) show an increase for external defenders, who participate more in the play of the team [16].

On the other hand, % OutDegree is increased in the 2nd half when fatigue is higher, and implies more mistakes by the players. The external defenders have less left back, while the midfielders have the greatest number of left back because they covered more distance than the rest of the tactical positions, taking more frequency of right back [30]. Therefore, midfielders have more % Betweeness [14] because the direct style of play decreases on the 2nd half.

Finally, the performance score has the same results than that of the volume of play because it is diminished for tactical positions, except for the forward, who gets goals because of the increase in his volume of play and chances for goals. Moreover, with a direct style of play, possession with long passing sequences will decrease and this may increase the chances of a goal [32].

In conclusion, this study constitutes a vision of the tactical/technical demands of the play on players of different tactical positions in relation to the heart rate response and collective behavior. For this reason, the practical applications of this study allow knowing the features of the system of the play depending on each moment of the match. Specifically, in relation with the volume of play, the efficiency index, and performance score, the tactical positions are more relevant in each feature. Furthermore, if we can control physiological parameter demands in soccer, we could analyze more deeply, such as economizing on energy or nutrient reserves. Moreover, other studies could use this investigation to go into detail for a specific tactical position, or to analyze a specific variable of the technical performance and their repercussion on each moment of the match.

On the other hand, this study has limitations in order to know the responses when the players participate in a competition match, where other factors like the concentration or vigor of the players can be altered. Another important limitation was the small sample used in this initial study. Moreover, it is recommended that investigations for other ages be conducted, in order to conclude results for other players' features. Furthermore, it is necessary the improvement of technology be in agreement with this area of research in order to strive for excellence in the exhaustive analysis of parameters.

5. Conclusions

The objective of this study was to analyze the influence of tactical positioning of the players in a friendly football match. Furthermore, different physiological and technical parameters were measured. The results suggest that fatigue is a component distinguished in the volume of play and efficiency index. When fatigue increases, the implication is that more mistakes are made by the players and these parameters decrease. Therefore, the study may suggest the relevance of measuring physiological, technical, and tactical parameters in order to apply a performance training and system knowledge of the game.

Acknowledgments: This work was supported by the FCT project PEst-OE/EEI/LA0008/2013.

Author Contributions: F.M.C. and S.G.-V. conceived and designed the experiments; J.I.O. and C.E. performed the experiments; F.M.L.M. analyzed the data; F.M.C., F.M.L.M. and S.G.-V. contributed materials/analysis tools; J.I.O., C.E. and F.M.C. wrote the paper.

Conflicts of Interest: The authors declare no conflict of interest.

Abbreviations

The following abbreviations are used in this manuscript: Heart Rate (HR), Maximum Heart rate (HRmax).

References

1. Gréhaigne, J.F.; Godbout, P.; Bouthier, D. The Foundations of Tactics and Strategy in Team Sports. *J. Teach. Phys. Educ.* **1999**, *18*, 159–174.
2. Bangsbo, J. Physiological demands of football. *Sports Sci. Exch.* **2014**, *27*, 1–6.
3. Clemente, F.M. *Small-Sided and Conditioned Games in Soccer Training: The Science and Practical Applications*; SpringerBriefs in Applied Sciences and Technology; Springer Singapore: Singapore, 2016.
4. Mohr, M.; Krustrup, P.; Bangsbo, J. Fatigue in soccer: A brief review. *J. Sports Sci.* **2005**, *23*, 593–599. [CrossRef] [PubMed]
5. Hoff, J.; Wisløff, U.; Engen, L.C.; Kemi, O.J.; Helgerud, J. Soccer specific aerobic endurance training. *Br. J. Sports Med.* **2002**, *36*, 218–221. [CrossRef] [PubMed]
6. Janssen, P. *Lactate Threshold Training*; Human Kinetics: Champaing, IL, USA, 2001.

7. Carling, C.; Bloomfield, J.; Nelsen, L.; Reilly, T. The role of motion analysis in elite soccer. *Sports Med.* **2008**, *38*, 839–862. [CrossRef] [PubMed]
8. Bangsbo, J.; Nørregaard, L.; Thorsø, F. Activity profile of competition football. *Can. J. Sports Sci.* **1991**, *16*, 110–116.
9. Gréhaigne, J.F.; Godbout, P.; Zerai, Z. How the "rapport de forces" evolves in a football match: The dynamics of collective decisions in a complex system. *Rev. Psicol. Deporte* **2011**, *20*, 747–765.
10. McGarry, T. Soccer as a Dynamical System: Some Theoretical Considerations. In *Science and Football V*; Reilly, T., Cabri, J., Araújo, D., Eds.; Routledge, Taylor & Francis Group: London, UK; New York, NY, USA, 2005; pp. 570–579.
11. Vilar, L.; Araújo, D.; Davids, K.; Button, C. The Role of Ecological Dynamics in Analysing Performance in Team Sports. *Sports Med.* **2012**, *42*, 1–10. [CrossRef] [PubMed]
12. Barreira, D.; Garganta, J.; Castellano, J.; Anguera, M.T. SoccerEye: A software solution to observe and record behaviours in sport settings. *Open Sports Sci. J.* **2013**, *6*, 47–55. [CrossRef]
13. Travassos, B.; Davids, K.; Araújo, D.; Esteves, P.T. Performance analysis in team sports: Advances from an Ecological Dynamics approach. *Int. J. Perform. Anal. Sport* **2013**, *13*, 83–95.
14. Duch, J.; Waitzman, J.S.; Amaral, L.A. Quantifying the performance of individual players in a team activity. *PLoS ONE* **2010**, *5*, e10937. [CrossRef] [PubMed]
15. Grund, T.U. Network structure and team performance: The case of English Premier League soccer teams. *Soc. Netw.* **2012**, *34*, 682–690. [CrossRef]
16. Clemente, F.M.; Martins, F.M.L.; Wong, D.P.; Kalamaras, D.; Mendes, R.S. Midfielder as the prominent participant in the building attack: A network analysis of national teams in FIFA World Cup 2014. *Int. J. Perform. Anal. Sport* **2015**, *15*, 704–722.
17. Malta, P.; Travassos, B. Characterization of the defense-attack transition of a soccer team. *Motricidade* **2014**, *10*, 27–37.
18. Krustrup, P.; Mohr, M.; Nybo, L.; Jensen, J.M.; Nielsen, J.J.; Bangsbo, J. The Yo-Yo IR2 test: Physiological response, reliability, and application to elite soccer. *Med. Sci. Sports Exerc.* **2006**, *38*, 1666–1673. [CrossRef] [PubMed]
19. Gréhaigne, J.F.; Godbout, P.; Bouthier, D. Performance assessment in team sports. *J. Teach. Phys. Educ.* **1997**, *16*, 500–516.
20. Gréhaigne, J.F.; Richard, J.F.; Griffin, L. *Teaching and Learning Team Sports and Games*; Routledge Falmar: New York, NY, USA, 2005.
21. Robinson, G.; O'Donoghue, P. A weighted kappa statistic for reliability testing in performance analysis of sport. *Int. J. Perform. Anal. Sport* **2007**, *7*, 12–19.
22. Cotta, C.; Mora, A.M.; Merelo, J.J.; Merelo-Molina, C. A network analysis of the 2010 FIFA world cup champion team play. *J. Syst. Sci. Complex.* **2013**, *26*, 21–42. [CrossRef]
23. Clemente, F.M.; Martins, F.M.L.; Kalamaras, D.; Wong, D.P.; Mendes, R.S. General network analysis of national soccer teams in FIFA World Cup 2014. *Int. J. Perform. Anal. Sport* **2015**, *15*, 80–96.
24. Opsahl, T.; Agneessens, F.; Skvoretz, J. Node centrality in weighted networks: Generalizing degree and shortest paths. *Soc. Netw.* **2010**, *32*, 245–251. [CrossRef]
25. Wasserman, S.; Faust, K. *Social Network Analysis: Methods and Applications*; Cambridge University Press: New York, NY, USA, 1994.
26. O'Donoghue, P. *Statistics for Sport and Exercise Studies: An Introduction*; Routledge Taylor & Francis Group: London, UK; New York, NY, USA, 2012.
27. Lakens, D. Calculating and reporting effect sizes to facilitate cumulative science: A practical primer for *t*-tests and ANOVAs. *Front. Psychol.* **2013**, *4*. [CrossRef] [PubMed]
28. Ogushi, T.; Ohashi, J.; Nagahama, H.; Isokawa, M.; Suzuki, S. Work intensity during soccer match-play (a case study). In *Science and Football II*; Reilly, T., Clarys, J., Stibbe, A., Eds.; E & FN Spon: London, UK, 1993; pp. 121–123.
29. Stølen, T.; Chamari, K.; Castagna, C.; Wisløff, U. Physiology of Soccer. *Sports Med.* **2005**, *35*, 501–536. [CrossRef] [PubMed]
30. Mohr, M.; Krustrup, P.; Bangsbo, J. Match performance of high-standard soccer players with special reference to development of fatigue. *J. Sports Sci.* **2003**, *21*, 519–528. [CrossRef] [PubMed]

31. Barreira, D.; Garganta, J.; Guimarães, P.; Machado, J.; Anguera, M.T. Ball recovery patterns as a performance indicator in elite soccer. *Proc. Inst. Mech. Eng. Part P J. Sports Eng. Technol.* **2014**, *228*, 61–72. [CrossRef]
32. Hughes, M.; Franks, I. Analysis of passing sequences, shots and goals in soccer. *J. Sports Sci.* **2005**, *23*, 509–514. [CrossRef] [PubMed]

11

ZumBeat: Evaluation of a Zumba Dance Intervention in Postmenopausal Overweight Women

Anja Rossmeissl [1,*], Soraya Lenk [1], Henner Hanssen [1], Lars Donath [2], Arno Schmidt-Trucksäss [1,*] and Juliane Schäfer [1,3]

1 Division of Sports and Exercise Medicine, Department of Sport, Exercise and Health, University of Basel, Birsstrasse 320 B, Basel 4052, Switzerland; soraya.lenk@unibas.ch (S.L.); henner.hanssen@unibas.ch (H.H.); juliane.schaefer@unibas.ch (J.S.)
2 Division of Movement and Exercise Science, Department of Sport, Exercise and Health, University of Basel, Birsstrasse 320 B, Basel 4052, Switzerland; lars.donath@unibas.ch
3 Basel Institute for Clinical Epidemiology and Biostatistics, University Hospital Basel, Spitalstrasse 12, Basel 4031, Switzerland
* Correspondence: anja.rossmeissl@unibas.ch (A.R.); arno.schmidt-trucksaess@unibas.ch (A.S.-T.)

Academic Editor: Eling de Bruin

Abstract: Physical inactivity is a major public health concern since it increases individuals' risk of morbidity and mortality. A subgroup at particular risk is postmenopausal overweight women. The aim of this study was to assess the feasibility and effect of a 12-week ZumBeat dance intervention on cardiorespiratory fitness and psychosocial health. Postmenopausal women with a body mass index (BMI) >30 kg/m^2 or a waist circumference >94 cm who were not regularly physically active were asked to complete a 12-week ZumBeat dance intervention with instructed and home-based self-training sessions. Before and after the intervention, peak oxygen consumption (VO_{2peak}) was assessed on a treadmill; and body composition and several psychometric parameters (including quality of life, sports-related barriers and menopausal symptoms) were investigated. Of 17 women (median age: 54 years; median BMI: 30 kg/m^2) enrolled in the study, 14 completed the study. There was no apparent change in VO_{2peak} after the 12-week intervention period (average change score: −0.5 mL/kg/min; 95% confidence interval: −1.0, 0.1); but, quality of life had increased, and sports-related barriers and menopausal symptoms had decreased. A 12-week ZumBeat dance intervention may not suffice to increase cardiorespiratory fitness in postmenopausal overweight women, but it increases women's quality of life.

Keywords: menopause; dance; cardiorespiratory fitness; Zumba; barriers; quality of life

---

1. Introduction

Many physiologic changes are brought about during menopause and the shifting levels of hormones, associated with a considerable increase in cardiovascular risk [1,2]. In addition to the health hazard associated with the metabolic changes and increasing abdominal fat commonly concurring with menopause, many women experience weight gain as a function of aging [3,4]. The weight gain is partly explained by decreasing basal metabolic rates and decreasing energy expenditure due to diminished physical activity [5,6]. Therefore, the observed decline in physical activity around the age of 55 years is a crucial issue in the postmenopausal phase [7,8], since inactive postmenopausal women who are overweight or obese have a substantially increased risk for cardiovascular diseases [9].

Much research has documented the tremendous benefits of physical activity on various health aspects [10]. Previous studies have additionally enhanced our understanding for the causes of inactivity and identified various categories of barriers associated with inactivity behavior in women at midlife [11–13]. Dance, on the other hand, is the second most popular leisure time physical activity after walking in women across all ages (25 to 75 years plus) [14]. Convincing benefits of dancing activities on physiologic, endocrine, cognitive and psychological levels have previously been shown [15–21]. Several studies revealed improved fitness, weight loss, reductions in cholesterol levels or inflammatory markers in women at risk after various forms of aerobic dancing [18,22–27], including "aerobics", "step aerobics" and "cultural dances". Zumba as a type of fitness dance that combines Latin rhythms and aerobics has rapidly reached tremendous popularity lately [28]. The first studies on Zumba revealed its sufficiency as a training method that is able to enhance cardiorespiratory fitness [29,30]. Moreover Zumba Gold has been shown to be safely applied in elderly or even chronically-ill people [31,32], although two studies warn of possible injuries associated with Zumba fitness and the wrong footwear [33,34]. In young normal weight females, Zumba improves fitness, trunk strength endurance, balance and quality of life [35]. Furthermore, Zumba has been shown to reduce neck-shoulder pain, as well as fat mass and to improve aerobic fitness in the setting of a workplace intervention [36–38]. A pilot study conducted at the same time as our study in a population of middle-aged obese women with metabolic syndrome reported weight reductions of 2.07 pounds on average, as well as improvements in systolic and diastolic blood pressure and fasting triglycerides after a 12-week intervention [39]. Quite recently, studies also started to examine aspects of motivation, self-perceived fitness and autonomy [40,41]. One of these studies published in 2015 found enhanced intrinsic motivation associated with fitness improvements, as well as reductions in body weight and fat mass after 16 weeks of Zumba dance in obese middle-aged women [40]. However, there is still a paucity of data on physical and mental health benefits from Zumba-style dancing activities in the older, sedentary overweight population. The aim of this study was to assess the feasibility of a 12-week ZumBeat dance intervention in sedentary, postmenopausal overweight women and to generate preliminary effect size estimates regarding cardiorespiratory fitness (primary outcome) and anthropometric and psychometric parameters (secondary outcomes).

2. Materials and Methods

2.1. Study Design

In this single-arm, monocentric, prospective interventional study, participants were examined before and after a 12-week Zumba dance intervention (ClinicalTrials.gov Identifier: NCT02384694). The 12-week intervention comprised a total of three planned weekly training sessions. Participants were asked to attend at least 2 out of 3 weekly sessions offered in-person at the facilities of the University of Basel. In addition, they were asked to complete at least one weekly session as home-based training. The study was approved by the local ethics committee (Ethikkommission Nordwest-und Zentralschweiz, Basel, Switzerland). Written informed consent was obtained from all participants prior to the start of the study.

2.2. Participants

Sedentary women were recruited from the community through leaflet advertisements in doctor's offices and pharmacies (700 pieces), on online marketplaces, University pin boards and during public talks. Moreover, heads of local clinics (e.g., endocrinology, internal medicine) were contacted via e-mail as mediators to address possible candidates. Potential participants contacted the study staff and were screened for eligibility. The inclusion criteria were: (1) postmenopausal woman between 45 and 65 years of age; (2) body mass index (BMI) >30 kg/m^2 or waist circumference >94 cm; and (3) not regularly physically active more than once a week. Subjects were excluded, when they: (1) were presently enrolled in another research study; (2) were unable to attend the training sessions; or (3) had medical contraindications for exercise (such as pulmonary and/or cardiovascular disease, epilepsy or an elevated risk of falls or other limitations for safe study participation). Women with renal dysfunctions, active malignancies or recent chemotherapies (<6 months) were also excluded. Contraindications for exercise were determined via assessment of medical history and clinical examination. The entire enrolment, intervention and measurement phase took 6 months. The study was conducted between May and October 2014. Participants were asked to maintain their usual dietary habits.

2.3. Measurements

At the initial visit, participants were interviewed and examined by an experienced physician. Anthropometric and psychometric parameters were collected before the exercise testing.

Demographic and anthropometric data, including height (in cm, stationary device, without shoes), weight (in kg, Inbody 720® Bioimpedanzmessgerät (JP Global Markets GmbH, Eschborn, Germany), in underwear), waist circumference (in cm, with tape directly above the iliac crest) and calculated BMI (in kg/m^2), were obtained. Blood pressure and heart rate at rest were recorded using an automated oscillometric device (Mobil-O-Graph NG, I.E.M., Stolberg, Germany) after 10 min of rest in supine position. The cuff was inflated 3 times to supra-systolic values (30 mmHg above the systolic blood pressure) automatically with a succeeding pressure release at a rate of 3 mmHg/ second.

We compiled a test battery consisting of common tests for the assessment of facets of psychosocial and physical health in association with being overweight, eating behavior, depression, menopausal symptoms, subjective health and quality of life, as well as sports-related barriers (Supplementary Materials, Table S1).

2.4. Exercise Testing

Peak oxygen consumption (VO_{2peak}) and maximum heart rate (HR_{max}) were assessed during spiroergometric cardiopulmonary exercise testing on a treadmill (H/P/Cosmos Pulsar 2005, H/P Cosmos Sports and Medical GmbH, Nussdorf-Traunstein, Germany) equipped with a suspension system and an emergency stop as routine safety measures. Participants were allowed to use handrails in case of instability and advised to look straight ahead during the testing. The space behind the treadmill was three meters; no sharp surfaces or material were in reach of the treadmill. One participant stumbled while stepping partly off the running belt, and the treadmill was stopped immediately (see flow chart Figure 1). As a consequence, safety measures were formally reinforced prior to the testing of the following participants. Before each exercise test, the spirometry system (Cortex Metalyzer® 3B (Cortex Biophysik GmbH, Leipzig, Germany)) was calibrated by two-point gas calibration with gases of known composition. After a 5-min period of familiarization and safety instruction while standing on the treadmill, participants performed a graded exercise test (pepper ramp protocol [42]). Throughout the entire duration of the test, cardiac function was recorded on a 12-lead electrocardiogram (custo cardio 100, CustoMed, Ottobrunn, Germany) under the supervision of a staff physician. Peak blood pressure values were obtained to rule out hypertensive blood pressure. To determine subjective effort, ratings of perceived exertion were acquired (Borg Scale [43]). The test was terminated upon reaching volitional exhaustion or fulfilment of absolute cardiorespiratory exhaustion criteria (2 or more out of the following: heart rate >80% of the predicted HR_{max} (= (220-age) $\pm$ 10%), ratings of perceived exertion $\geqslant$18 (Borg scale: 6 to 20), respiratory exchange ratio $\geqslant$1.05, no further increment in VO_{2peak}, supervisor's impression).

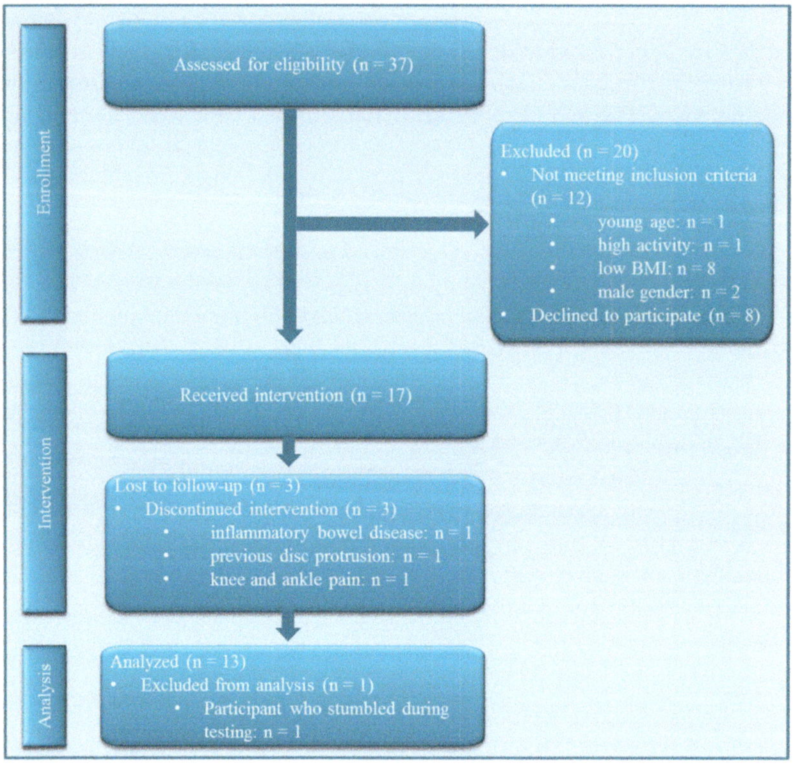

Figure 1. Flow of participants through the trial. Abbreviations: BMI, body mass index.

2.5. Dance Intervention

We modified the original higher impact Zumba-style and composed a set of ZumBeat choreographies aiming at a reduced strain for the musculoskeletal system by avoiding high impact jumping movements, appropriate for an overweight population (Supplementary Materials, Figures S1 and S2), similar to Zumba Gold®. During the 12-week intervention period, 3 instructed 60-min classes were provided per week, of which participants were instructed to attend a minimum of 2. Participants were allowed to join the in-person training up to three times per week and, thus, compensate for missed trainings in earlier or later weeks. Positive feedback and verbal encouragement were used to enhance adherence during the in-person sessions. Participants also received a DVD with dance moves, recorded by our team, for the home-based self-trainings. Participants were instructed to perform home-based self-trainings at least once a week by choosing from a set of 10 dances on a menu plus additional warm-up and cool-down sections. Self-monitoring is considered the cornerstone of behavioral obesity treatment as it enhances self-awareness and self-regulatory capabilities [44,45]. Although a causal relationship has not been established, the literature suggests that consistent self-monitoring of exercise is associated with a greater amount of exercise and weight loss, as well as fewer difficulties with exercise [46]. We therefore instructed our participants to record their home-based training sessions on a log.

During 3 instructed training sessions in Weeks 1, 5 and 12, heart rate was recorded on a Polar watch (RS 400, Polar Electro Oy, Kempele, Finland) during the whole course of the session. Training heart rates were calculated from dancing periods only (40 to 45 min).

2.6. Statistical Analyses

The primary outcome of this study was the change in VO_{2peak} (in mL/kg/min) after the 12-week intervention period; secondary outcomes were changes in BMI, weight, waist circumference, percent body fat, visceral fat mass, muscle mass, systolic blood pressure, diastolic blood pressure, resting heart rate, quality of life, sports-related barriers, menopausal symptoms, depression, psychiatric symptoms, impulsivity and eating behavior. Paired *t*-tests were used to assess changes in outcome after the intervention period. In sensitivity analyses, we removed a few unusual data points to see whether our analyses were robust to outliers. For each analysis, we report the estimated change in outcome with its 95% confidence interval in order to emphasize clinical relevance over statistical significance. To facilitate use of our data for planning future studies, we also report Cohen's d as an effect size measure, which can be readily interpreted as the percentage of the standard deviation of the change scores (such that a Cohen's d of 0.5 means the difference equals half a standard deviation). We used R Version 3.1.2 (R Foundation for Statistical Computing, Vienna, Austria) and the R add-on package lattice Version 0.20–30 for our analyses and graphics [47].

2.7. Power Calculation

Based on previous literature [18,22,25,48,49], we assumed a mean VO_{2peak} of 25 to 35 mL/kg/min in women between 45 and 65 years of age, a standard deviation of 5 mL/kg/min and a correlation between baseline and follow-up VO_{2peak} of 0.7. A 3.5-mL/kg/min (= 1 MET, metabolic equivalent) higher fitness level was associated with a 13% risk reduction of all-cause mortality and a 15% lower risk for cardiovascular disease events or death in men and women according to epidemiological data [50]. A large scale longitudinal study observed a risk reduction of 15% all-cause and 19% cardiovascular mortality with each MET increment in fitness [51]. Based on these previous findings, we aimed at a risk reduction of at least 10% for cardiovascular disease events and, therefore, considered an improvement in VO_{2peak} of 3 mL/kg/min as clinically meaningful. With 17 study participants, the power was 85% to detect such improvement (using a paired *t*-test at a 2-sided significance level of 0.05).

3. Results

3.1. Participant Characteristics

Thirty-seven subjects responded to our advertisements. Twenty of them did not start the intervention because of failure to meet the eligibility criteria or refusal to participate (Figure 1). Seventeen overweight women were enrolled in the study, with a mean age of 55 years, median BMI of 30 kg/m^2 and median waist circumference of 103 cm (Table 1). Out of the 17 participants, 13 were on oral medications; six took antihypertensive drugs (two β-blockers); two antidepressants; one a long-acting β_2 agonist.

Table 1. Participant baseline characteristics.

Characteristic	All Participants (*n* = 17)
Female sex, *n*	17
Age, years	55 (6)
Height, cm	167 (9)
Weight, kg	85 (79, 94)
BMI, kg/m^2	30 (29, 33)
Waist circumference, cm	103 (102, 114)
Percent body fat, %	39 (8)
Visceral fat mass [1], cm^2	130 (118, 156)
Systolic blood pressure [2], mmHg	126 (12)
Diastolic blood pressure [2], mmHg	80 (10)
Smoking, n	–
Non-smoker	13
Ex-smoker	3
Current smoker	1

Abbreviations: BMI, body mass index; data are the mean (standard deviation) or median (interquartile range) if not stated otherwise; [1] Available in 16/17 participants; [2] after excluding one participant who forgot to take relevant medication on the day of the baseline visit, available in 16/17 participants.

3.2. *Training Completion and Intensity*

Out of the 17 participants, three were lost to follow-up. The remaining 14 participants attended a median of 20 of the recommended 24 instructed training sessions (interquartile range (IQR) 14, 24) and completed a median of seven of the recommended 12 home-based self-training sessions (IQR 4, 9), where one participant did not provide information on the number of completed home-based trainings. The overall median training performance was 30 of the recommended 36 training sessions (IQR 20, 34). In detail: two participants completed eight and 12 instructed sessions (corresponding to an average of ⩽1 attendance per week); nine completed between 13 and 24 instructed sessions (corresponding to an average of one to two attendances per week); and three participants completed 30 instructed sessions (corresponding to an average of >2 attendances per week). Regarding home-based self-training, there were 10 participants that completed between two and nine sessions (corresponding to an average of <1 completion per week); two completed 18 sessions (corresponding to an average of 1.5 completions per week); and one participant completed 20 sessions (corresponding to an average of >1.5 completions per week). Overall, five participants completed between eight and 24 instructed or home-based self-training sessions (corresponding to an average of ⩽2 trainings per week); six completed between 25 and 34 sessions (corresponding to an average of two to three trainings per week); and three participants completed between 37 and 41 sessions (corresponding to an average of >3 sessions per week).

During the instructed training sessions in Weeks 1, 5 and 12, participants spent ⩽5% of the time at 50% to 59% of a participant's individual HR_{max}, while the remaining time of the training sessions was spent at heart rate zones ⩾60% of the HR_{max} (Figure 2). Participants performed the instructed training sessions in Weeks 1, 5 and 12 at a median of 69% (IQR 65, 74), 75% (IQR 69, 78) and 72% (IQR 67, 74) of the HR_{max} (Supplementary Materials, Figure S3).

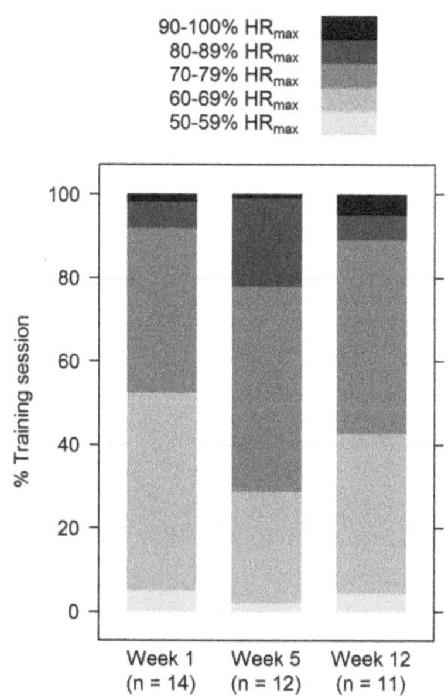

Figure 2. Average percentage of time spent at certain heart rate zones during three (instructed) training sessions in Weeks 1, 5 and 12. Heart rate zones were calculated individually based on the maximum heart rate (HR_{max}) during baseline exercise testing.

3.3. *Effect of the Intervention on Cardiorespiratory Fitness*

One participant stumbled during treadmill testing and did not complete the test protocol. We therefore excluded this participant from the analysis of both the VO_{2peak} and HR_{max}. For each participant considered for analysis, Figure 3 shows the change in VO_{2peak} after the 12-week intervention period. On average, there was no apparent change in VO_{2peak} (−0.5 mL/kg/min, 95% confidence interval (CI) −1.0, 0.1; $p = 0.114$, Table 2), where all participants considered for analysis fulfilled at least two objective exertion criteria at baseline and follow-up testing.

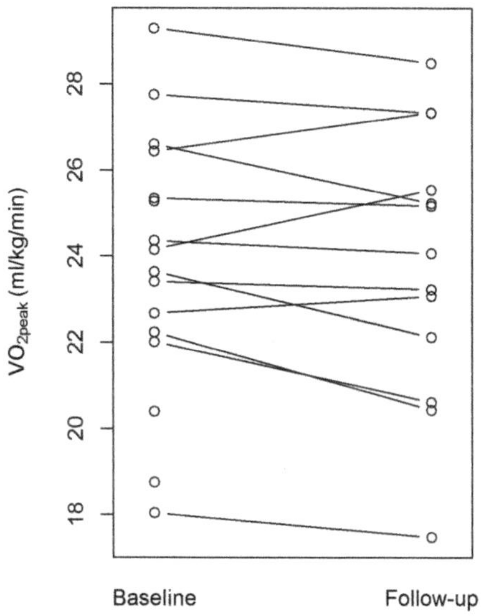

Figure 3. Individual responses in peak oxygen consumption (VO_{2peak}) showing the direction of change.

Table 2. Effect of the 12-week ZumBeat dance intervention on cardiorespiratory fitness, anthropometry and cardiovascular parameters.

Parameter	N [1]	Intervention (n = 17)		Change from Baseline (95% CI)	p-Value	Cohen's d
		Baseline (Mean (SD))	Follow-up (Mean (SD))			
VO_{2peak}, mL/kg/min	13	24.3 (2.9)	23.9 (3.2)	−0.5 (−1.0, 0.1)	0.114	−0.47
HR_{max}, bpm	12	161.8 (15.5)	164.5 (17.0)	2.7 (−2.8, 8.1)	0.305	0.31
Anthropometry						
Weight, kg	14	91.0 (13.1)	90.4 (11.6)	−0.6 (−2.4, 1.3)	0.509	−0.18
BMI, kg/m^2	14	32.7 (4.9)	32.5 (4.2)	−0.2 (−0.9, 0.4)	0.444	−0.21
Waist circumference, cm	14	108.8 (9.2)	107.2 (8.5)	−1.6 (−3.3, 0.2)	0.072	−0.52
Percent body fat, %	14	39.5 (8.2)	38.1 (7.4)	−1.3 (−3.6, 0.9)	0.210	−0.35
Fat mass, kg	14	36.1 (10.2)	34.7 (9.0)	−1.4 (−3.7, 0.9)	0.200	−0.36
Visceral fat mass, cm^2	13	140.7 (25.6)	138.4 (27.1)	−2.2 (−9.6, 5.1)	0.523	−0.18
Muscle mass, kg	14	30.3 (5.3)	31.0 (5.0)	0.7 (−0.3, 1.7)	0.162	0.40
Cardiovascular parameters						
SBP, mmHg	12	126.6 (14.2)	131.0 (12.3)	4.4 (−1.4, 10.2)	0.124	0.48
DBP, mmHg	12	80.4 (9.9)	83.3 (9.8)	2.9 (−1.2, 6.9)	0.146	0.45
Resting heart rate, bpm	13	63.5 (7.5)	62.3 (6.5)	−1.2 (−5.5, 3.2)	0.578	−0.16

Abbreviations: VO_{2peak}, peak oxygen consumption; HR_{max}, maximum heart rate; BMI, body mass index; SBP, systolic blood pressure; DBP, diastolic blood pressure; SD, standard deviation; CI, confidence interval; [1] Number of participants with baseline and follow-up data available.

3.4. *Effect of the Intervention on Anthropometric Parameters*

On average, anthropometric parameters showed small changes in the expected direction, though associated with considerable uncertainty (Table 2). Data on visceral fat mass were only available in 13 participants at baseline and follow-up. There were no changes in medication between the baseline and follow-up visit, except for two women who forgot to take their antihypertensive medications at the day of either the baseline or follow-up visit and who were therefore excluded from the blood pressure analyses. One of them was also excluded from the heart rate analyses (β-blocking agents) (Table 2).

3.5. Effect of the Intervention on Psychometric Parameters

3.5.1. Quality of Life

At the end of the 12-week intervention period, participants' overall self-rated quality of life had increased by 9.2 out of 100 points (95% CI 1.6, 16.8) on the Impact of Weight on Quality of Life (IWQOL) questionnaire [52]; and self-esteem and work-related quality of life had increased by 15.6 points (95% CI 2.8, 28.4) and 10.3 points (95% CI 0.1, 20.4) (Table 3).

Table 3. Effect of the 12-week ZumBeat dance intervention on psychometry.

Questionnaire	N [1]	Intervention (n = 17)		Change from Baseline (95% CI)	p-Value	Cohen's d	+/− [2]	Norm [3]
		Baseline (Mean (SD))	Follow-up (Mean (SD))					
IWQOL (0–100)	14	–	–	–	–	–	–	–
Total score	–	79.4 (17.2)	88.7 (8.8)	9.2 (1.6, 16.8)	0.022	0.70	+	91.8
Physical function	–	75.5 (17.9)	83.6 (13.3)	8.1 (−1.2, 17.4)	0.082	0.50	+	90.0
Self-esteem	–	68.1 (29.0)	83.7 (19.5)	15.6 (2.8, 28.4)	0.021	0.70	+	87.5
Sexual life	–	86.2 (25.4)	92.9 (18.2)	6.7 (−2.0, 15.3)	0.119	0.45	+	95.1
Public distress	–	91.9 (14.7)	96.1 (5.3)	4.2 (−2.3, 10.7)	0.189	0.37	+	96.5
Work	–	87.5 (18.0)	97.8 (5.2)	10.3 (0.1, 20.4)	0.048	0.58	+	95.4
SBB (0 to 4)	14	2.5 (0.5)	2.1 (0.6)	−0.4 (−0.7, −0.2)	0.001	−1.09	+	2.2
MRS(0 to 44)	14	11.9 (7.6)	9.5 (7.1)	−2.4 (−4.6, −0.2)	0.036	−0.62	+	8.8
BDI (0 to 63)	14	7.2 (7.8)	4.8 (5.3)	−2.4 (−5.6, 0.7)	0.118	−0.45	+	7.7
ISR (0 to 4)	14	0.5 (0.5)	0.4 (0.4)	−0.1 (−0.2, 0.0)	0.216	−0.35	+	0.4
I-8 (0 to 4)	14	–	–	–	–	–	–	–
Urgency	–	2.3 (0.6)	2.2 (0.8)	−0.1 (−0.4, 0.1)	0.314	−0.28	+	2.5
Intention	–	3.6 (1.0)	4.0 (0.6)	0.4 (−0.1, 0.9)	0.094	0.48	+	3.8
Endurance	–	4.1 (0.6)	3.9 (0.9)	−0.2 (−0.6, 0.2)	0.254	−0.32	–	4.3
Risk	–	3.6 (0.8)	3.2 (0.8)	−0.4 (−0.9, 0.2)	0.156	−0.40	+	2.8
FEV	14	–	–	–	–	–	–	–
Dietary restraint (0 to 21)	–	9.1 (3.8)	9.8 (4.4)	0.7 (−2.0, 3.4)	0.582	0.15	+	8.2
Disinhibition (0 to 16)	–	8.2 (3.6)	7.1 (3.2)	−1.1 (−2.5, 0.4)	0.132	−0.43	+	7.1
Hunger (0 to 14)	–	7.2 (3.8)	5.0 (3.7)	−2.2 (−4.2, −0.3)	0.028	−0.66	+	5.7

Abbreviations: IWQOL, Impact of Weight on Quality of Life; SBB, Sports-related Situational Barriers Scale; MRS, Menopause Rating Scale; BDI, Beck Depression Inventory; ISR, ICD-10-Symptom-Rating; I-8, German Version of the UPPS Impulsive Behavior Scale; FEV, German Version of the Dutch Eating Behavior Questionnaire (DEBQ); SD, standard deviation; CI, confidence interval; [1] Number of participants with baseline and follow up data available; [2] "+" symbolizes improvement of the test result, "−" symbolizes deterioration; [3] normative values for the general population.

3.5.2. Menopausal Symptoms

Symptoms that are frequently encountered during menopausal transition had decreased by 2.4 out of 44 points (95% CI 0.2, 4.6) on the Menopause Rating Scale (MRS) [53] (Table 3).

3.5.3. Sports-Related Barriers

Barriers towards exercise had decreased by 0.4 out of four points (95% CI 0.2, 0.7) on the Sports-related Situational Barriers (SBB) scale [54] (Table 3).

3.5.4. Psychiatric Symptoms

Levels of depression on the Beck Depression Inventory II (BDI) had improved slightly [55]. Other psychiatric complaints, such as anxiety, compulsion, somatization or eating disorders, were not prevalent among the study participants and were essentially unchanged after the end of the intervention period, based on the results of the ICD-10 Symptom Rating (ISR) scale [56] (Table 3).

3.5.5. Impulsivity and Eating Behavior

While most impulsivity sub-scales were essentially unchanged after the end of the intervention period, intentional behavior had increased slightly, with an average change from baseline of 0.4 out of four points (95% CI −0.1, 0.9) on the I-8 questionnaire (German Version of the UPPS Impulsive Behavior Scale) [57]. Dietary restraint and disinhibition towards food had not changed after the end of the intervention period. However, feelings of hunger were reduced by 2.2 out of 14 points (95% CI 0.3, 4.2) on the German Version of the Dutch Eating Behavior Questionnaire [58] (Table 3).

3.6. Sensitivity Analyses

Compared to the main analysis of the VO_{2peak}, exclusion of two participants who stopped exercise testing prior to having reached (subjective) exertion led to a similar pattern of change after the 12-week intervention period (average change score: −0.2 mL/kg/min, 95% CI −0.8, 0.3; $p = 0.382$). Estimated changes from baseline were generally decreased after excluding a few outliers with unusually strong improvements in outcome (Supplementary Materials, Table S2). For example, changes in percent body fat and muscle mass were decreased after excluding two outliers with an unusually strong decrease in percent body fat and one outlier with an unusually strong increase in muscle mass, respectively.

4. Discussion

Developing, piloting, evaluating, reporting and implementing are important steps for interventions, as suggested by the Medical Research Council [59]. Generally, studies can be declared as feasible when they fulfil the criteria of successful recruitment, retention/compliance/adherence and safety.

With regard to feasibility assessment in the process of evaluating and developing a future intervention, one result of this study is that the intervention itself appears to be feasible: in our study, only three participants (equaling 18%) discontinued the study participation. Previous literature suggests drop-out rates due to orthopedic problems of 25% [41]. We attribute the relative success to the low hazardous style of the ZumBeat dance moves. Most Zumba classes demand high coordination and experience with the choreographies. Assuming a lack of the above, the likelihood for musculoskeletal injury is increased. The small number of complications from the training, the small drop-out rate and good adherence in this study suggest the feasibility of the intervention itself.

We observed no benefit for cardiorespiratory fitness following a 12-week ZumBeat dance intervention in postmenopausal overweight women and only small benefits, if any, for body composition. However, single items of health-related quality of life may be enhanced and menopausal symptoms and sports-related barriers reduced. This implies possible reductions of problems often encountered in the field of activity promotion and might contribute to a better understanding in this important public health area. Future projects should implement and thoroughly assess this topic.

The literature suggests that Zumba dance is a suitable training method to enhance cardiovascular fitness and strength [29,35,38]. However, older, overweight populations have rarely been studied. A recent publication by Dalleck *et al.* shows that Zumba Gold® training can be categorized as moderate exercise and is in line with current guidelines for improving and maintaining cardiorespiratory fitness [60]. While on average, women in this study did not improve their VO_{2peak}, Krishnan *et al.* found an improvement in VO_{2peak} of 1 mL/kg/min in a similar study population after a 16-week, three times weekly, 60-min per session Zumba intervention [40]. In their study, VO_{2peak} was not measured, but calculated after conducting a walking test. A quality criterion for our study is the direct measurement of VO_{2peak}. Another study among female hospital workers indicated an improvement in VO_{2peak} of 1.46 mL/kg/min (95% CI 0.17, 2.75) after 12 weeks of training and a reduction in fat mass comparable to that observed in our study [60]. However, the participants were younger (mean age: 46 years), had a lower BMI (mean BMI: 26 kg/m^2) and, therefore, might have adapted to the training more easily. Moreover, this might have allowed them to exercise at greater training intensities right from the start. The reported change in VO_{2peak} corresponds to improvements between 0.9% and 9%, 5% on average only. This still lies in the range possible of retest adaption effects [61] or corresponds to a 3% to 5% reduction of the relative risk for cardiovascular events [51]. The great variability in study participation with a lack of continuity of exercise over the summer period in our study may explain why we were not able to add to the growing body of evidence for an effect of Zumba on fitness. This might have diminished measurable improvements and be explanatory for the missing increment in VO_{2peak}, but clearly reflects real-life circumstances. The endurance section of the lessons (excluding warm-up and cool-down) evoked a rise in heart rates above the level necessary to acquire training adaptions and gains in fitness, with median heart rates ranging between 69% and 75% of the HR_{max} (Supplementary Materials, Figure S3) and the main portion of the lesson at heart rate zones between 60% and 79% of the participants' HR_{max} (Figure 2). Exercise intensity progressed from moderate to higher intensities over the time-course of the intervention, as recommended in exercise training guidelines [62]. According to the subjective impression of the instructor, the training sessions were all well tolerated. This confirms that the intensity of the training itself meets current recommendations and, therefore, should have been sufficient to positively influence fitness [63]. Moreover, a pilot study suggests that Zumba® dance classes might allow greater energy expenditure, but Zumba® DVD workouts might be suitable to maintain fitness [64].

On average, participants did not show a large benefit in anthropometric parameters after the 12-week intervention period. Single participants, however, showed extreme changes in body composition, with one participant losing 7.4% and another losing 10.8% body fat. There was no evidence for a change in blood pressure, but both systolic and diastolic average levels in this small sample appeared slightly higher after the intervention. This is in line with results from an eight-week Zumba® intervention, which did not result in relevant changes in body composition [41]. A recent publication by Cugusi *et al.* showed significant weight and fat mass reductions, as well as gains in muscle mass after a 12-week Zumba dance intervention similar to ours, in a younger overweight population (mean age 38.9 $\pm$ 9.7 years) [65]. They also reported decreases in blood pressure levels. This indicates that Zumba may contribute to significant improvement in body composition, but whether this is possible in an elderly overweight population with appropriate training time and effort remains to be proven.

Cugusi *et al.* investigated quality of life in relation to Zumba dancing [65]. In their study, physical functioning and emotional role were the only two out of eight domains assessed that showed significant amelioration. Our study suggests improvements in quality of life scores associated with being overweight. At baseline, scores were ranging between normal values for healthy people and participants in weight reduction programs in each subscale. After the intervention, the scores appeared improved, but a causal attribution to the intervention cannot be made due to the study design. Larger scaled controlled trials are needed for confirmation.

Our results suggest a reduction in sports-related barriers (0.4 out of four points (95% CI 0.2, 0.7) on the SBB scale). Sedentariness implies the existence of manifold barriers and a lack of motivation. One major factor accounting for inactivity is the lack of self-motivation. Greater self-efficacy, on the other hand, has been identified as key determinant in increasing physical activity [13,66]. Studies show that a recent exercise experience or mastery can improve self-efficacy beliefs and increase exercise adherence in the maintenance phase [67]. Therefore, an increase in self-esteem and a decrease in barriers as observed in this study could be a first step towards greater activity participation. Future controlled studies are required to confirm our exploratory results regarding barriers and should simultaneously monitor associated self-motivation and self-efficacy beliefs.

Average baseline values of all sub-scores and the total MRS score were above the healthy European norm [68]. While previous research has revealed ambiguous results of exercise on menopausal symptoms, menopausal symptoms seemed lower post-intervention in this study and may be worth future exploration.

Two participants showed elevated levels of depression on the BDI-II at baseline, beyond the cut-off for moderate depression; both of them had reduced their depression scores after the end of the intervention (one of them by more than eight points, representing a clinically-relevant improvement). Average depression levels in our study were not elevated and remained essentially unchanged after the intervention, whereas other studies have reported higher depression levels among diabetic and obese people [69–72]. Furthermore, we did not find symptoms suggestive of other psychiatric disorders nor did they change over the course of the intervention, but due to the small sample size and single-arm design, a generalization of these results in not feasible.

While impulsivity as a construct is strongly associated with behavioral control and adaptive regulations to the individual's surroundings, it is often more pronounced in patients with binge eating disorders or obesity [73]. Physical activity, on the other hand, has been shown to moderate impulsive behavior in addition to behavioral therapy [74]. In this study, impulsive behavior was more prevalent at baseline compared to normative values on all four sub-scores of the I-8 questionnaire, but did not seem to be affected by the intervention.

In addition, this study revealed encouraging results suggesting a reduction in hunger perceptions, which could lead to a more stable eating behavior, but still needs to be proven through further research.

Limitations

This study presents some limitations. First, due to recruitment problems, our study has a small sample size and lacks a control group. We originally designed this study as a randomized controlled trial, but were only able to recruit 17 participants and, therefore, changed the study design, with approval from the ethics committee, to a prospective, interventional single-arm study. Despite our great efforts in terms of recruitment, we were not able to meet the target total sample size as determined for a two-arm trial, including a control group. Interested women were too young or active, while the targeted participants did not respond to our advertisements. The advertisements might have been more successful if more research personnel had approached potential candidates verbally in person or via local media. We were unable to place costly advertisements in newspapers or distribute leaflets to private households for this study, as it was only funded by internal resources. Moreover, future studies might consider a matching of the contact person with participants (older, overweight woman), a more convenient location and closer telephone follow-up in order to enhance recruitment efficiency [66]. In addition, incentives for study participation should be reconsidered. Given the low response to advertisement in this study and even lower eligibility rates, careful reconsideration of the strict inclusion criteria might be another approach, but simultaneously changes the purpose of the study. Our practical experience is comparable to the Zumba pilot study reported by Araneta *et al.* in which 35 women completed eligibility screening by phone, 23 were eligible for a first visit, 18 met eligibility criteria, 16 initiated Zumba classes and 13 completed the study. Therefore, these response and retention rates may be characteristic for this type of study in a similar population. Our recruitment strategies were insufficient to generate a sample large enough for a randomized controlled trial, and therefore, this part of the project was not feasible. Recruitment strategies need to be carefully reconsidered before starting a large randomized controlled trial. This may include the option of multi-center studies. With the above-mentioned limitation (lacking a control group) in mind, all resulting data and their interpretations below need to be handled with caution. They should rather be interpreted as exploratory indicators serving to generate effect sizes for future controlled trials.

Secondly, the study has a short length of follow-up, limiting the strength of findings on the mid- to long-term effects of the ZumBeat dance intervention.

Thirdly, participants who dropped out of the intervention could not be included in the final results, raising issues of effectiveness among those who stop exercising.

In sum, our study suggests a decrease in sports-related barriers, better attitudes towards exercise and improvements in weight-adjusted quality of life following a 12-week ZumBeat dance intervention. As a result, individuals may be more active in the post-intervention period, so that cardiorespiratory fitness and weight are then steadily improved. This has important public health implications, since current literature suggests that postmenopausal sedentary women who are overweight have an increased cardiovascular risk, which can be modified by physical activity [9]. A short-term ZumBeat dance intervention may offset initially small, but steadily-increasing changes in cardiovascular risk factors for those who eventually make long-term behavioral changes. Future studies should modify the length of the intervention, which might result in larger fitness improvements. While our study has a short length of follow-up, limiting the strength of findings on the mid- to long-term effects of the ZumBeat dance intervention, prospective research should examine participants' appraisal of the program and physical activity levels in the follow-up period after the intervention.

5. Conclusions

A 12-week ZumBeat dance intervention may not suffice to improve cardiorespiratory fitness or substantially improve body composition in sedentary postmenopausal overweight women. However, it shows good feasibility in terms of adherence and safety, helps to improve weight-related quality of life and to reduce sports-related barriers. Future studies are needed to evaluate whether the psychosocial improvements are persistent after the intervention and whether these are transformable into additional health gains.

Acknowledgments: The authors thank all participants for their time and effort, which were vital to the completion of this research project. The authors would also like to thank the personnel of the Division of Sports and Exercise Medicine at the Department of Sport, Exercise and Health for their technical, logistical and mental support.

Author Contributions: Contributions to authorship: Anja Rossmeissl, Juliane Schäfer and Arno Schmidt-Trucksäss designed this study. Anja Rossmeissl, Soraya Lenk and Henner Hanssen were responsible for data collection at the Department of Sport, Exercise and Health. Anja Rossmeissl and Soraya Lenk designed and delivered the ZumBeat dance intervention. Anja Rossmeissl, Arno Schmidt-Trucksäss and Juliane Schäfer carried out the statistical analyses and created the graphs. Anja Rossmeissl wrote the first draft of the manuscript. Anja Rossmeissl, Lars Donath, Arno Schmidt-Trucksäss and Juliane Schäfer revised the manuscript. All authors reviewed, commented on and approved the final version of the manuscript.

Conflicts of Interest: The authors declare no conflict of interest.

References

1. Lentz, G.M.; Lobo, R.A.; Gershenson, D.M.; Katz, V.L. *Comprehensive Gynecology: Expert Consult Online and Print*, 6th ed.; Elsevier Health Sciences: Philadelphia, PA, USA, 2012; pp. 273–299.
2. Lobo, R.A.; Davis, S.R.; de Villiers, T.J.; Gompel, A.; Henderson, V.W.; Hodis, H.N.; Lumsden, M.A.; Mack, W.J.; Shapiro, S.; Baber, R.J. Prevention of diseases after menopause. *Climacteric* **2014**, *17*, 540–556. [CrossRef] [PubMed]
3. Al-Safi, Z.A.; Polotsky, A.J. Obesity and menopause. *Best Pract. Res. Clin. Obstet. Gynaecol.* **2014**, *29*, 548–553. [CrossRef] [PubMed]
4. Lovejoy, J.C. Weight gain in women at midlife: The influence of menopause. *Obes. Manag.* **2009**, *5*, 52–56. [CrossRef]
5. Duval, K.; Prud'homme, D.; Rabasa-Lhoret, R.; Strychar, I.; Brochu, M.; Lavoie, J.M.; Doucet, E. Effects of the menopausal transition on energy expenditure: A monet group study. *Eur. J. Clin. Nutr.* **2013**, *67*, 407–411. [CrossRef] [PubMed]
6. Lovejoy, J.C.; Champagne, C.M.; de Jonge, L.; Xie, H.; Smith, S.R. Increased visceral fat and decreased energy expenditure during the menopausal transition. *Int. J. Obes. Lond.* **2008**, *32*, 949–958. [CrossRef] [PubMed]
7. Sun, F.; Norman, I.J.; While, A.E. Physical activity in older people: A systematic review. *BMC Public Health* **2013**, *13*, 1–17. [CrossRef] [PubMed]

8. Sui, X.; Zhang, J.; Lee, D.C.; Church, T.S.; Lu, W.; Liu, J.; Blair, S.N. Physical activity/fitness peaks during perimenopause and bmi change patterns are not associated with baseline activity/fitness in women: A longitudinal study with a median 7-year follow-up. *Br. J. Sports Med.* **2013**, *47*, 77–82. [CrossRef] [PubMed]
9. Chomistek, A.K.; Manson, J.E.; Stefanick, M.L.; Lu, B.; Sands-Lincoln, M.; Going, S.B.; Garcia, L.; Allison, M.A.; Sims, S.T.; LaMonte, M.J.; *et al.* Relationship of sedentary behavior and physical activity to incident cardiovascular disease: Results from the women's health initiative. *J. Am. Coll. Cardiol.* **2013**, *61*, 2346–2354. [CrossRef] [PubMed]
10. Lee, I.M.; Shiroma, E.J.; Lobelo, F.; Puska, P.; Blair, S.N.; Katzmarzyk, P.T.; Lancet Physical Activity Series Working Group. Effect of physical inactivity on major non-communicable diseases worldwide: An analysis of burden of disease and life expectancy. *Lancet* **2012**, *380*, 219–229. [CrossRef]
11. McArthur, D.; Dumas, A.; Woodend, K.; Beach, S.; Stacey, D. Factors influencing adherence to regular exercise in middle-aged women: A qualitative study to inform clinical practice. *BMC Womens Health* **2014**, *14*. [CrossRef] [PubMed]
12. Bruner, B.; Chad, K. Physical activity attitudes, beliefs, and practices among women in a woodland cree community. *J. Phys. Act. Health* **2013**, *10*, 1119–1127. [PubMed]
13. Im, E.O.; Lee, B.; Chee, W.; Stuifbergen, A. eMAPA Research Team. Attitudes toward physical activity of white midlife women. *J. Obstet. Gynecol. Neonatal Nurs.* **2011**, *40*, 312–321. [CrossRef] [PubMed]
14. Fan, J.X.; Kowaleski-Jones, L.; Wen, M. Walking or dancing: Patterns of physical activity by cross-sectional age among u.S. Women. *J. Aging Health* **2013**, *25*, 1182–1203. [CrossRef] [PubMed]
15. Kattenstroth, J.C.; Kalisch, T.; Holt, S.; Tegenthoff, M.; Dinse, H.R. Six months of dance intervention enhances postural, sensorimotor, and cognitive performance in elderly without affecting cardio-respiratory functions. *Front. Aging Neurosci.* **2013**, *5*. [CrossRef] [PubMed]
16. Belardinelli, R. Exercise training in chronic heart failure: How to harmonize oxidative stress, sympathetic outflow, and angiotensin II. *Circulation* **2007**, *115*, 3042–3044. [CrossRef] [PubMed]
17. Kim, S.H.; Kim, M.; Ahn, Y.B.; Lim, H.K.; Kang, S.G.; Cho, J.H.; Park, S.J.; Song, S.W. Effect of dance exercise on cognitive function in elderly patients with metabolic syndrome: A pilot study. *J. Sports Sci. Med.* **2011**, *10*, 671–678. [PubMed]
18. Shimamoto, H.; Adachi, Y.; Takahashi, M.; Tanaka, K. Low impact aerobic dance as a useful exercise mode for reducing body mass in mildly obese middle-aged women. *Appl. Hum. Sci.* **1998**, *17*, 109–114. [CrossRef]
19. Murrock, C.J.; Graor, C.H. The effects of dance on depression, physical function, and disability in underserved adults. *J Aging Phys Act* **2014**, *22*, 380–385. [CrossRef] [PubMed]
20. Coubard, O.A.; Duretz, S.; Lefebvre, V.; Lapalus, P.; Ferrufino, L. Practice of contemporary dance improves cognitive flexibility in aging. *Front. Aging Neurosci.* **2011**, *3*. [CrossRef] [PubMed]
21. Duberg, A.; Hagberg, L.; Sunvisson, H.; Moller, M. Influencing self-rated health among adolescent girls with dance intervention: A randomized controlled trial. *JAMA Pediatr.* **2013**, *167*, 27–31. [CrossRef] [PubMed]
22. Gillett, P.A.; Eisenman, P.A. The effect of intensity controlled aerobic dance exercise on aerobic capacity of middle-aged, overweight women. *Res. Nurs. Health* **1987**, *10*, 383–390. [CrossRef] [PubMed]
23. Murrock, C.J.; Gary, F.A. Culturally specific dance to reduce obesity in african american women. *Health Promot. Pract.* **2010**, *11*, 465–473. [CrossRef] [PubMed]
24. Gullu, E.; Gullu, A.; Cicek, G.; Yamaner, F.; Imamoglu, O.; Gumusdag, H. The effects of aerobic exercises on cardiovascular risk factors of sedentary women. *Int. J. Acad. Res.* **2013**, *5*, 160–167. [CrossRef]
25. Okura, T.; Nakata, Y.; Ohkawara, K.; Numao, S.; Katayama, Y.; Matsuo, T.; Tanaka, K. Effects of aerobic exercise on metabolic syndrome improvement in response to weight reduction. *Obesity* **2007**, *15*, 2478–2484. [CrossRef] [PubMed]
26. Mosher, P.E.; Ferguson, M.A.; Arnold, R.O. Lipid and lipoprotein changes in premenstrual women following step aerobic dance training. *Int. J. Sports Med.* **2005**, *26*, 669–674. [CrossRef] [PubMed]
27. Williford, H.N.; Blessing, D.L.; Barksdale, J.M.; Smith, F.H. The effects of aerobic dance training on serum lipids, lipoproteins and cardiopulmonary function. *J. Sports Med. Phys. Fit.* **1988**, *28*, 151–157.
28. Thomson, W.R. Worldwide survey of fitness trends for 2013. *ACSMs Health Fit. J.* **2012**, *16*, 8–17.
29. Luettgen, M.; Foster, C.; Doberstein, S.; Mikat, R.; Porcari, J. Zumba(®): Is the "fitness-party" a good workout? *J. Sports Sci. Med.* **2012**, *11*, 357–358. [PubMed]
30. Otto, R.M.; Maniguet, E.; Peters, A.; Boutagy, N.; Gabbard, A.; Wygand, J.W.; Yoke, M. The Energy Cost of Zumba Exercise. *Med. Sci. Sports Exerc.* **2011**, *43*. [CrossRef]

31. Bennett, P.; Corradini, A.; Ockerby, C.; Cossich, T. Exercise during hemodialysis the intradialytic Zumba Gold. *Nephrol. News Issues* **2012**, *26*, 31–32. [PubMed]
32. Sanders, M.E.; Prouty, J. Zumba® fitness is gold for all ages. *Acsms Health Fit. J.* **2012**, *16*, 25–28.
33. Inouye, J.; Nichols, A.; Maskarinec, G.; Tseng, C.W. A survey of musculoskeletal injuries associated with zumba. *Hawaii J. Med. Public Health* **2013**, *72*, 433–436. [PubMed]
34. Schrimpf, C.; Haastert-Talini, K.; von Falck, C.; Rustum, S.; Wilhelmi, M.; Teebken, O.E. High sport sneakers may lead to peripheral artery occlusion in Zumba® dancers. *Vasa* **2014**, *43*, 78–80. [CrossRef] [PubMed]
35. Donath, L.; Roth, R.; Hohn, Y.; Zahner, L.; Faude, O. The effects of zumba training on cardiovascular and neuromuscular function in female college students. *Eur. J. Sport Sci.* **2014**, *14*, 569–577. [CrossRef] [PubMed]
36. Barene, S.; Krustrup, P.; Brekke, O.L.; Holtermann, A. Soccer and Zumba as health-promoting activities among female hospital employees: A 40-weeks cluster randomised intervention study. *J. Sports Sci.* **2014**, *32*, 1539–1549. [CrossRef] [PubMed]
37. Barene, S.; Krustrup, P.; Holtermann, A. Effects of the workplace health promotion activities soccer and Zumba on muscle pain, work ability and perceived physical exertion among female hospital employees. *PLoS ONE* **2014**, *9*, e115059. [CrossRef] [PubMed]
38. Barene, S.; Krustrup, P.; Jackman, S.R.; Brekke, O.L.; Holtermann, A. Do soccer and Zumba exercise improve fitness and indicators of health among female hospital employees? A 12-week rct. *Scand. J. Med. Sci. Sports* **2014**, *24*, 990–999. [CrossRef] [PubMed]
39. Araneta, M.R.; Tanori, D. Benefits of zumba fitness among sedentary adults with components of the metabolic syndrome: A pilot study. *J. Sports Med. Phys. Fit.* **2015**, *55*, 1227–1233.
40. Krishnan, S.; Tokar, T.N.; Boylan, M.M.; Griffin, K.; Feng, D.; McMurry, L.; Esperat, C.; Cooper, J.A. Zumba® dance improves health in overweight/obese or type 2 diabetic women. *Am. J. Health Behav.* **2015**, *39*, 109–120. [CrossRef] [PubMed]
41. Delextrat, A.A.; Warner, S.; Graham, S.; Neupert, E. An 8-week exercise intervention based on Zumba® improves aerobic fitness and psychological well-being in healthy women. *J. Phys. Act. Health* **2015**, epub ahead of print. [CrossRef] [PubMed]
42. Peterson, M.J.; Pieper, C.F.; Morey, M.C. Accuracy of $VO_{2(max)}$ prediction equations in older adults. *Med. Sci. Sports Exerc.* **2003**, *35*, 145–149. [CrossRef] [PubMed]
43. Borg, G. Perceived exertion as an indicator of somatic stress. *Scand. J. Rehabil. Med.* **1970**, *2*, 92–98. [PubMed]
44. Dalle Grave, R.; Calugi, S.; Centis, E.; El Ghoch, M.; Marchesini, G. Cognitive-behavioral strategies to increase the adherence to exercise in the management of obesity. *J. Obes.* **2011**, *2011*, 348293. [CrossRef] [PubMed]
45. Woodard, C.M.; Berry, M.J. Enhancing adherence to prescribed exercise: Structured behavioral interventions in clinical exercise programs. *J. Cardiopulm. Rehabil.* **2001**, *21*, 201–209. [CrossRef] [PubMed]
46. Carels, R.A.; Darby, L.A.; Rydin, S.; Douglass, O.M.; Cacciapaglia, H.M.; O'Brien, W.H. The relationship between self-monitoring, outcome expectancies, difficulties with eating and exercise, and physical activity and weight loss treatment outcomes. *Ann. Behav. Med.* **2005**, *30*, 182–190. [CrossRef] [PubMed]
47. Sarkar, D. *Lattice: Multivariate Data Visualization with R*; Springer: New York, NY, USA, 2008; p. 265.
48. Garber, C.E.; McKinney, J.S.; Carleton, R.A. Is aerobic dance an effective alternative to walk-jog exercise training? *J. Sports Med. Phys. Fit.* **1992**, *32*, 136–141.
49. Leelarungrayub, D.; Saidee, K.; Pothongsunun, P.; Pratanaphon, S.; YanKai, A.; Bloomer, R.J. Six weeks of aerobic dance exercise improves blood oxidative stress status and increases interleukin-2 in previously sedentary women. *J. Bodyw. Mov. Ther.* **2011**, *15*, 355–362. [CrossRef] [PubMed]
50. Kodama, S.; Saito, K.; Tanaka, S.; Maki, M.; Yachi, Y.; Asumi, M.; Sugawara, A.; Totsuka, K.; Shimano, H.; Ohashi, Y.; *et al.* Cardiorespiratory fitness as a quantitative predictor of all-cause mortality and cardiovascular events in healthy men and women: A meta-analysis. *JAMA* **2009**, *301*, 2024–2035. [CrossRef] [PubMed]
51. Lee, D.C.; Sui, X.; Artero, E.G.; Lee, I.M.; Church, T.S.; McAuley, P.A.; Stanford, F.C.; Kohl, H.W., 3rd; Blair, S.N. Long-term effects of changes in cardiorespiratory fitness and body mass index on all-cause and cardiovascular disease mortality in men: The aerobics center longitudinal study. *Circulation* **2011**, *124*, 2483–2490. [CrossRef] [PubMed]
52. Kolotkin, R.L.; Crosby, R.D. Psychometric evaluation of the impact of weight on quality of life-lite questionnaire (iwqol-lite) in a community sample. *Qual. Life Res.* **2002**, *11*, 157–171. [CrossRef] [PubMed]
53. Potthoff, P.; Heinemann, L.A.; Schneider, H.P.; Rosemeier, H.P.; Hauser, G.A. [The menopause rating scale (MRS II): Methodological standardization in the German population]. *Zentralbl. Gynakol.* **2000**, *122*, 280–286. [PubMed]

54. Krämer, L.; Fuchs, R. Barrieren und Barrierenmanagement im Prozess der Sportteilnahme. Zwei neue Messinstrumente. *Z. Gesundheitspsychol.* **2010**, *18*, 170–182. [CrossRef]
55. Beck, A.T.; Steer, R.A.; Ball, R.; Ranieri, W. Comparison of beck depression inventories -ia and -ii in psychiatric outpatients. *J. Pers. Assess.* **1996**, *67*, 588–597. [CrossRef] [PubMed]
56. Tritt, K.; von Heymann, F.; Zaudig, M.; Zacharias, I.; Sollner, W.; Loew, T. [Development of the "Icd-10-Symptom-Rating"(ISR) questionnaire]. *Z. Psychosom. Med. Psychother.* **2008**, *54*, 409–418. [PubMed]
57. Kovaleva, A.; Beierlein, C.; Schmitt, M.; Kemper, C.J. Eine Kurzskala zur Messung von Impulsivität nach dem UPPSs-Ansatz: Die Skala impulsives Verhalten (I-8). In *GESIS Working Papers*; GESIS: Köln, Geramny, 2012; Volume 20.
58. Pudel, D.; Westenhöfer, J. *Fragebogen zum Essverhalten (FEV), Handanweisung*; Hogrefe: Göttingen, Geramny, 1989.
59. Craig, P.; Dieppe, P.; Macintyre, S.; Michie, S.; Nazareth, I.; Petticrew, M. Developing and evaluating complex interventions: The new medical research council guidance. *Int. J. Nurs. Stud.* **2013**, *50*, 587–592. [CrossRef] [PubMed]
60. Dalleck, L.C.; Roos, K.A.; Byrd, B.R.; Weatherwax, R.M. Zumba Gold(®): Are the physiological responses sufficient to improve fitness in middle-age to older adults? *J. Sports Sci. Med.* **2015**, *14*, 689–690. [PubMed]
61. Scharhag-Rosenberger, F.; Walitzek, S.; Kindermann, W.; Meyer, T. Differences in adaptations to 1 year of aerobic endurance training: Individual patterns of nonresponse. *Scand. J. Med. Sci. Sports* **2012**, *22*, 113–118. [CrossRef] [PubMed]
62. American College of Sports Medicine. *Acsm's Guidelines for Exercise Testing and Prescription*, 8th ed.; Lippincott Williams & Wilkins: Philadelphia, PA, USA, 2010; p. 380.
63. Garber, C.E.; Blissmer, B.; Deschenes, M.R.; Franklin, B.A.; Lamonte, M.J.; Lee, I.M.; Nieman, D.C.; Swain, D.P. American college of sports medicine position stand. Quantity and quality of exercise for developing and maintaining cardiorespiratory, musculoskeletal, and neuromotor fitness in apparently healthy adults: Guidance for prescribing exercise. *Med. Sci. Sports Exerc.* **2011**, *43*, 1334–1359. [CrossRef] [PubMed]
64. Delextrat, A.; Neupert, E. Physiological load associated with a Zumba fitness workout: A comparison pilot study between classes and a DVD. *J. Sports Sci.* **2015**, *34*, 1–9. [CrossRef] [PubMed]
65. Cugusi, L.; Wilson, B.; Serpe, R.; Medda, A.; Deidda, M.; Gabba, S.; Satta, G.; Chiappori, P.; Mercuro, G. Cardiovascular effects, body composition, quality of life and pain after a Zumba® fitness program in italian overweight women. *J. Sports Med. Phys. Fit.* **2015**. epub ahead of print.
66. Bauman, A.E.; Reis, R.S.; Sallis, J.F.; Wells, J.C.; Loos, R.J.; Martin, B.W.; Lancet Physical Activity Series Working, G. Correlates of physical activity: Why are some people physically active and others not? *Lancet* **2012**, *380*, 258–271. [CrossRef]
67. Wilbur, J.; Vassalo, A.; Chandler, P.; McDevitt, J.; Miller, A.M. Midlife women's adherence to home-based walking during maintenance. *Nurs. Res.* **2005**, *54*, 33–40. [CrossRef] [PubMed]
68. Heinemann, K.; Ruebig, A.; Potthoff, P.; Schneider, H.P.; Strelow, F.; Heinemann, L.A.; Do, M.T. The menopause rating scale (MRS) scale: A methodological review. *Health Qual. Life Outcomes* **2004**, *2*, 1–8.
69. Anderson, R.J.; Freedland, K.E.; Clouse, R.E.; Lustman, P.J. The prevalence of comorbid depression in adults with diabetes: A meta-analysis. *Diabetes Care* **2001**, *24*, 1069–1078. [CrossRef] [PubMed]
70. Violante, R.; Santoro, S.; Gonzalez, C. [Prevalence of depression and anxiety in a cohort of 761 obese patients: Impact in adherence to therapy and its outcome]. *Vertex* **2011**, *22*, 85–93. [PubMed]
71. Zeman, M.; Jirak, R.; Zak, A.; Jachymova, M.; Vecka, M.; Tvrzicka, E.; Stankova, B.; Dusejovska, M. Metabolic syndrome and depression—Clinical relations. *Cas. Lek. Cesk.* **2008**, *147*, 75–80. [PubMed]
72. Almeida, O.P.; Calver, J.; Jamrozik, K.; Hankey, G.J.; Flicker, L. Obesity and metabolic syndrome increase the risk of incident depression in older men: The health in men study. *Am. J. Geriatr. Psychiatry* **2009**, *17*, 889–898. [CrossRef] [PubMed]
73. Schag, K.; Schonleber, J.; Teufel, M.; Zipfel, S.; Giel, K.E. Food-related impulsivity in obesity and binge eating disorder—A systematic review. *Obes. Rev.* **2013**, *14*, 477–495. [CrossRef] [PubMed]
74. Pendleton, V.R.; Goodrick, G.K.; Poston, W.S.; Reeves, R.S.; Foreyt, J.P. Exercise augments the effects of cognitive-behavioral therapy in the treatment of binge eating. *Int. J. Eat. Disord.* **2002**, *31*, 172–184. [CrossRef] [PubMed]

12

Optimal Timing for Post-Activation Potentiation in Women Collegiate Volleyball Players

Robert Ah Sue [1], Kent J. Adams [2] and Mark DeBeliso [1,*]

[1] Department of Physical Education and Human Performance, Southern Utah University, Cedar City, UT 84720, USA; robertahsue@gmail.com

[2] Kinesiology Department California State University Monterey Bay, Seaside, CA 93955, USA; kadams@csumb.edu

* Correspondence: markdebeliso@suu.edu

Academic Editor: Eling Douwe de Bruin

Abstract: Post-activation potentiation (PAP) has been shown to acutely amplify muscular power output and may be advantageous for athletes looking to improve performance. PAP may have an acute window of effectiveness between 2 to 20 min. With correct timing and implementation it may be possible to induce PAP in competitive situations. The purpose of this study was to examine the time frame of potentiation following a PAP warm-up in collegiate female volleyball players. In this study, nine female collegiate volleyball players completed three laboratory sessions over the course of 10 days. During the first session, the athlete's 5-RM back squat was determined for subsequent use as the conditioning activity to initiate PAP. A repeated measures experimental design was then employed for Sessions 2 and 3 where half of the participants alternately performed either a dynamic or PAP warm-up prior to performing a standing long jump (SLJ) at 2, 6, 10, 14, and 18 min. A mixed-factor repeated measures ANOVA was used to determine the effects of the two warm-up strategies (PAP *vs.* dynamic) on standing long jump (SLJ) performance across time. There was a significant effect for time ($p < 0.01$) and warm-up strategy ($p < 0.01$). Bonferroni *post hoc* techniques determined that the SLJs that followed the PAP warm-up were significantly greater at 2 (4.8%), 6 (3.6%), and 10 (3.6%) min compared to SLJs post-dynamic warm-up ($p < 0.05$). However, those differences did not persist at 14 or 18 min ($p > 0.05$). Further analysis included non-parametric pairwise comparisons (Wilcoxon signed-rank tests) between the SLJ scores at 2, 6, 10, 14, and 18 min (PAP *vs.* dynamic). The non-parametric results were consistent with the parametric results. Within the parameters of this study, it is concluded that performing a 5-RM back squat induces a measureable PAP effect for up to 10 min.

Keywords: back squat; standing long jump; post-activation potentiation (PAP)

---

1. Introduction

Evidence suggests that muscular power output can be increased by inducing a post-activation potentiation (PAP) effect with heavy resistance exercises (e.g., 5-RM back squat) [1–6]. PAP is defined as an increase in muscle performance after a conditioning contraction [7]. More specifically, PAP is an increase in muscle isometric twitch and low frequency titanic force following a conditioning activity [8]. With the appropriate conditioning activity and correct timing of the subsequent athletic action, it may be possible to induce PAP in competitive situations. However, when attempting to apply PAP to improve performance in a competitive environment, the interplay between stimulus and fatigue must be considered. With that said, a practical challenge in using PAP is to determine the optimal conditions in which stimulus and fatigue can coexist to benefit the athlete's performance [9]. Specifically, if the PAP conditioning activity is too great (volume and/or intensity), or if there is not sufficient recovery time following the conditioning activity, the associated fatigue of the conditioning activity may not be measurably expressed.

Despite evidence supporting the effectiveness of PAP for increasing power output, finding the precise time window of effectiveness post-PAP remains vague [1–5]. Identifying the window of time that muscular power is increased from PAP is a key next step in making PAP principles more applicable to use in an applied setting. In doing so, it is essential to consider two possible reasons for muscular power decline: decay of the physiological mechanisms responsible for PAP and increasing levels of muscular fatigue. Following a maximal strength exercise the effects of PAP will eventually diminish, which makes the specifics of timing that much more important [8,10]. Studies that show no increase in jumping performance often have multiple measuring points within 4 min, which suggest fatigue as a potential contributor [8,11]. An intense activity that might activate a high degree of PAP result might also produce greater fatigue [8]. Suggested modalities of the PAP as a conditioning activity include the back squat and the bench press at intensities ranging from 60%–90% of 1-RM [12]. The National Strength and Conditioning Association (NSCA) suggests that elite athletes may experience positive muscle enhancement from 2 to 20 min following a PAP conditioning activity and that PAP should be reserved for resistance-trained power athletes with high relative strength [12]. Hence, indicating a large variability in the period of a potentiating effect (coexistence with fatigue), which is dependent on the potentiating modality, intensity employed, the potentiated exercise/movement, training status, relative strength, and rest period following the PAP event.

The purpose of this study was to examine the time frame of potentiation following a PAP warm-up in collegiate female volleyball players. We hypothesized that, when athletes used a warm-up (WU) that included a PAP stimulus, they would perform better in the standing long jump (SLJ) than when the athletes used only a dynamic WU. Additionally, it was of primary importance to determine how long the PAP WU advantage lasted.

2. Materials and Methods

2.1. Participants

Participants were a convenience sample of female volleyball athletes at Salt Lake Community College, Utah (SLCC). Permission from the head coach and school administration was granted prior to the study. Student athletes were asked to volunteer for the study. Permission from the Institutional Review Board to use human subjects was obtained before conducting any training or assessments of the student athlete participants. Participants were given a written consent to read and sign before any action in the study was taken. All athletes were 18 years or older. Table 1 provides participant descriptive information.

Table 1. Participant descriptive information *.

N	Age (years)	Height (cm)	Mass (kg)	5-RM BSQ (kg)	Est 1-RM BSQ (kg)
9	18.3 ± 0.5	179.2 ± 5.3	68.8 ± 7.9	62.9 ± 11.1	70.6 ± 12.5

* Participant means and standard deviations for descriptive information; BSQ-back squat; 5-RM-five repetition maximum; Est 1-RM BSQ-estimated one repetition maximum (Brzycki equation).

2.2. Instruments and Apparatus

All sessions were held in the Lifetime Activities Center at SLCC. Equipment necessary to conduct this study included a squat rack, a 20.45 kg barbell, weighted plates (ranging from 1.14 to 20.45 kg), measuring tape, blue painter masking tape to set up jump markers (see Figure 1), and a measuring stick.

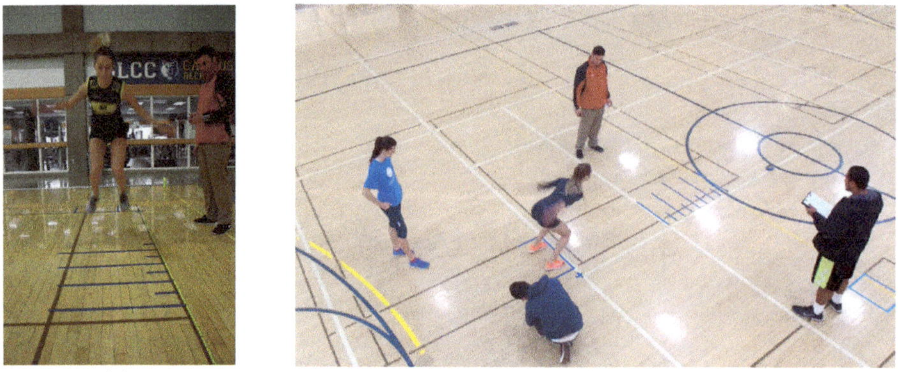

(a) (b)

Figure 1. (**a**) Athlete attempting a standing long jump; (**b**) Set up of standing long jump area adjacent to the weight room where 5-RM was performed.

2.3. Procedures

2.3.1. Assessment

Session 1 consisted of a 45-min study orientation. Participant age, height, and weight were recorded. The investigator then reviewed the proper technique for the execution of the back squat and SLJ with the participants. Following the orientation, the 5-RM back squat was assessed per the recommendations of Baechle and Earle [13] as described below. The 5-RM back squat would later serve as the conditioning activity to induce PAP (modality and intensity) during Sessions 2 and 3 (Figure 2).

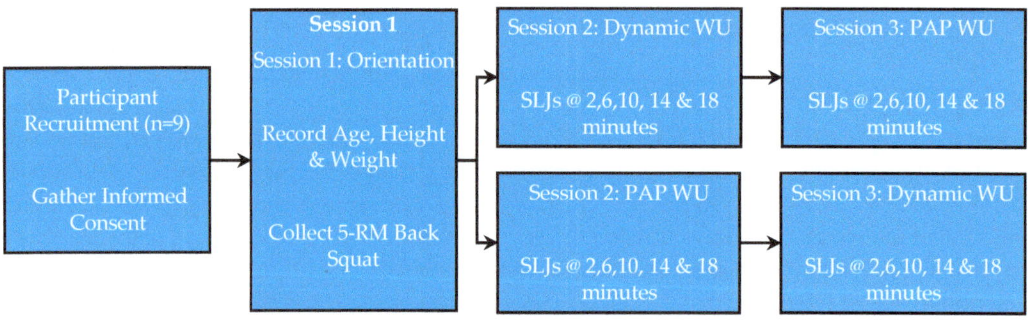

Figure 2. Study time line overview of events. PAP: post-activation potentiation; WU: warm-up; 5-RM back squat used as the PAP WU conditioning activity.

Sessions 2 and 3 were held on two consecutive days. During Session 2, all athletes performed the identical dynamic warm-up protocol and then were randomly divided into two groups: PAP and non-PAP. The participants in the non-PAP group rested for 5 min and then proceeded to have SLJs recorded. Those in the PAP group performed back squat sets culminating in a 5-RM set as described below. Two minutes following the 5-RM back squat, the participants started the SLJ trials. During Session 3, the participants crossed-over with regard to the WU procedures, and SLJs were again recorded (Figure 2). The study utilized a randomized repeated measures cross-over design in order to guard against the effects of learning (or testing), which is known to be a threat to internal validity. Further, repeated measures designs are more economical with regard to participant numbers and statistical power.

In order to simulate an "active" athletic setting, instead of a seated rest between jumps, athletes alternated between walking and jogging the length of the basketball court. Thirty seconds prior to their jump, athletes were notified to prepare for their SLJ. SLJs were strictly regulated to the 5 established time markers (2, 6, 10, 14, and 18 min).

2.3.2. Dynamic Warm-Up

The dynamic WU protocol was identical to the WU protocol applied in the athlete's regular season strength and condition program; this helped maintain consistency/specificity. The standard warm-up consisted of (in specific order): 20 high knees, 20 buttock kickers, 20 lunges, 20 karaoke, 20 A-skips, 20 side shuffle, 30 s of line hops (both feet), 15 s of line hops (one set each leg), 10 broad jumps, 10 squat hops, 10 leg sweeps (hamstring warm up), 20 reverse lunges, 20 walking quad/hamstring stretch, 20 straight leg bounding, 10 leg swings, 10 medium arm circles, and 10 large arm circles.

2.3.3. Standing Long Jump (SLJ)

Athletes started in a standstill position with toes just behind the starting line [13]. The athlete then performed a countermovement and jumped forward as far as possible [13]. The athlete was required to land on their feet for the jump to be scored; otherwise, the trial was repeated [13]. In the event of a fault, the athlete was allowed only one immediate re-jump to avoid fatigue or hindrance of another athlete's timing. A mark was placed at the back edge of the athlete's rear most heel, and the tape measure determined the distance between the starting line and the mark [13]. The standing long jump has been shown to be a reliable field test for estimation of muscular power of the lower limbs (ICC = 0.95) [14].

2.3.4. PAP Warm-Up

Athletes performed three warm-up sets of back squats in 8 min (8–10 receptions @ unloaded Olympic bar, 6–8 repetitions @ 30% 1-RM, and 5 repetitions @ 50% 1-RM). Following the WU back squats, athletes were instructed to perform 1 set of 5 repetitions of the back squat using their 5-RM weight (considered the PAP conditioning activity). The reliability of the 1-RM back squat has been reported as ICC = 0.91–0.99 [15].

2.3.5. Dynamic Warm-Up (Non-PAP) Trials

Following the standard warm-up the non-PAP group went directly into SLJ measurements at 2, 6, 10, 14, and 18 min intervals.

2.3.6. Post-Activation Potentiation (PAP) Warm-Up Trials

Following the standard warm-up, the PAP group then performed 3 sets of warm-up back squats followed by 1 set of 5 repetitions of back squats using their current 5-RM. Athletes then performed SLJs on the basketball court (10 feet adjacent from the weight room, Figure 1) at 2, 6, 10, 14, and 18 min intervals. For the purpose of contrasting the results of this study, 1-RM back squat estimates were calculated using the Brzycki equation [16].

2.3.7. Design and Analysis

A mixed-factor repeated measures ANOVA (2X5) was used to determine the effects of the 2 WU strategies (PAP *vs.* dynamic) on SLJ performance at 5 points in time (2, 6, 10, 14, and 18 min). *Post hoc* procedures included single-factor repeated measures ANOVAs and Bonferroni technique paired *t*-tests. ICCs were calculated to determine reliability of the SLJ measures. Effect sizes were also calculated as Cohen's pair wise effect size (d) = (mean PAP WU SLJ-mean Non-PAP WU SLJ)/Non-PAP WU SLJ SD. Further statistical analysis included non-parametric pairwise Wilcoxon signed-rank tests between the SLJ scores at 2, 6, 10, 14, and 18 min between the two warm-up strategies (PAP *vs.* dynamic). Statistical analysis was conducted using IBM SPSS software (version 24).

3. Results

There was a significant effect for time ($p < 0.01$) and warm-up strategy ($p < 0.01$). Repeated ANOVA measures indicated that the SLJs were not significantly different at any point in time following the PAP WU ($p > 0.05$), whereas the SLJs following the Dynamic WU (non-PAP) did vary significantly over time ($p < 0.01$). Bonferroni *post hoc* techniques (paired *t*-tests) determined that the SLJs that followed the PAP WU were significantly greater at 2, 6, and 10 min when compared to the SLJ scores following the dynamic WU ($p < 0.05$). However, those differences did not persist at 14 or 18 min ($p > 0.05$) (see Table 2). It should be noted that the ICC for the SLJ trials following the dynamic WU recorded during the current study was ICC = 0.88 (90% CI: 0.75–0.96).

Table 2. Standing long jump (SLJ) performance at 5 points in time following PAP and Non-PAP warm-ups.

PAP *vs.* Non-PAP SLJ					
	2 min	**6 min**	**10 min**	**14 min**	**18 min**
Non-PAP WU (cm)	191.4 ± 10.1	196.1 ± 10.2	199.9 ± 10.3	199.6 ± 11.8	200.7 ± 9.6
PAP WU (cm)	200.5 ± 13.9 *	203.3 ± 14.1 *	207.1 ± 13.3 *	202.6 ± 13.5	205.2 ± 13.4
%Δ	4.8%	3.6%	3.6%	1.5%	2.2%
p-value	0.02	0.03	0.04	0.40	0.09
Effect Size (ES)	0.90	0.71	0.70	0.25	0.47

Participant means and standard deviations (SD) for descriptive information; * PAP WU significantly greater than Non-PAP WU ($p < 0.05$). Paired *t*-test *p*-values; %Δ = (PAP WU SLJ-Non-PAP WU SLJ)/Non-PAP WU SLJ.

Due to the small sample size and the potential violations of normality, a nonparametric test was conducted between SLJs at each measurement time interval using the Wilcoxon signed-rank test, as recommended in [17]. The Wilcoxon signed-rank test provides a comparison of the difference in median scores between paired trails, whereas the paired *t*-test compares mean scores between paired trails. The results of the pairwise Wilcoxon signed-rank tests were as follows: 2 min: $p < 0.05$, 6 min: $p = 0.011$, 10 min: $p = 0.043$, 14 min: $p = 0.26$, and 18 min: $p = 0.12$—consistent with the initial statistical analysis.

4. Discussion

The objective of this study was to determine if a conditioning activity consisting of a single 5-RM set of the back squat was effective at inducing PAP and increasing SLJ performance and, if so, for what duration. SLJs were performed following two WU scenarios (dynamic and PAP). The SLJs that followed the PAP warm-up were significantly greater at 2, 6, and 10 min when compared to the SLJ scores following the non-PAP warm-up (effect size range 0.70–0.90 SD). However, those differences did not persist at 14 or 18 min. These data suggest that use of a single 5-RM set of the back squat induced PAP and increased SLJ for up to 10 min following the lift (*i.e.*, the conditioning activity). Jumps increased in each of the first three points in time (2, 6, and 10 min) before decreasing, suggesting that the optimal window of time for utilizing the PAP is around 10 min. With that said, the SLJs following the PAP stimuli were on average greater at all time intervals, ranging from 1.5%–4.8%. Hence, the data collected supported the study hypothesis at time intervals 2, 6, and 10 min, but not at 14 or 18 min.

The 5-RM back squats recorded during this study were equated to 1-RM estimates using the Brzycki equation [16]. The 1-RM estimates were 70.6 ± 12.5 kg which is approximately the 60th percentile for NCAA Division I female volleyball players [18]. Multiple studies have used heavy-load back squats as a conditioning activity to increase muscle power through PAP [1–4,19]. Kilduff *et al.* examined the effects of PAP on a counter jump movement and ballistic bench throws in sample of professional rugby players ($n = 23$) and reported that 8–12 min of recovery time was required between the conditioning activity and the subsequent explosive activity in order to enhance muscle power output [4]. Jenson and Ebben [11] examined the effects of PAP on vertical jump (VJ) performance in a sample of NCAA Division I male and female athletes ($n = 21$) at 10 s and 1, 2, 3, and 4 min following a 5-RM back squat and found decreased performance. In a study comparing VJs at 15 s, 2, 4, 6, 8, 10, 12, 14, and 16 min following a 5 repetition deadlift at 85% of 1-RM, Arias *et al.* demonstrated that PAP was not measurably induced [20]. The data from the Arias study suggest that a high frequency of jumps following a heavy-load conditioning activity may impede PAP [20]. Further, the Arias study used relatively untrained young men ($n = 15$), where training status was suspected to have interfered with the expression of PAP. Ebben suggested improved performance might require 3 to 4 min of rest between the use of a heavyweight training load and plyometrics [21]. In terms of optimal recovery for PAP, this study showed the highest SLJ at 10 min following the back squat. Kilduff *et al.* noted optimal recovery time required for enhanced muscle performance was also in the 8–12 min window [4]. This study, along with previous literature, suggests minimizing fatigue in the first 4 min, and a recovery period of at least 8 min will capture the benefits of an induced PAP more efficiently [1–5,11,21]. It is also important to note that a dynamic warm-up was used prior to the PAP stimulus used in the current study (*i.e.*, a 5-RM back squat). Dynamic warm-ups are shown to enhance performance and should be considered along with PAP [22].

Data suggest that PAP manifests to a greater degree in athletes and highly trained individuals compared to recreationally trained individuals [13,23–25]. The NSCA recommends that PAP should be reserved for those with "very high relative strength" [12]. Participants in this study were collegiate female athletes. However, the athlete's strength to body mass ratios were on average 1.03 kg Est 1-RM back squat/kg body mass, which cannot be considered high relative strength. This is the third such study that has demonstrated that PAP can be effective in individuals with lower relative body strength [26,27]. However, we acknowledge that the effects of the PAP stimulus used in this study may be amplified in participants with higher relative strength. One study comparing PAP in female NCAA athletes called for individual strength considerations along with specific rest times for optimizing power [28]. Xenofondos *et al.* and others suggest that PAP is affected by the training background of individuals and not their gender [7,13]. This suggests the procedures applied in this study may be relevant to male athletes as well. In terms of specific muscle composition, the proportion of fast-twitch motor units might also be related to the effectiveness of neuromuscular activation [7,29]. Again, the participants in this study were collegiate volleyball players, suggesting they have proficient jumping skills, which is typically due to the presence of a higher proportion of fast-twitch motor units. It is vital to contemplate the variety of factors that can affect PAP (training status, potentiating stimulus, fatigue, rest period, window of excitation, muscle fiber composition, *etc.*). As such, we suggest that strength and conditioning coaches follow an individualized approach to implementing PAP training protocols.

In the current study, eight of the nine participants experienced a measureable potentiation as measured by the SLJ as a result of the PAP WU. Following the SLJ assessment collected at the 10 min interval, seven of the nine participants had lower SLJ scores. During the initial 10 min, it appears that fatigue and potentiation coexisted (exhibited by the significantly greater SLJ measures). Fatigue was likely the main contributor to the decrease in SLJs at the 14- and 18-min trials. A recent study examined the effects of PAP (conditioning activity was 3 repetitions of the back squat at 90% 1-RM) on VJ performance in female division II NCAA athletes [28]. VJ performance was assessed prior to, and 5 min after, the PAP back squat set. Collectively, the athletes did not experience a measureable PAP effect. Further, a subset of the participants was volleyball players, and they experienced a reduction in VJ performance. Clearly, fatigue and potentiation did not coexist in this study [28]. We found a comparison of the current study with Sygulla and Fountaine's study [28] to be revealing. Participants in both studies were female collegiate volleyball players (non-division I), approximately the same age (18–19 years), with similar relative body strength (1.03–1.20 1-RM back squat kg/kg body mass). Conversely, the current study used a 5-RM back squat followed by SLJs initiated 2 min after the PAP conditioning activity, whereas Sygulla and Fountaine's study [28] used a back squat set of three repetitions at 90% 1-RM followed by VJs initiated 5 min post-PAP conditioning activity. Yet, the results of Sygulla and Fountaine's study [28] are in direct contrast to the results of our study in regard to jumping performance. It is possible that their study design [28], which measured pre- and post-PAP VJs on the same day in a non-cross over design, is responsible for the discrepant results. Specifically, based on the results and their study design, there is no way to tell if the pre-PAP VJs confounded the effects of the PAP stimulus (conditioning activity). If Sygulla and Fountaine's study had used a same-day cross-over study design or assessed PAP and non-PAP WUs on separate days, their results may have been more consistent with our study. While the current study did employ a cross-over design, an obvious limitation was the small sample size of $n = 9$. The current study used an intact team of nine female collegiate volleyball players, and the team only had nine players at the time of the study. A future study should attempt to replicate the findings of the current study; otherwise, the results of the current study should be included in a subsequent meta-analysis.

The improvement in the SLJ noted in the current study as a result of the PAP WU is consistent with previous studies that have demonstrated that a PAP WU can significantly increase both upper and lower body power output [26,27,30–35]. The SLJ is a full-body coordinated movement driven by lower-body muscle power. It is not certain that the improvements in SLJ ability noted in this study as a result of a PAP WU would be specific and transferable to the unpredictable factors in volleyball competition. However, it is reasonable to think that an elevated physical state induced by a PAP WU (*i.e.*, conditioning activity) may well lead to a slight edge over the competition for the early minutes of a volleyball contest. With that said, a PAP WU strategy might be better utilized when applied as a conditioning activity for predictable performance tests. For example, every year NCAA eligible athletes compete in the NFL combine for an assessment of their athletic ability [36]. The SLJ and VJ are used as an overall indicator of power in these athletes [13,36]. Athletes competing in such assessments could potentially use heavy back squats to induce PAP and improve performance. Long jumpers and triple jumpers are also examples of athletes looking for acute enhancement of muscular power output in predictable competition scenarios. Future research should focus on the effects of a PAP WU on specific sport competitions such as the long jump, the triple jump, and various throwing events.

5. Conclusions

Within the parameters of this study: (1) There was an improvement in SLJ following a conditioning activity that combined a dynamic warm-up with a 5-RM back squat; (2) the effects of PAP resulted in significant improvement in SLJ for up to 10 min; (3) therefore, the results of this study suggest that, if the conditioning activity is performed correctly per the specific applied context, PAP may be used to improve power in predictable situations. We suggest further research should be geared towards implementation of PAP in competitive situations.

Acknowledgments: We would like to thank Coach Sue Dulaney for allowing the facilities and equipment of Salt Lake Community College to be used freely during the study. The primary investigator (Robert Ah Sue) thanks his wife-to-be for her encouragement and support through the process.

Author Contributions: Robert Ah Sue and Mark DeBeliso conceived and designed the experiments; Robert Ah Sue performed the experiment; Robert Ah Sue, Mark DeBeliso, and Kent J. Adams analyzed the data; Robert Ah Sue wrote the initial draft of the paper. All authors contributed to the revisions of the manuscript and have approved the final manuscript.

Conflicts of Interest: The authors declare no conflict of interest.

References

1. Mitchell, C.J.; Sale, D.G. Enhancement of jump performance after a 5-RM squat is associated with postactivation potentiation. *Eur. J. Appl. Physiol.* **2011**, *111*, 1957–1963. [CrossRef] [PubMed]
2. Weber, K.R.; Brown, L.E.; Coburn, J.W.; Zinder, S.M. Acute Effects of Heavy-Load Squats on Consecutive Squat Jump Performance. *J. Strength Cond. Res.* **2009**, *22*, 726–730. [CrossRef] [PubMed]
3. Mangus, B.C.; Takahashi, M.; Mercer, J.A.; Holcomb, W.R.; McWhorter, J.W.; Sanchez, R. Investigation of vertical jump performance after completing heavy squat exercises. *J. Strength Cond. Res.* **2006**, *20*, 597–600. [PubMed]

4. Kilduff, L.P.; Bevan, H.R.; Kingsley, M.I.; Owen, N.J.; Bennett, M.A.; Bunce, P.J.; Hore, A.M.; Maw, J.R.; Cunningham, D.J. Postactivation potentiation in professional rugby players: Optimal recovery. *J. Strength Cond. Res.* **2007**, *21*, 1134–1138. [CrossRef] [PubMed]
5. Sotiropoulos, K.; Smilios, I.; Christou, M.; Barzouka, K.; Spaias, A.; Douda, H.; Tokmakidis, S.P. Effects of warm-up on vertical jump performance and muscle electrical activity using half-squats at low and moderate intensity. *J. Sports Sci. Med.* **2010**, *9*, 326–331. [PubMed]
6. Lima, L.C.; Oliveira, F.B.; Oliveira, T.P.; Assumpcao, C.O.; Greco, C.C.; Cardozo, A.C.; Denadai, B.S. Postactiation potentiation biases maximal isometric strength assessment. *Biomed. Res. Int.* **2014**. [CrossRef] [PubMed]
7. Xenofondos, A.; Laparidis, K.; Kyranoudis, A.; Galazoulas, C.; Bassa, E.; Kotzamanidis, C. Post-Activation Potentiation: Factors Affecting it and the Effect on Performance. *JPES* **2010**, *28*, 32–39.
8. Sale, D. Postactivation potentiation: Role in performance. *Br. J. Sports Med.* **2004**, *38*, 386–387. [CrossRef] [PubMed]
9. Rassier, D.E.; MacIntosh, B.R. Coexistence of potentiation and fatigue in skeletal muscle. *Braz. J. Med. Biol. Res.* **2000**, *33*, 499–509. [PubMed]
10. Gilbert, G.; Lees, A. Changes in the force development characteristics of muscle following repeated maximum force and power exercise. *SLE* **2005**, *48*, 1576–1584. [CrossRef] [PubMed]
11. Jensen, R.L.; Ebben, W.P. Kinetic analysis of complex training rest interval effect on vertical jump performance. *J. Strength Cond. Res.* **2003**, *17*, 345–349. [CrossRef] [PubMed]
12. NSCA Hot Topic: Post-Activation Potentiation (PAP). Available online: https://www.nsca.com/Education/Articles/Hot-Topic-Post-Activation-Potentiation-%28PAP%29/ (accessed on 5 May 2016).
13. Baechle, T.R.; Earle, R.W. Resistance training and spotting techniques. In *Essentials of Strength and Conditioning*, 3rd ed.; Baechle, T.R., Earle, R.W., Eds.; Human Kinetics: Champaign, IL, USA, 2008; pp. 350–351.
14. Markovic, G.; Dizdar, D.; Jukic, I.; Cardinale, M. Reliability and Factorial Validity of Squat and Countermovement Jump Tests. *J. Strength Cond. Res.* **2004**, *18*, 551–555. [CrossRef] [PubMed]
15. McMaster, D.T.; Gill, N.; Cronin, J.; McGuigan, M. A brief review of strength and ballistic assessment methodologies in sport. *Sports Med.* **2014**, *44*, 603–623. [CrossRef] [PubMed]
16. Brzycki, M. Strength testing—Predicting a one-rep max from reps-to-fatigue. *J. Phys. Educ. Recreat. Dance* **1993**, *64*, 88–90. [CrossRef]
17. McDonald, J.H. *Handbook of Biological Statistics*, 3rd ed.; Sparky House Publishing: Baltimore, MD, USA, 2014; pp. 183–189.
18. Hoffman, J. *Norms for Fitness, Performance, and Health*; Human Kinetics: Champaign, IL, USA, 2006.
19. Baker, D. Acute effect of alternating heavy and light resistances on power output during upper-body complex power training. *J. Strength Cond. Res.* **2003**, *17*, 493–497. [CrossRef] [PubMed]
20. Arias, J.C.; Coburn, J.W.; Brown, L.E.; Galpin, A.J. The acute effects of heavy deadlifts on vertical jump performance in men. *Sports* **2016**, *4*, 22. [CrossRef]
21. Ebben, W.P. Complex Training: A Brief Review. *J. Sports Sci. Med.* **2002**, *1*, 42–46. [PubMed]
22. McMillian, D.J.; Moore, J.H.; Hatler, B.S.; Taylor, D.C. Dynamic *vs.* static-stretching warm-up: The effect on power and agility performance. *J. Strength Cond. Res.* **2006**, *20*, 492–499. [CrossRef] [PubMed]
23. Chiu, Z.F.; Fry, A.C.; Weiss, L.W.; Schilling, B.K.; Brown, L.E.; Smith, S.L. Postactivation potentiation response in athletic and recreationally trained individuals. *J. Strength Cond. Res.* **2003**, *17*, 671–677. [CrossRef] [PubMed]
24. Gourgoulis, V.; Aggeloussis, N.; Kasimatis, P.; Mavromatis, G.; Garas, A. Effect of a submaximal half-squats warm-up program on vertical jumping ability. *J. Strength Cond. Res.* **2003**, *17*, 342–344. [CrossRef] [PubMed]
25. Duthie, G.M.; Young, W.B.; Aitken, D.A. The acute effects of heavy loads on jump squat performance: An evaluation of the complex and contrast methods of power development. *J. Strength Cond. Res.* **2002**, *16*, 530–538. [CrossRef] [PubMed]
26. Tano, G.; Bishop, A.; Berning, J.M.; Adams, K.J.; DeBeliso, M. Post activation potentiation in north american high school football players. *J. Sports Sci.*. in press.
27. Hamilton, C.; Berning, J.M.; Sevene, T.G.; Adams, K.J.; DeBeliso, M. The effects of post activation potentiation on the hang power clean. *JOPER* **2016**, *3*, 1–9.
28. Sygulla, K.S.; Fountaine, C.J. Acute post-activation potentiation in NCAA division II female athletes. *Int. J. Exer. Sci.* **2014**, *7*, 212–219.

29. Gullich, A.; Schmidtbleicher, D. MVC-induced short-term potentiation of explosive force. *New Stud. Athl.* **1996**, *11*, 67–81.
30. Harris, C.; Dolny, D.; Browder, K.; Adams, K.J.; DeBeliso, M. The effect of prior contractile activity on power output. *Med. Sci. Sports Exerc.* **2004**, *36*, S2379.
31. Harris, C.; Moore, J.; DeBeliso, M.; Adams, K.J.; Berning, J.; Hansen, C. The effects of heavy squats on potentiating 30 second Wingate test performance. *Med. Sci. Sports Exerc.* **2006**, *38*, S292. [CrossRef]
32. Mallander, S.; Berning, J.; Pederson, S.; Adams, K.J.; DeBeliso, M.; Stamford, B.; Maud, P. 5RM bench increases medicine ball put distance in trained males and females. *Med. Sci. Sports Exerc.* **2008**, *40*, S262. [CrossRef]
33. Berning, J.M.; Adams, K.J.; DeBeliso, M.; Sevene-Adams, P.G.; Harris, C.; Stamford, B.A. Effect of functional isometric squats on vertical jump in trained and untrained men. *J. Strength Cond. Res.* **2010**, *24*, 2285–2289. [CrossRef] [PubMed]
34. Harris, C.; Kipp, K.; Adams, K.J.; DeBeliso, M.; Berning, J.M. The effects of high intensity warm-up on shot put performance. *Med. Sci. Sports Exerc.* **2011**, *43*, S600. [CrossRef]
35. Dove, B.C.; Sevene, T.G.; Harris, C.; DeBeliso, M.; Adams, K.J.; Carson, C.A.; Berning, J.M. 5RM bench press increases medicine ball put distance in untrained males but not untrained females. *Med. Sci. Sports Exerc.* **2013**, *45*, S597.
36. Verderame, M. NFL Combine Drills Explained: Broad Jump. Available online: http://www.sbnation.com/nfl/2014/2/22/5406020/nfl-combine-2014-drills-broad-jump (accessed on 5 May 2016).

13

Differences in Spatial Physical Activity Patterns between Weekdays and Weekends in Primary School Children: A Cross-Sectional Study Using Accelerometry and Global Positioning System

Rahel Bürgi * and Eling D. de Bruin

Department of Health Sciences and Technology, Institute of Human Movement Sciences and Sport, ETH Zürich, Leopold-Ruzicka-Weg 4, Zurich 8093, Switzerland; eling.debruin@hest.ethz.ch

* Correspondence: rahel.buergi@hest.ethz.ch

Academic Editor: Michael Duncan

Abstract: Targeting the weekend to promote physical activity (PA) in children seems to be promising given that they tend to be less physically active and, particularly, as the age-related decline in PA is more marked during weekends. Considering the ambiguity of why children are not able to maintain their PA level on weekends, the aim of the present study was to objectively investigate differences in children's spatial PA patterns between week and weekend days using the combination of Global Positioning System (GPS) and accelerometry. Seventy-four second graders (aged 7–9 years) and 98 sixth graders (aged 11–14 years) wore an accelerometer and GPS sensor for seven consecutive days to determine where children spend time and engage in PA. Time-matched accelerometer and GPS data was mapped with a geographic information system and multilevel analyses accounting for the hierarchical structure of the data were conducted. Differences between weekdays and weekends regarding the total time spent and the absolute and relative level of PA in various settings were found in both age groups. The findings support previous research pointing to the importance of targeting weekend PA, especially when children grow older. Future interventions should encourage children to use outdoor spaces more frequently on weekends, rather than stay at home, and to commute actively to destinations other than school.

Keywords: physical activity; accelerometer; GPS; children; location; weekend; weekday

---

1. Introduction

Regular physical activity (PA) in children is associated with many physical and psychological health benefits, and there is a widespread belief that PA contributes to children's social development [1–3]. Evidence is present that PA performed during childhood may also contribute to an active lifestyle in adulthood [4,5]. Current international public health guidelines for children recommend at least one hour of moderate-vigorous PA (MVPA) per day [6]. However, only a small percentage of school-aged children achieve these recommendations [7,8]. In Switzerland, only one in five boys and just only one in ten girls aged 11 are adequately physically active according to these PA recommendations [8]. In light of this evidence, the promotion of an active and healthy lifestyle during childhood and adolescence should be an urgent public health priority.

In order to develop effective evidence-based public health interventions, it is essential to have a clear understanding of children's PA patterns and its influencing factors [9]. A large number of studies have been conducted in the last ten years to assess patterns and correlates of children's PA, in which gender, age, socioeconomic status, and parental and peer influences were among the most investigated correlates [10]. However, since previous studies mostly rely on subjective assessment methods that are subject to recall bias, knowledge on children's PA is still incomplete [11]. Using objective high-frequency accelerometry, which facilitates the analysis of temporal correlates, previous studies were able to find notable differences in PA level between weekdays and weekends [12–14]. Given that school-aged children generally accumulated more health-enhancing PA on weekdays than on weekends, Brooke and colleagues [12] pointed to the importance of targeting weekend PA for future interventions. Moreover, different studies showed that the well-investigated decline in MVPA across age groups between childhood and adolescence is more marked on weekends than weekdays [14–16], which also supports interventions focusing on PA maintenance on weekend days.

Although there is growing evidence about the discrepancy in PA level between weekdays and weekends, it is still unclear why children are not able to maintain their weekday PA level on weekends. It is suggested that the low accumulation of MVPA during weekends can partly be explained by the absence of the structured school environment, a greater television viewing time, or a more significant familial influence [17–19]. The longer sleep duration at weekends, which limits waking hours available for recreational pursuits and PA, may also be an influential factor [20]. To shed light on this issue, future studies encompassing multidimensional correlates have to investigate differences in activity patterns between weekdays and weekends in more detail [12,21].

Along with the increased use of ecological models in public health, also the environment in which PA takes place has become a stronger focus of attention [22]. Primarily, environmental interventions and changes are thought to have a high potential for sustained impact on populations, especially on those groups that are hard to reach with PA promotion programs [23]. A growing body of research emphasises that environmental factors may have a crucial influence on children's PA patterns [24], but this influence seems to be highly context-specific [25,26]. Therefore, to guide more targeted PA promotion programs, knowledge on differences in context-specific PA between weekdays and weekends may be a promising step.

Recent technological advances have led to the advent of Global Positioning System (GPS) in PA related studies [27,28]. The development of lightweight, accurate, and affordable GPS devices has opened up new possibilities to investigate how people move within their neighbourhood [27,29]. When combining these devices with accelerometers, objectively measured PA can be linked to the location in which the activity takes place, thereby providing a spatial context of PA. Given that the combination of GPS and accelerometry provides objective, reliable, and accurate measurements of context-specific PA [30,31], studies using this objective approach are increasing in numbers and new evidence about context-specific activity patterns is being generated. A review by McCrorie and colleagues [28], which summarises the current literature about using the combination of GPS and accelerometry in children and adolescents, has indicated that objectively measured environmental characteristics can significantly influence children's PA levels. Moreover, they showed that roads, school grounds, and the home environment are particularly important for both total PA and MVPA [28]. However, nearly none of the studies using GPS and accelerometry examined if there were any differences in the context-specific PA patterns between week and weekend days in primary school children. Klinker and colleagues [32] provided baseline results on both the use of different domains and the time spent in these domains separately for week and weekend days. However, neither did they conduct formal statistical tests of differences between weekdays and weekends nor did they investigate whether there are differences between these time segments relating to the accumulation of MVPA.

Using the combination of GPS and accelerometry, the aim of the current study therefore was to assess objectively the spatial PA patterns during weekdays and weekends in school-aged children living in an urban area in Switzerland. In particular, the goal was to investigate if there were any significant differences in context-specific PA between week and weekend days in both second- and sixth-grade children. In addition to existing literature, we aimed to consider not only the use of and total time spent in different settings, but also the time spent in health-enhancing MVPA. Given that reporting both relative and absolute amounts of PA can provide complementary information [12,33], we used the amount of MVPA in minutes as an absolute outcome and the proportion of MVPA in %

as a relative outcome to examine differences in the context-specific PA behaviour between week and weekend days.

2. Materials and Methods

2.1. Setting

To investigate spatial activity patterns of Swiss primary school children in relation to gender and socioeconomic differences, we previously conducted two cross-sectional studies in two different municipalities in the German-speaking part of Switzerland. During January and April 2013, a convenience sample of sixth-grade children participated in a first study carried out in Winterthur [33]. Winterthur is the sixth largest city in Switzerland, with a population of over 100,000 residents. One year later, between February and June 2014, a convenience sample of second-grade children participated in a second study conducted in the municipality of Zurich [34]. With a population of over 400,000 residents, Zurich is the largest city in Switzerland. Both cities represent an urban area, which is representative in relation to various demographic values (e.g., unemployment rate, foreign nationals, or social assistance rate) [35]. In both years, the same recruitment and data collection procedures were applied, which enabled us to aggregate the data for the current study to investigate differences in the spatial PA behaviour between week and weekend days in a sample of both second- and sixth-grade children.

2.2. Participant Recruitment

After approval of the school authorities, relevant teachers from public schools in one of the two municipalities were informed in cooperation with the local office of sports by an information letter. If a teacher agreed to take part, his class was visited by a trained study team consisting of the first author [RB] and a student research assistant during a lesson. The study team briefed the class about the study and provided all children with an information letter and an entry form for their parents. To be eligible to participate, children had to be free from any severe disability which prevented them from engaging in routine everyday PA. For every pupil in a participating class, the participation was voluntary and parental written informed consent was obtained. Ethical approval for both studies was obtained from the Ethics Committee of the ETH Zurich (EK 2012-N-62; EK 2013-N-66).

2.3. Data Collection and Measures

Data were collected in Winterthur during March and April 2013 and in Zurich during May and June 2014, respectively. It was ensured that all measurements took place within a regular school week without irregular days off from school or school excursions. One day before the start of the measurements, the study team visited the corresponding class again and fitted each registered child with an elastic belt equipped with a tri-axial accelerometer (GT3X, Actigraph, Pensacola, FL, USA) to measure PA and a GPS receiver (BT-Q1000XT, QStarz, Taipei, Taiwan) to record the geographical location (Circular Error Probability, CEP, (50%) < 3 m). Both devices offer accurate measures and are suitable for use in larger population studies with a data collection period of seven or more days [36,37]. The study team configured the devices for each child in advance setting them to record at ten second intervals with their internal clocks synchronized. This rather high sampling frequency was used to reflect children's PA pattern accurately, which is spontaneous and intermittent in its nature [38]. All children were given a detailed verbal and written instruction on belt wear which involved wearing the belt around the waist from waking to bedtime on seven consecutive days starting the next day. Due to the limited battery life of the GPS receiver, each child was provided with a charger and was instructed to recharge the receiver during each night when asleep. Children further received a small diary in which they had to report times they woke up and went to bed and times and reasons when the belt was not worn throughout the week. To obtain information on children's age, sex, home address, and sports club membership, a short parental questionnaire was handed out. The same instrument served to assess factors of children's individual socio-economic status (e.g., nationality, language spoken at home, parental education and income). In addition, height and weight were measured using a stadiometer (seca 213, Seca AG, Hamburg, Germany) and a digital scale (Beurer GS 12, Beurer GmbH, Ulm, Germany) with participants wearing light indoor clothing and shoes removed. Daily meteorological data, such as mean temperatures (in °C), sum of precipitation (in mm), and the sum of sunshine duration (in min), were provided by MeteoSwiss for each measurement week [39]. One day after the last day of measurements, children had to bring all instruments back to school, where they were collected by the study team. Figure 1 gives an overview on the data collection during the measurement week.

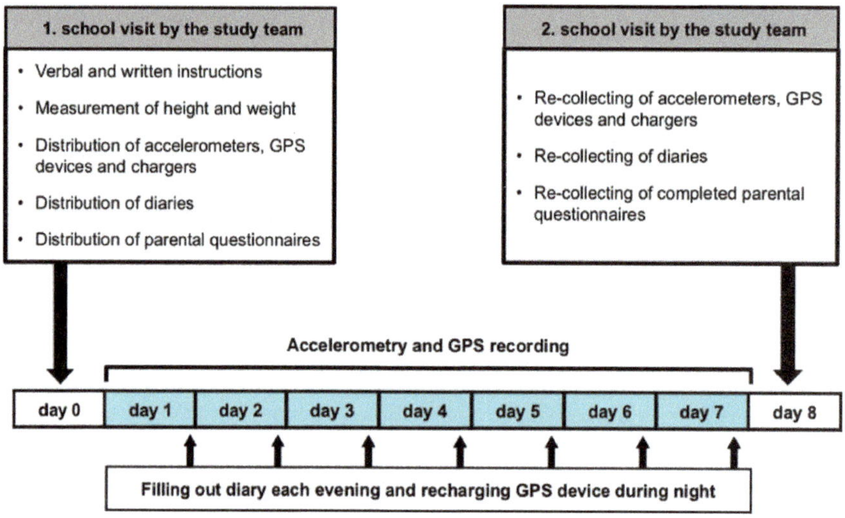

Figure 1. Overview on the data collection during the measurement week. GPS = global positioning system.

2.4. Data Merging and Processing

After manually reviewing each participant's GPS and accelerometer data file to ensure that they contained no incomplete or erroneous data, GPS and accelerometer data were matched by date and time. We used existing software (Actilife 6.5.2, Actigraph, Pensacola, FL, USA) for this process producing for each recorded GPS point a measure of activity and location. Only accelerometer data from the vertical axis was considered for further analysis since current accelerometer cut points for different activity levels are based on vertical axis counts. The processing of the matched data was performed using MATLAB R2012a (MathWorks, Natick, MA, USA) and R 3.1.2 (R Development Core Team, Vienna, Austria). Intervals with >60 min of consecutive zero activity counts were classified as non-wear time and excluded from analysis [40]. Activity records >5461 counts per 10 s were identified as outliers [41] and replaced with the mean of the previous and the following value. Based on age-appropriate cut-points [42,43], each data point was then classified as sedentary (<101 counts per minute (CPM)), light (101–2295 CPM), moderate (2296–4011 CPM) or vigorous (⩾4012 CPM) activity. To remove GPS outliers from the data, we processed the data by visual observation as well as automatic identification of invalid GPS data points using extreme changes in distance (>500 m per 10 s) and invalid values of altitude, which are not possible for the respective regions.

The location-based categorisation of the matched data points was conducted in ArcGIS 10 (ESRI, Redlands, CA, USA). Each participant's data points were imported into ArcGIS and plotted on their own point layer. We chose to define the seven activity settings presented in Figure 2 to assign each data point to a location. The settings used are based on similar studies in this field of research [44–46] and the ability to clearly assign each point to a location within ArcGIS. The assignment process was conducted in a hierarchical order using the point-in-polygon overlay, which is a spatial operation in ArcGIS. During this process described in Figure 2, each participant's data layer was overlaid on five different polygon layers to determine which data points are contained within which polygons. The creation of the five polygon layers was done using further geospatial data (land-use data, register data, points-of-interest, and satellite imagery) provided by the Land Surveying Office of Winterthur and the Office for Geomatics and Surveying of the City of Zurich and has been described elsewhere [33]. To take the GPS measurement error into account, a buffer zone of ten meters was drawn around the school, recreation, and street polygons [30,36,47].

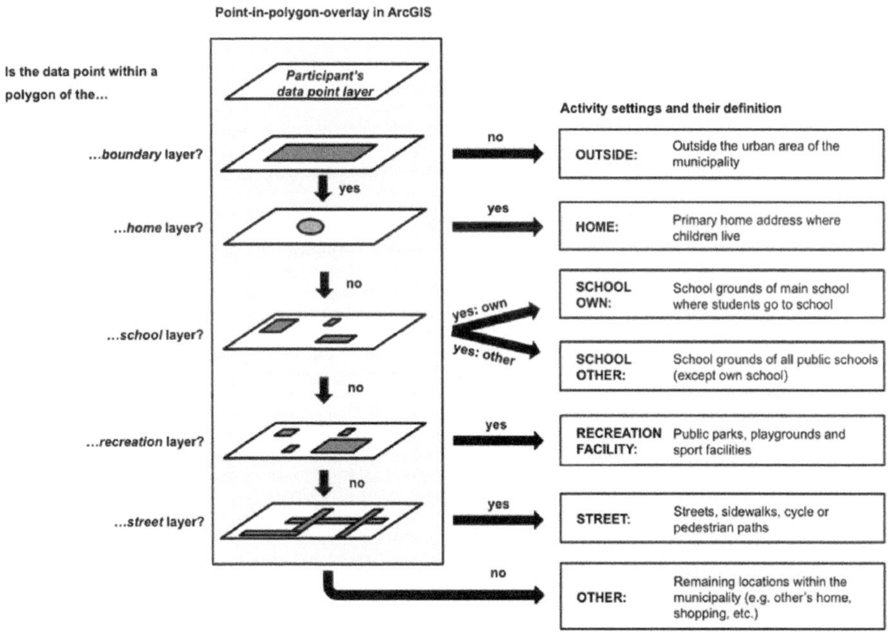

Figure 2. Definitions of activity settings and overview of the hierarchical assignment process in the geographic information system ArcGIS. The assignment process was conducted using the point-in-polygon-overlay, which is a spatial operation in ArcGIS. The creation of the five polygon layers *boundary, home, school, recreation,* and *street* was done using further geospatial data provided by the Land Surveying Office of Winterthur and the Office for Geomatics and Surveying of the City of Zurich.

2.5. Data Analysis

Children had to provide at least one weekday and one weekend day with four full hours of matched data to be included in the analysis [33]. To improve the data quality, we only considered matched wear time data on valid days from locations in which the participant spent ⩾2 min during this day.

Statistical analyses were performed using *R*. Descriptive statistics to calculate frequency distributions (number (*n*) and proportion (%)) for categorical data, mean and standard deviation (SD) for normally distributed variables, or median and interquartile ranges (IQR) for non-normally distributed data were used to describe the general characteristics of the two groups. Univariate analysis using χ^2-test, *t*-test, or Mann-Whitney-*U*-test was performed to test differences in general characteristics between age groups.

Differences in spatial PA patterns between week and weekend days within the two age groups were examined by using the total time spent in a setting and both an absolute (amount of MVPA in min) and relative (proportion of MVPA in %) outcome measure of MVPA, as this can provide complementary information. Mean daily minutes of total time and MVPA that a participant spent in each setting were calculated as outcomes separately for week and weekend days. From these values, we further calculated the proportion of time spent in MVPA out of the total time spent in each setting separately for weekdays and weekends based on children who visited the corresponding setting. As these variables were not normally distributed, median and IQR were used to present the outcome measures stratified by age group.

For the three outcomes and separated by age group, we conducted multilevel analyses based on individual scores across days and locations to provide results on differences between week and weekend days. Models were transformed by log transformation to fulfil the model assumptions and individuals and classes were included as random effects accounting for the hierarchical structure of the data [48]. To adjust for individual differences, sex, BMI, sports club membership, total matched wear time, weather conditions (mean temperature, sum of precipitation, and sum of sunshine duration), and socioeconomic characteristics (language spoken at home, highest parental education, parental income and nationality) were included as potential confounders, as these parameters may have an influence on children's activity patterns [49,50]. A backward elimination algorithm with Akaike's information criterion (AIC) as a goodness-of-fit measure was applied to test the contribution of the entered predictors and to determine the final models. For each model, we used a single-step method calculating interaction contrasts to investigate differences between week and weekend days across settings. Differences were provided by the transformed and adjusted *p*-values, which were calculated from F-tests based on Sattethwaite's or Kenward-Roger approximation.

3. Results

3.1. General Characteristics

A total of 86 second graders and 123 sixth graders out of 407 invited children provided consent and wore a measurement belt during one week. One second grader and two sixth graders returned a malfunctioning accelerometer, and one second grader lost both devices during the week. One further second grader had to be excluded due to illness which prevented him from engaging in routine everyday PA. Another 32 participants did not fulfil the inclusion criteria of at least one weekday and one weekend day with four full hours of matched data. Thus, the final study population consisted of 74 second and 98 sixth graders (Figure 3). Table 1 presents the general characteristics of the study population separated by age group. Participants wore the devices during a median time of 12.8 h per day at a median of seven days. During this time, valid GPS data was available for a median of 9.7 h per day, which is equal to a median of 77.2% of the total accelerometer wear time data. In total, children reached a median of five valid weekdays and two valid weekend days. The two age groups showed similar wear time characteristics and did not differ in relation to the available amount of daily combined data.

Table 1. General characteristics of the study population, stratified by age.

Characteristic	Second Graders	Sixth Graders	*p*-Value
Age in years, mean (SD)	8.5 (0.3)	12.5 (0.4)	**<0.001** **
Gender, boys, *n* (%)	38 (51.4)	45 (45.9)	0.480 *
Gender, girls, *n* (%)	36 (48.6)	53 (54.1)	–
Body height in cm, mean (SD)	133.4 (5.6)	154.7 (7.7) [1]	**<0.001** **
Body weight in kg, median (IQR)	28.4 (25.6–32.1)	44.2 (38.2–53.8) [1]	**<0.001** ***
BMI in kg/m^{-2}, median (IQR)	15.9 (15.1–17.5)	18.3 (16.5–20.7) [1]	**<0.001** ***
Daily wear time in min, median (IQR)	754.6 (702.6–799.5)	772.4 (727.1–810.4)	**0.029** ***
Daily combined data in min, median (IQR)	575.4 (493.4–621.6)	579.0 (498.6–659.7)	0.435 ***
Availability of GPS data in %, median (IQR)	76.8 (68.6–84.6)	78.1 (68.1–86.8)	0.569 ***
Wear days, median (IQR)	7.0 (7.0–7.0)	7.0 (7.0–7.0)	0.264 ***
Valid weekdays, median (IQR)	5.0 (5.0–5.0)	5.0 (4.0–5.0)	0.301 ***
Valid weekend days, median (IQR)	2.0 (2.0–2.0)	2.0 (2.0–2.0)	**0.031** ***

Bold: significant difference at $p < 0.05$; [1] Missing values from 5 participants; * χ^2-test; ** *t*-test; *** Mann-Whitney-*U*-test; SD = Standard Deviation; BMI = Body Mass Index; IQR = Interquartile Range.

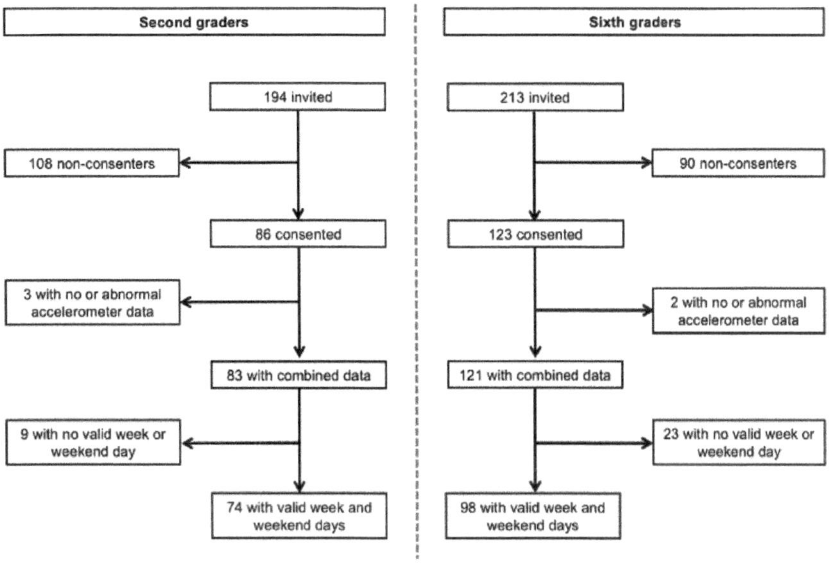

Figure 3. Study flow chart.

3.2. *Daily Minutes of Total Time Spent in Settings*

3.2.1. Second Graders

Table 2 provides results on the median time accumulated by the children in settings separately for weekdays and weekend days and stratified by age group. During weekdays, second graders accumulated most of their time at own school (42.4%), at home (22.5%), and on streets (14.9%), whereas home (35.2%), streets (19.2%), and other places (16.0%) were the most visited settings on weekend days (Table 2). Compared to the weekend, second-grade children recorded slightly more minutes of total matched wear time on regular school days (+42.9 min, $p = 0.047$). In nearly all settings, except for streets, we further found significant differences in daily minutes of total time between week and weekend days: While second graders spent significantly more time at both their own school and other schools on weekdays (+244.6 min, $p < 0.001$; resp. +19.6 min, $p = 0.02$), home (+38.3 min, $p < 0.001$), recreational facilities (+3.9 min, $p < 0.001$), other places (+7.4 min, $p = 0.032$), and the area outside their home city (+5.7 min, $p < 0.001$) were significantly more frequently used on weekends.

3.2.2. Sixth Graders

Consistent with children from second grade, own school (35.2%), home (35.2%), and streets (14.3%) were the most visited settings among sixth-grade children on weekdays, and home (54.5%), streets (17.2%), and other places (15.0%) on weekend days, respectively (Table 2). Furthermore, this age group also recorded significantly more minutes of total matched wear time on weekdays compared to weekend days (+75.6 min, $p = 0.003$). Within the different settings, sixth graders spent significantly more time on weekdays at their own school (+226.7 min, $p < 0.001$) and in recreational facilities (+2.9 min, $p = 0.022$), while significantly more time was accumulated at home (+76.8 min, $p < 0.001$) and in other places (+18.8 min, $p < 0.001$) on weekend days.

Table 2. Daily minutes of total time spent in settings, by weekday and weekend day, stratified by age.

Setting	Weekday			Weekend Day			*p*-Value *
	n	Median	IQR	*n*	Median	IQR	
Second Graders							
Total	74	597.2	540.2–668.0	74	554.3	464.2–604.2	**0.047**
Home	74	134.0	71.4–171.9	74	172.3	85.4–302.3	**<0.001**
Own school	74	244.6	204.7–285.0	74	0.0	0.0–0.0	**<0.001**
Other school	74	19.6	4.6–31.8	74	0.0	0.0–4.8	**0.020**
Recreation	74	14.5	3.4–37.1	74	18.4	0.0–71.8	**<0.001**
Street	74	83.6	63.1–116.3	74	92.4	60.4–137.1	0.234
Other	74	58.5	41.9–79.0	74	65.9	26.9–121.7	**0.032**
Outside	74	0.0	0.0–2.4	74	5.7	0.0–97.8	**<0.001**
Sixth Graders							
Total	98	610.6	551.2–695.9	98	535.0	479.0–622.6	**0.003**
Home	98	216.3	169.4–283.4	98	293.1	164.1–412.8	**<0.001**
Own school	98	226.7	152.9–283.1	98	0.0	0.0–0.0	**<0.001**
Other school	98	1.6	0.0–27.9	98	0.0	0.0–2.6	0.355
Recreation	98	2.9	0.0–18.2	98	0.0	0.0–7.1	**0.022**
Street	98	78.0	62.8–105.9	98	81.2	47.2–121.0	0.490
Other	98	51.5	37.2–82.0	98	70.3	40.1–99.2	**<0.001**
Outside	98	0.0	0.0–0.0	98	0.0	0.0–51.8	0.052

Bold: significant difference at $p < 0.05$; * *p*-values are calculated from F-test based on Sattethwaite's or Kenward-Roger approximation; IQR = Interquartile Range.

3.3. Daily Minutes of MVPA Spent in Settings

3.3.1. Second Graders

Table 3 provides results on the median daily minutes of MVPA spent in different settings separated for weekdays and weekend days. In total, second-grade children spent a median time of 68.9 min in MVPA on a regular school day, whereby most of their MVPA was accumulated at own school (40.0%), on streets (21.1%) and at home (13.3%). On weekend days, second graders accumulated a total median of 59.6 min in MVPA, whereof 21.4% was spent on streets, 21.3% at home and 17.8% in other places. Significantly more MVPA on weekdays was recorded at own school (+24.6 min, $p < 0.001$), at other school (+2.6 min, $p < 0.001$) and on streets (+2.7 min, $p < 0.001$), whereas on weekend days, a significantly greater amount of MVPA was accumulated at home (+3.1 min, $p < 0.001$), in recreational facilities (+0.1 min, $p < 0.001$) and outside the city (+0.1 min, $p < 0.001$).

Table 3. Daily minutes of MVPA in settings, by weekday and weekend day, stratified by age.

Setting	Weekday			Weekend Day			*p*-Value *
	n	Median	IQR	*n*	Median	IQR	
Second Graders							
Total	74	68.9	53.6–83.1	74	59.6	40.3–82.4	0.313
Home	74	7.7	4.4–12.3	74	10.8	4.2–21.8	**<0.001**
Own school	74	24.6	17.3–37.8	74	0.0	0.0–0.3	**<0.001**
Other school	74	2.6	0.8–5.0	74	0.0	0.0–0.5	**<0.001**
Recreation	74	2.5	0.6–7.4	74	2.6	0.0–13.3	**<0.001**
Street	74	13.6	9.6–18.7	74	10.9	3.7–18.3	**<0.001**
Other	74	6.1	3.4–9.4	74	7.5	1.9–15.8	0.573
Outside	74	0.0	0.0–0.1	74	0.1	0.0–11.5	**<0.001**
Sixth Graders							
Total	98	52.7	44.6–65.1	98	27.2	18.2–48.2	**<0.001**
Home	98	5.8	4.0–9.2	98	6.4	4.5–11.2	0.063
Own school	98	17.1	13.7–23.1	98	0.0	0.0–0.0	**<0.001**
Other school	98	0.3	0.0–5.2	98	0.0	0.0–0.1	0.482
Recreation	98	0.4	0.0–3.0	98	0.1	0.0–1.2	0.812
Street	98	16.4	12.2–23.3	98	8.3	2.4–16.0	**<0.001**
Other	98	4.1	2.2–5.8	98	3.5	1.6–6.5	0.977
Outside	98	0.0	0.0–0.0	98	0.0	0.0–1.5	0.825

Bold: significant difference at $p < 0.05$; * *p*-values are calculated from F-test based on Sattethwaite's or Kenward-Roger approximation; IQR = Interquartile Range; MVPA = Moderate to Vigorous Physical Activity.

3.3.2. Sixth Graders

Sixth graders accumulated the majority of their MVPA on weekdays at own school (33.9%), on streets (33.8%) and at home (11.9%), and during weekends on streets (32.0%), at home (22.4%) and in other places (16.6%), respectively (Table 3). Sixth-grade children achieved a significantly higher amount of MVPA on weekdays than they did on weekend days (+25.5 min, $p < 0.001$). Within settings, significant differences with children spending more minutes in MVPA during the school week than on weekend days were only found at own school (+17.1 min, $p < 0.001$) and on streets (+8.1 min, $p < 0.001$).

3.4. Proportion of Time Spent in MVPA in Settings

3.4.1. Second Graders

Table 4 provides results on the proportion of time spent in MVPA in total and across settings by week and weekend days. To indicate how many children visited the correspondent setting, the number of children (*n*) is presented. Overall, the second-grade children recorded 11.3% of their total time in MVPA on weekdays and 10.8% on weekend days, respectively ($p > 0.05$). On weekdays, the highest proportions of time spent in MVPA were observed on streets (17.6%), in recreational facilities (17.4%) and at other schools (17.2%), while on weekend days, children were most active at own school (39.4%), in recreational facilities (16.1%) and at other schools (12.6%). Significantly higher proportions on weekdays compared to weekend days were found at other schools (+4.6%, $p = 0.025$), on streets (+6.9%, $p < 0.001$) and in other places (+1.9%, $p = 0.043$). In contrast, own school was the only setting in which second-grade children recorded a considerably higher proportion of time spent in MVPA on weekend days (+29.4%, $p < 0.001$). Both on week and weekend days, the smallest proportion of time spent in MVPA was observed in the home environment (6.0% and 5.5%, respectively).

Table 4. Proportion of time spent in MVPA in settings based on children who visited the corresponding setting (*n*), by weekday and weekend day, stratified by age.

Setting	Weekday			Weekend Day			*p*-Value *
	n	Median	IQR	*n*	Median	IQR	
Second Graders							
Total	74	11.3	9.1–13.6	74	10.8	7.5–15.5	0.852
Home	74	6.0	4.7–9.1	69	5.5	4.1–8.8	0.438
Own school	74	10.0	8.2–13.2	19	39.4	17.6–48.3	**<0.001**
Other school	64	17.2	10.2–23.8	29	12.6	5.7–24.3	**0.025**
Recreation	67	17.4	9.3–27.7	56	16.1	7.2–27.0	0.272
Street	74	17.6	11.9–22.7	73	10.7	7.5–15.8	**<0.001**
Other	74	11.2	7.3–14.7	72	9.3	6.4–15.5	**0.043**
Outside	24	8.6	3.4–12.6	37	8.4	2.8–16.3	0.871
Sixth Graders							
Total	98	8.6	7.2–10.4	98	5.3	3.4–9.4	**<0.001**
Home	98	3.0	2.1–4.1	98	2.6	1.6–4.4	0.747
Own school	98	8.8	5.9–11.7	21	16.3	8.0–38.7	0.437
Other school	65	21.9	9.5–30.0	32	13.6	4.5–35.3	**<0.001**
Recreation	70	19.8	8.5–36.3	54	9.2	3.3–30.8	**0.003**
Street	98	20.5	14.0–28.9	97	9.7	3.4–16.6	**<0.001**
Other	98	7.4	4.8–10.1	96	5.1	2.6–8.8	**<0.001**
Outside	17	5.1	2.8–11.8	31	5.3	1.9–12.3	**0.035**

Bold: significant difference at $p < 0.05$; * *p*-values are calculated from F-test based on Sattethwaite's or Kenward-Roger approximation; IQR = Interquartile Range; MVPA = Moderate to Vigorous Physical Activity.

3.4.2. Sixth Graders

Among sixth graders, the proportion of time spent in MVPA on weekdays were largest at other school (21.9%), on streets (20.5%), and in recreational facilities (19.8%), whereas the highest relative activity level on weekend days was observed at own school (16.3%), at other school (13.6%), and on streets (9.7%). In contrast to second graders, sixth-grade children showed a significantly more active behaviour on weekdays compared to weekend days (+3.3%, $p < 0.001$). Accordingly, they recorded significantly higher MVPA-proportions on weekdays compared to weekends at other schools (+8.3%, $p < 0.001$), in recreational facilities (+10.6%, $p = 0.003$), on streets (+10.8%, $p < 0.001$), and in other places (+2.3%, $p < 0.001$). A significantly more active behaviour on weekend days was only found outside the city (+0.2%, $p < 0.035$). Consistent with second graders, the smallest proportion of time spent in MVPA on weekdays as well as on weekend days was found at home in this age group (3.0% and 2.6%, respectively).

4. Discussion

The aim of the present study was to investigate differences in the spatial PA patterns between weekdays and weekends in second and sixth-grade children living in two urban areas in Switzerland. In both age groups, we found several differences between week and weekend days in relation to the total time spent as well as to the absolute and relative level of PA in total and within various settings. While second graders did not show a significant difference in their absolute or relative PA level between week and weekend days over all settings, sixth-grade children were significantly less active on weekend days. On weekdays, the school environment was the most frequently used setting in which both age groups accumulated more than one third of their total MVPA. Although significantly less time was spent at their own school on weekend days, the proportion of time spent in MVPA was much higher during this time of the week compared to school days, especially among second-grade children. In contrast, second and sixth graders spent most of their weekend time at home where they engaged in significantly more MVPA on weekend days compared to weekdays. Nevertheless, the proportion of time spent in MVPA at home did not differ significantly between time segments and was generally low in both age groups. Furthermore, we found a significantly higher PA level in the street environment on weekdays compared to weekend days in both age groups, although second and sixth graders spent a similar amount of time there on week and weekend days.

4.1. Differences in General Physical Activity Patterns between Weekdays and Weekends

Both second and sixth graders recorded significantly more minutes of matched wear time data on weekdays compared to weekend days. However, while sixth-grade children also engaged in significantly more MVPA and showed a higher proportion of time spent in MVPA during the school week compared to weekend days, second graders did not show a significant difference between time segments in relation to their absolute or relative PA level over all settings. A study by Trost and colleagues showed that younger children exhibited higher levels of PA on weekends, whereas older children and adolescents were more active on weekdays relative to weekends [51]. This is somewhat consistent with the findings in the present study. Moreover, previous studies further reported that the decline in MVPA with age is consistently higher on weekends than on weekdays [14,16]. Although we did not statistically prove differences between age groups, this finding is approximately congruent with our study results: second graders were engaging in more MVPA than sixth graders on both week and weekend days, whereby this difference was particularly accentuated on weekend days. Thus, in line with previous research [12], our findings support the promotion of weekend PA, especially when children grow older.

4.2. Differences in Context-Specific Physical Activity Patterns between Weekdays and Weekends

When focusing on the various settings, the school environment was the most used setting on weekdays in both age groups and therefore significantly more time in MVPA was then accumulated within this setting compared to weekend days. This finding is in line with other studies which already reported that children spent the majority of time on weekdays at school and that this environment is an important setting regarding the daily accumulation of MVPA [32,47,52]. However, only a few studies at present have investigated how this environment is used by children outside scheduled school hours during weekdays and, especially, during weekend days. Klinker and colleagues [32] found that school grounds are important places to spend time on weekdays during after school hours but less so on weekend days. Only 34.5% of the participants used a school ground during weekends and the median time they spent at school was zero minutes [32]. In the present study, slightly more children (47.3% second graders and 43.9% sixth graders, respectively) used either the school grounds of their own school or those of another school on a weekend day, but the median time spent in both settings was also zero minutes among all participants. Despite this low use of school grounds during weekends, the high MVPA-proportion recorded by children who spent time there during this time segment may still indicate the potential importance of the school setting as an activity-promoting environment. Accordingly, both age groups also recorded noticeably high MVPA-proportions when spending time at other schools. These results confirm a previous study that indicated that an open and unrestricted access to school grounds during leisure time for organized sports and unstructured play is an urgent need [32]. However, further studies should gain more knowledge on what children are doing when staying on school grounds. It can be hypothesized that one reason for the high relative PA level is that the school infrastructure is often used for organized PA in the context of sports clubs as well as voluntary sports at school. To conclude, findings in the present study potentially suggest that targeting a broader use of school grounds during non-school hours on week and weekend days for both organized and unstructured PA could be a promising avenue for future interventions.

The home environment was the only setting in which children from both age groups accumulated significantly more time in MVPA on weekend days compared to weekdays or showed a trend to do so. The higher absolute amount of MVPA recorded on weekend days can mostly be attributed to the more frequent use of this setting during this part of the week. It is hardly surprising that children are spending more time at home when the structured school routine is absent, which probably leads to more opportunities to accumulate health-enhancing PA in this setting. However, when considering the relative MVPA outcome, a similar and particularly small MVPA-proportion was recorded at home on week and weekend days and across both age groups. This finding supports previous research that identified home as an environment in which children are less active than when they are out of it [53,54]. The increasing range of screen-based technologies has led to a higher engagement in sedentary activities such as TV viewing, playing computer games, or surfing the internet and may attract children to stay at home rather than using outdoor spaces which are more conducive for PA [53–55]. Therefore, interventions which encourage children to go out more for walking and playing outdoors, especially on weekends when they have a greater choice in how they spend their time, would be an important approach to promote PA among primary school children, particularly the older ones.

Although both age groups spent a similar amount of time during week and weekend days on streets, they showed a significantly higher absolute and relative level of PA in this setting on weekdays compared to weekend days. This different behaviour in the street environment can partly be explained by the absence of ways to and from schools during non-school days. Previous studies showed the significant contribution of the journey to school to total PA [46,56,57] and that children who walk or cycle to school have a greater overall PA level than those who are driven to school or take public transportation [58]. Furthermore, given that peer support is particularly relevant on school days [59], children probably are more likely to use the street environment for informal PA with their friends such as playing tag, skipping, or ball games on weekdays than on weekend days. In contrast, the higher time spent in motorised transport may be a reason for the more sedentary behaviour within this setting during non-school days [60]. Accordingly, the promotion of active commuting to other destinations than school could contribute toward achieving higher PA levels [61], which would be of particular value for weekend days in both age groups. To reach this goal, safe residential streets and neighbourhoods are required, especially as the lack of perceived neighbourhood safety seems to be associated with lower levels of active transport [62,63].

Other places were significantly more visited by both age groups on weekend days than on weekdays, which is obvious when time-consuming school-related activities are absent. However, second as well as sixth graders showed a significantly higher relative PA level when visiting this setting during school days. Similar to the street environment, the more pronounced peer influence during weekdays may be responsible for this difference [59]. It can be hypothesized that during weekdays, other places such as the near neighbourhood, private gardens, or other's home are rather visited in the company of peers or close friends engaging in active free-play. Appropriately, different studies could show that presence of peers and friends is associated with higher activity levels [64,65]. In contrast, during weekend days, children are more likely to use this setting together with family members engaging in more sedentary activities. Dunton and colleagues [66] found that although most of the parent-child pairs performed some joint MVPA, the duration of these activities was short. Moreover, this low activity behaviour was particularly accentuated in parents with older children as they spent more time in sedentary activities and less time in PA together [66]. The same authors therefore concluded that the promotion of joint parent-child PA in families with older children may be a promising method to combat the age-related decline in PA [66]. In accordance with this conclusion, our results further indicate that the promotion of joint parent-child PA would predominantly be useful during weekend days.

The use of recreational facilities such as parks, playgrounds, and sport facilities was generally low during week and weekend days and among both age groups. This result is in line with previous research reporting that the use of green space as an absolute measure of time is low [28,46]. In addition to other studies, we could further observe a tendency that second graders compared to sixth graders spent more time in recreational facilities, which was particularly true for weekend days. Second-grade children further achieved significantly more minutes of MVPA on weekend days compared to weekdays in this setting, while sixth graders were significantly less active in parks and sport facilities during weekends. In line with a recent study reporting that open spaces and parks offer a common setting for joint parent-child PA [67], we can consider that second-grade children rather tended to visit parks and sport facilities accompanied by their parents and were engaging together in PA. Furthermore, the sixth graders' low use of parks and sport facilities can partly be explained by the fact that this setting is more likely to be visited in summer months than during winter and early spring, which is when the study of the sixth graders was conducted [44]. Nevertheless, the high proportion of time spent in MVPA recorded in both age groups confirms previous research that already established that green space is highly conducive for PA even though rarely visited [28,46]. Therefore, future interventions should target the more frequent use of recreational facilities, especially in older children and during weekend days. This also includes the promotion of organized PA in the context of sports clubs or commercial sports providers as the benefits of structured activities have been well proven and joining organized sports during childhood appears to increase the chance for an active lifestyle in young adulthood [68,69].

4.3. Limitations

The present study has several limitations. We assessed the PA patterns of a convenience sample of second and sixth graders from two urban regions and surveyed them during early spring and in summer months, respectively. Therefore, findings are not generalizable to other populations and seasons. Given that the participation was voluntary for every pupil in a participating class, we cannot exclude certain effects due to selection bias. As both the city and season differed between second and sixth graders for administrative reasons, we decided not to investigate differences between age groups, although this comparison would represent an important issue and should be considered in future research. The combination of accelerometry and GPS is a promising method to gain further insights in children's PA patterns and studies using this approach are increasing in number. However, the use of GPS and accelerometry is associated with several problems. The accuracy of the GPS signal varies with the environment. Urban canyons, vegetative cover, or indoors within structures impermeable to satellite signals are associated with inaccurate and missing GPS positions and therefore can lead to misclassification errors and under- or overrepresentations of certain settings [45]. Although we did not impute missing data, we tried to reduce issues with spatial inaccuracy by identifying invalid GPS points and choosing buffer zones around polygons. However, misclassification bias remains possible. Moreover, accelerometer-based measurements of PA also have limitations, predominantly consisting of the inability to assess activities accurately in which the body's centre of gravity is relatively fixed such as cycling [70], the absence of a universal consensus on processing methods and accelerometer cut points for determining MVPA [71], and reactivity issues [72]. The inclusion criterion of at least one valid week and weekend day of four full hours of combined data was chosen to maximize data retention for analysis. This criterion is rather low in comparison with other studies [32,41], and might limit the reliability of the presented results. However, with a daily median of more than nine hours of combined data in both age groups, we still reached a satisfying amount of data that enabled us to conduct a full day pattern analysis.

5. Conclusions

To the best of our knowledge this is the first study which objectively assessed by means of accelerometry and GPS and by using both an absolute and relative outcome measure of MVPA the spatial PA behaviour in primary school children and investigated whether there are differences between week and weekend days in two different age groups. In both second and sixth-grade students we could find several differences in the spatial PA patterns between week and weekend days. These differences emphasise the need of targeting weekend PA for future interventions, especially when children grow older. Future interventions should encourage children to use outdoor spaces, such as parks and sport facilities, more frequently on weekends rather than stay at home and should also encourage children to commute actively on weekend days in the absence of the daily journey to school. Further studies need to confirm whether the present findings also apply in rural and suburban populations and in different seasons of the year. Furthermore, future cross-sectional and longitudinal studies should investigate age differences in the spatial PA behaviour between week and weekend days to shed light on the age-related decline in PA when children grow older.

Acknowledgments: The authors would like to thank all the school children and their parents, as well as all teachers, for their participation in the study. We would also like to thank everyone who helped with the recruitment of teachers and the data collection. Moreover, we would like to acknowledge the Land Surveying Office of Winterthur and the Office for Geomatics and Surveying of the City of Zurich for providing the geospatial data. Thanks also to H.P. Stamm for proofreading the manuscript and providing valuable inputs.

Author Contributions: R.B. and E.D.B. conceived and designed the experiments; R.B. performed the experiments; R.B. and E.D.B. analysed the data; R.B. and E.D.B. wrote the paper. All authors have read and approved the final manuscript.

Conflicts of Interest: The authors declare no conflict of interest.

References

1. Andersen, L.B.; Riddoch, C.; Kriemler, S.; Hills, A. Physical activity and cardiovascular risk factors in children. *Br. J. Sports Med.* **2011**, *45*, 871–876. [CrossRef] [PubMed]
2. Biddle, S.J.; Asare, M. Physical activity and mental health in children and adolescents: A review of reviews. *Br. J. Sports Med.* **2011**, *45*, 886–895. [CrossRef] [PubMed]
3. Janssen, I.; LeBlanc, A.G. Systematic review of the health benefits of physical activity and fitness in school-aged children and youth. *Int. J. Behav. Nutr. Phys. Act.* **2010**, *7*. [CrossRef] [PubMed]
4. Kjonniksen, L.; Torsheim, T.; Wold, B. Tracking of leisure-time physical activity during adolescence and young adulthood: A 10-year longitudinal study. *Int. J. Behav. Nutr. Phys. Act.* **2008**, *5*. [CrossRef] [PubMed]
5. Hallal, P.C.; Victora, C.G.; Azevedo, M.R.; Wells, J.C. Adolescent physical activity and health: A systematic review. *Sports Med.* **2006**, *36*, 1019–1030. [CrossRef] [PubMed]
6. World Health Organization. *Global Recommendations on Physical Activity for Health*; World Health Organization Press: Geneva, Switzerland, 2010.

7. Verloigne, M.; Van Lippevelde, W.; Maes, L.; Yildirim, M.; Chinapaw, M.; Manios, Y.; Androutsos, O.; Kovacs, E.; Bringolf-Isler, B.; Brug, J.; et al. Levels of physical activity and sedentary time among 10- to 12-year-old boys and girls across 5 European countries using accelerometers: An observational study within the ENERGY-project. *Int. J. Behav. Nutr. Phys. Act.* **2012**, *9*. [CrossRef] [PubMed]
8. Currie, C.; Zanotti, C.; Morgan, A.; Currie, D.; de Looze, M.; Roberts, C.; Samdal, O.; Smith, O.; Barnekow, V. *Social Determinants of Health and Well-Being Among Young People*; Health Behaviour in School-aged Children (HBSC) study: International report from the 2009/2010 survey; WHO Regional Office for Europe: Copenhagen, Danmark, 2012.
9. Sallis, J.F.; Owen, N.; Fotheringham, M.J. Behavioral epidemiology: A systematic framework to classify phases of research on health promotion and disease prevention. *Ann. Behav. Med.* **2000**, *22*, 294–298. [CrossRef] [PubMed]
10. Craggs, C.; Corder, K.; van Sluijs, E.M.; Griffin, S.J. Determinants of change in physical activity in children and adolescents: A systematic review. *Am. J. Prev. Med.* **2011**, *40*, 645–658. [CrossRef] [PubMed]
11. Ekelund, U.; Tomkinson, G.R.; Armstrong, N. What proportion of youth are physically active? Measurement issues, levels and recent time trends. *Br. J. Sports Med.* **2011**, *45*, 859–865. [CrossRef] [PubMed]
12. Brooke, H.L.; Corder, K.; Atkin, A.J.; van Sluijs, E.M. A systematic literature review with meta-analyses of within- and between-day differences in objectively measured physical activity in school-aged children. *Sports Med.* **2014**, *44*, 1427–1438. [CrossRef] [PubMed]
13. Moses, S.; Meyer, U.; Puder, J.; Roth, R.; Zahner, L.; Kriemler, S. Das Bewegungsverhalten von Primarschulkindern in der Schweiz. *Schweiz. Z. Sportmed. Sporttraumatol.* **2007**, *55*, 62–68.
14. Nader, P.R.; Bradley, R.H.; Houts, R.M.; McRitchie, S.L.; O'Brien, M. Moderate-to-vigorous physical activity from ages 9 to 15 years. *JAMA* **2008**, *300*, 295–305. [CrossRef] [PubMed]
15. Wong, S.L.; Colley, R.; Connor Gorber, S.; Tremblay, M. Actical accelerometer sedentary activity thresholds for adults. *J. Phys. Act. Health* **2011**, *8*, 587–591. [PubMed]
16. Brooke, H.L.; Atkin, A.J.; Corder, K.; Ekelund, U.; van Sluijs, E.M. Changes in time-segment specific physical activity between ages 10 and 14 years: A longitudinal observational study. *J. Sci. Med. Sport Sports Med. Aust.* **2016**, *19*, 29–34. [CrossRef] [PubMed]
17. Treuth, M.S.; Catellier, D.J.; Schmitz, K.H.; Pate, R.R.; Elder, J.P.; McMurray, R.G.; Blew, R.M.; Yang, S.; Webber, L. Weekend and weekday patterns of physical activity in overweight and normal-weight adolescent girls. *Obesity (Silver Spring)* **2007**, *15*, 1782–1788. [CrossRef] [PubMed]
18. Fairclough, S.J.; Ridgers, N.D.; Welk, G. Correlates of children's moderate and vigorous physical activity during weekdays and weekends. *J. Phys. Act. Health* **2012**, *9*, 129–137. [PubMed]
19. McMinn, A.M.; Griffin, S.J.; Jones, A.P.; van Sluijs, E.M. Family and home influences on children's after-school and weekend physical activity. *Eur. J. Public Health* **2013**, *23*, 805–810. [CrossRef] [PubMed]
20. Thorleifsdottir, B.; Bjornsson, J.K.; Benediktsdottir, B.; Gislason, T.; Kristbjarnarson, H. Sleep and sleep habits from childhood to young adulthood over a 10-year period. *J. Psychosom. Res.* **2002**, *53*, 529–537. [CrossRef]
21. Fairclough, S.J.; Boddy, L.M.; Mackintosh, K.A.; Valencia-Peris, A.; Ramirez-Rico, E. Weekday and weekend sedentary time and physical activity in differentially active children. *J. Sci. Med. Sport Sports Med. Aust.* **2015**, *18*, 444–449. [CrossRef] [PubMed]
22. Bauman, A.E.; Reis, R.S.; Sallis, J.F.; Wells, J.C.; Loos, R.J.F.; Martin, B.W. Correlates of physical activity: Why are some people physically active and others not? *Lancet* **2012**, *380*, 258–271. [CrossRef]
23. Giles-Corti, B.; Timperio, A.; Bull, F.; Pikora, T. Understanding physical activity environmental correlates: Increased specificity for ecological models. *Exerc. Sport Sci. Rev.* **2005**, *33*, 175–181. [CrossRef] [PubMed]
24. Ding, D.; Sallis, J.F.; Kerr, J.; Lee, S.; Rosenberg, D.E. Neighborhood environment and physical activity among youth a review. *Am. J. Prev. Med.* **2011**, *41*, 442–455. [CrossRef] [PubMed]
25. Klinker, C.D.; Schipperijn, J.; Kerr, J.; Ersboll, A.K.; Troelsen, J. Context-specific outdoor time and physical activity among school-children across gender and age: Using accelerometers and GPS to advance methods. *Front. Public Health* **2014**, *2*. [CrossRef] [PubMed]
26. Ferreira, I.; van der Horst, K.; Wendel-Vos, W.; Kremers, S.; van Lenthe, F.J.; Brug, J. Environmental correlates of physical activity in youth—A review and update. *Obes. Rev.* **2007**, *8*, 129–154. [CrossRef] [PubMed]
27. Jankowska, M.M.; Schipperijn, J.; Kerr, J. A framework for using GPS data in physical activity and sedentary behavior studies. *Exerc. Sport Sci. Rev.* **2015**, *43*, 48–56. [CrossRef] [PubMed]

28. McCrorie, P.R.W.; Fenton, C.; Ellaway, A. Combining GPS, GIS, and accelerometry to explore the physical activity and environment relationship in children and young people—A review. *Int. J. Behav. Nutr. Phys. Act.* **2014**, *11*. [CrossRef] [PubMed]
29. Maas, J.; Sterkenburg, R.P.; de Vries, S.I.; Pierik, F. Using GPS to measure the interaction between individuals and their neighbourhood. In *Neighbourhood Structure and Health Promotion*; Stock, C., Ellaway, A., Eds.; Springer US: Boston, MA, USA, 2013; pp. 153–175.
30. Kerr, J.; Duncan, S.; Schipperjin, J. Using global positioning systems in health research: A practical approach to data collection and processing. *Am. J. Prev. Med.* **2011**, *41*, 532–540. [CrossRef] [PubMed]
31. Rodriguez, D.A.; Brown, A.L.; Troped, P.J. Portable global positioning units to complement accelerometry-based physical activity monitors. *Med. Sci. Sport Exerc.* **2005**, *37*, 572–581. [CrossRef]
32. Klinker, C.D.; Schipperijn, J.; Toftager, M.; Kerr, J.; Troelsen, J. When cities move children: Development of a new methodology to assess context-specific physical activity behaviour among children and adolescents using accelerometers and GPS. *Health Place* **2015**, *31*, 90–99. [CrossRef] [PubMed]
33. Bürgi, R.; Tomatis, L.; Murer, K.; de Bruin, E.D. Localization of physical activity in primary school children using accelerometry and global positioning system. *PLoS ONE* **2015**, *10*, e0142223. [CrossRef] [PubMed]
34. Bürgi, R.; Tomatis, L.; Murer, K.; de Bruin, E.D. Spatial physical activity patterns among primary school children living in neighbourhoods of varying socioeconomic status: A cross-sectional study using accelerometry and Global Positioning System. *BMC Public Health* **2016**, *16*. [CrossRef] [PubMed]
35. Statistik Schweiz. *Statistisches Lexikon der Schweiz*. Available online: http://www.bfs.admin.ch/bfs/portal/de/index/infothek/lexikon.html (accessed on 3 October 2012).
36. Schipperijn, J.; Kerr, J.; Duncan, S.; Madsen, T.; Klinker, C.D.; Troelsen, J. Dynamic accuracy of GPS receivers for use in health research: A novel method to assess GPS accuracy in real-world settings. *Front. Public Health* **2014**, *2*. [CrossRef] [PubMed]
37. Freedson, P.S.; Melanson, E.; Sirard, J. Calibration of the Computer Science and Applications, Inc. accelerometer. *Med. Sci. Sports Exerc.* **1998**, *30*, 777–781. [CrossRef] [PubMed]
38. Nilsson, A.; Ekelund, U.; Yngve, A.; Sjöström, M. Assessing physical activity among children with accelerometers using different time sampling intervals and placements. *Pediatr. Exerc. Sci.* **2002**, *14*, 87–96.
39. Federal Office of Meteorology and Climatology. *MeteoSwiss*. Available online: http://www.meteoschweiz.admin.ch (accessed on 14 July 2014).
40. Troiano, R.P.; Berrigan, D.; Dodd, K.W.; Masse, L.C.; Tilert, T.; McDowell, M. Physical activity in the United States measured by accelerometer. *Med. Sci. Sport Exerc.* **2008**, *40*, 181–188. [CrossRef] [PubMed]
41. Almanza, E.; Jerrett, M.; Dunton, G.; Seto, E.; Pentz, M.A. A study of community design, greenness, and physical activity in children using satellite, GPS and accelerometer data. *Health Place* **2012**, *18*, 46–54. [CrossRef] [PubMed]
42. Evenson, K.R.; Catellier, D.J.; Gill, K.; Ondrak, K.S.; McMurray, R.G. Calibration of two objective measures of physical activity for children. *J. Sports Sci.* **2008**, *26*, 1557–1565. [CrossRef] [PubMed]
43. Trost, S.; Loprinzi, P.; Moore, R.; Pfeiffer, K. Comparison of accelerometer cut points for predicting activity intensity in youth. *Med. Sci. Sport Exerc.* **2011**, *43*, 1360–1368. [CrossRef] [PubMed]
44. Oreskovic, N.M.; Blossom, J.; Field, A.E.; Chiang, S.R.; Winickoff, J.P.; Kleinman, R.E. Combining global positioning system and accelerometer data to determine the locations of physical activity in children. *Geospat. Health* **2012**, *6*, 263–272. [CrossRef] [PubMed]
45. Rainham, D.G.; Bates, C.J.; Blanchard, C.M.; Dummer, T.J.; Kirk, S.F.; Shearer, C.L. Spatial classification of youth physical activity patterns. *Am. J. Prev. Med.* **2012**, *42*, e87–e96. [CrossRef] [PubMed]
46. Klinker, C.D.; Schipperijn, J.; Christian, H.; Kerr, J.; Ersboll, A.K.; Troelsen, J. Using accelerometers and global positioning system devices to assess gender and age differences in children's school, transport, leisure and home based physical activity. *Int. J. Behav. Nutr. Phys. Act.* **2014**, *11*. [CrossRef] [PubMed]
47. Dessing, D.; Pierik, F.H.; Sterkenburg, R.P.; van Dommelen, P.; Maas, J.; de Vries, S.I. Schoolyard physical activity of 6–11 year old children assessed by GPS and accelerometry. *Int. J. Behav. Nutr. Phys. Act.* **2013**, *10*. [CrossRef] [PubMed]
48. Cerin, E. Statistical approaches to testing the relationships of the built environment with resident-level physical activity behavior and health outcomes in cross-sectional studies with cluster sampling. *J. Plan. Lit.* **2011**, *26*, 151–167. [CrossRef]

49. Lamprecht, M.; Fischer, A.; Wiegand, D.; Stamm, H.P. *Sport Schweiz 2014: Kinder-und Jugendbericht*; Bundesamt für Sport BASPO: Magglingen, Switzerland, 2015.
50. Duncan, J.S.; Hopkins, W.G.; Schofield, G.; Duncan, E.K. Effects of weather on pedometer-determined physical activity in children. *Med. Sci. Sports Exerc.* **2008**, *40*, 1432–1438. [CrossRef] [PubMed]
51. Trost, S.G.; Pate, R.R.; Freedson, P.S.; Sallis, J.F.; Taylor, W.C. Using objective physical activity measures with youth: How many days of monitoring are needed? *Med. Sci. Sports Exerc.* **2000**, *32*, 426–431. [CrossRef] [PubMed]
52. Maddison, R.; Jiang, Y.; Vander Hoorn, S.; Exeter, D.; Mhurchu, C.N.; Dorey, E. Describing patterns of physical activity in adolescents using global positioning systems and accelerometry. *Pediatr. Exerc. Sci.* **2010**, *22*, 392–407. [PubMed]
53. Kneeshaw-Price, S.; Saelens, B.E.; Sallis, J.F.; Glanz, K.; Frank, L.D.; Kerr, J.; Hannon, P.A.; Grembowski, D.E.; Chan, K.C.; Cain, K.L. Children's objective physical activity by location: Why the neighborhood matters. *Pediatr. Exerc. Sci.* **2013**, *25*, 468–486. [PubMed]
54. Mackett, R.L.; Paskins, J. Children's physical activity: The contribution of playing and walking. *Child. Soc.* **2008**, *22*, 345–357. [CrossRef]
55. Oreskovic, N.M.; Perrin, J.M.; Robinson, A.I.; Locascio, J.J.; Blossom, J.; Chen, M.L.; Winickoff, J.P.; Field, A.E.; Green, C.; Goodman, E. Adolescents' use of the built environment for physical activity. *BMC Public Health* **2015**, *15*, 251. [CrossRef] [PubMed]
56. Southward, E.F.; Page, A.S.; Wheeler, B.W.; Cooper, A.R. Contribution of the school journey to daily physical activity in children aged 11–12 years. *Am. J. Prev. Med.* **2012**, *43*, 201–204. [CrossRef] [PubMed]
57. Van Sluijs, E.M.; Fearne, V.A.; Mattocks, C.; Riddoch, C.; Griffin, S.J.; Ness, A. The contribution of active travel to children's physical activity levels: Cross-sectional results from the ALSPAC study. *Prev. Med.* **2009**, *48*, 519–524. [CrossRef] [PubMed]
58. Davison, K.K.; Werder, J.L.; Lawson, C.T. Children's active commuting to school: Current knowledge and future directions. *Prev. Chronic Dis.* **2008**, *5*, A100. [PubMed]
59. Corder, K.; Craggs, C.; Jones, A.P.; Ekelund, U.; Griffin, S.J.; van Sluijs, E.M. Predictors of change differ for moderate and vigorous intensity physical activity and for weekdays and weekends: A longitudinal analysis. *Int. J. Behav. Nutr. Phys. Act.* **2013**, *10*. [CrossRef] [PubMed]
60. Biddle, S.J.; Gorely, T.; Marshall, S.J.; Cameron, N. The prevalence of sedentary behavior and physical activity in leisure time: A study of Scottish adolescents using ecological momentary assessment. *Prev. Med.* **2009**, *48*, 151–155. [CrossRef] [PubMed]
61. Smith, L.; Sahlqvist, S.; Ogilvie, D.; Jones, A.; Griffin, S.J.; van Sluijs, E. Is active travel to non-school destinations associated with physical activity in primary school children? *Prev. Med.* **2012**, *54*, 224–228. [CrossRef] [PubMed]
62. Jones, A.P.; Coombes, E.G.; Griffin, S.J.; van Sluijs, E.M.F. Environmental supportiveness for physical activity in English schoolchildren: A study using Global Positioning Systems. *Int. J. Behav. Nutr. Phys. Act.* **2009**, *6*. [CrossRef] [PubMed]
63. Carver, A.; Timperio, A.; Crawford, D. Playing it safe: The influence of neighbourhood safety on children's physical activity. A review. *Health Place* **2008**, *14*, 217–227. [CrossRef] [PubMed]
64. Salvy, S.J.; Bowker, J.W.; Roemmich, J.N.; Romero, N.; Kieffer, E.; Paluch, R.; Epstein, L.H. Peer influence on children's physical activity: An experience sampling study. *J. Pediatr. Psychol.* **2008**, *33*, 39–49. [CrossRef] [PubMed]
65. Sallis, J.F.; Taylor, W.C.; Dowda, M.; Freedson, P.S.; Pate, R.R. Correlates of vigorous physical activity for children in grades 1 through 12: Comparing parent-reported and objectively measured physical activity. *Pediatr. Exerc. Sci.* **2002**, *14*, 30–44.
66. Dunton, G.F.; Liao, Y.; Almanza, E.; Jerrett, M.; Spruijt-Metz, D.; Chou, C.P.; Pentz, M.A. Joint physical activity and sedentary behavior in parent-child pairs. *Med. Sci. Sports Exerc.* **2012**, *44*, 1473–1480. [CrossRef] [PubMed]
67. Dunton, G.; Liao, Y.; Almanza, E.; Jerrett, M.; Spruijt-Metz, D.; Pentz, M. Locations of joint physical activity in parent–child pairs based on accelerometer and GPS monitoring. *Ann. Behav. Med.* **2013**, *45*, 162–172. [CrossRef] [PubMed]
68. Fletcher, A.C.; Nickerson, P.; Wright, K.L. Structured leisure activities in middle childhood: Links to well-being. *J. Commun. Psychol.* **2003**, *31*, 641–659. [CrossRef]

69. Kjonniksen, L.; Anderssen, N.; Wold, B. Organized youth sport as a predictor of physical activity in adulthood. *Scand. J. Med. Sci. Sports* **2009**, *19*, 646–654. [CrossRef] [PubMed]
70. Welk, G.J. Use of accelerometry-based activity monitors to assess physical activity. In *Physical Activity Assessments for Health-Related Research*; Welk, G.J., Ed.; Human Kinetics: Champaign, IL, USA, 2002; pp. 125–141.
71. Corder, K.; Ekelund, U.; Steele, R.M.; Wareham, N.J.; Brage, S. Assessment of physical activity in youth. *J. Appl. Physiol.* **2008**, *105*, 977–987. [CrossRef] [PubMed]
72. Dossegger, A.; Ruch, N.; Jimmy, G.; Braun-Fahrlander, C.; Mader, U.; Hanggi, J.; Hofmann, H.; Puder, J.J.; Kriemler, S.; Bringolf-Isler, B. Reactivity to accelerometer measurement of children and adolescents. *Med. Sci. Sports Exerc.* **2014**, *46*, 1140–1146. [CrossRef] [PubMed]

14

Structural Analysis of Women's Heptathlon

Freya Gassmann [1,*], Michael Fröhlich [2] and Eike Emrich [1]

[1] Department of Economics and Sociology of Sport, Institute for Sport Science, Saarland University, Campus Gebäude B8 1, Saarbrücken 66123, Germany; e.emrich@mx.uni-saarland.de

[2] Department of Sports Science, University of Kaiserslautern, Erwin-Schrödinger-Street, Kaiserslautern 67663, Germany; michael.froehlich@sowi.uni-kl.de

* Correspondence: f.gassmann@mx.uni-saarland.de

Academic Editor: Eling Douwe de Bruin

Abstract: The heptathlon comprises the results of seven single disciplines, assuming an equal influence from each discipline, depending on the measured performance. Data analysis was based on the data recorded for the individual performances of the 10 winning heptathletes in the World Athletics Championships from 1987 to 2013 and the Olympic Games from 1988 to 2012. In addition to descriptive analysis methods, correlations, bivariate and multivariate linear regressions, and panel data regressions were used. The transformation of the performances from seconds, centimeters, and meters into points showed that the individual disciplines do not equally affect the overall competition result. The currently valid conversion formula for the run, jump, and throw disciplines prefers the sprint and jump disciplines but penalizes the athletes performing in the 800 m run, javelin throw, and shotput disciplines. Furthermore, 21% to 48% of the variance of the sum of points can be attributed to the performances in the disciplines of long jump, 200 m sprint, 100 m hurdles, and high jump. To balance the effects of the single disciplines in the heptathlon, the formula to calculate points should be reevaluated.

Keywords: athletics; rule change; cluster analysis; factor analysis; competitive performance

---

1. Introduction and Theoretical Framework

The women's heptathlon is an additive competition consisting of seven disciplines. Within two competition days, the women perform (in order) the disciplines of 100 m hurdles, high jump, shotput, and a 200 m run on the first day and a long jump, javelin throw, and 800 m run on the second day. The result in points achieved in the seven disciplines based on individual performances is determined by a points system that was changed last in 1985 [1,2]. The idea of the heptathlon implicitly assumes a relative balance of the single disciplines on the overall performance. Therefore, a conversion formula for the run, jump, and throw disciplines has been developed by Karl Ulbrich and applied for almost 30 years according to the International Association of Athletics Federations (IAAF). The conversion formula contains the following components:

(1) Run competitions (200 m, 800 m, and 100 m hurdles) = $P = A \times (B - T)^C$; T = time in seconds;
(2) Jump competitions (high jump and long jump) = $P = A \times (M - B)^C$; M = measurement result in centimeters;
(3) Throw competitions (shotput and javelin throw) = $P = A \times (D - B)^C$; D = distance in meters.

These components result in a power function with the constants A, B, and C with discipline-specific constants. In this context, Pitsch *et al.* [3] noted that the disciplines are not weighted equally. Increasing performance in some disciplines is reflected in only a slightly progressive increase in points.

The general problem in determining the sum of points achieved in the heptathlon is that, on the one hand, the evaluation of the individual performance in a discipline follows normative assumptions about the transformation rules, and on the other hand, linearity between performances measured and points achieved is impossible [3,4]. Letzelter [5] already noted this source of error by stating that the linear transformation of performances into points negates the "law of quantity" of training and denies the "principle of progressive load". Hence, normative assumptions per se influence the required equal weighting of individual disciplines [6] and contradict the principle of equally weighted balance between the disciplines, as formulated by Trkal [1] for example:

> " ... that the new tables should be developed according to the following nine principles: ... 3). The tables in all disciplines should be: a modification of current tables, linear in all disciplines, very slightly progressive in all disciplines [...] 9) As far as possible, the tables should eliminate the possibility that an athlete specializing in one discipline is able to acquire sufficient points in that disciplines to overcome a low scores in weaker disciplines and beat more versatile all-round athletes."

Concerning the general principles of balance as expressed explicitly in Principle 9, Kenny *et al.* [7], Westera [6] and others noted within the context of the decathlon that further analyses are required. In particular, the questions arise regarding the extent to which performances in single disciplines are included in the total result in an equally weighted form and the contribution of each discipline to the overall result.

Regarding the single heptathlon disciplines, Westera [2] further notes the following:

> "When starting from the principle of all roundness, the ideal score distribution should be uniform over the disciplines. The large deviations from uniformity prompt for a revision of the current scoring method."

Therefore, analogous to the studies about the influence of a single discipline on the total result in the men's decathlon [8–10], the following questions are examined.

(1) The extent to which a specific discipline and/or cluster of disciplines determines the total number of points to a more than random high scale in the women's heptathlon [2,5,11,12],
(2) The extent to which, at an individual level, strengths and weaknesses in individual disciplines or clusters of disciplines can be balanced and/or overcompensated.

We will examine the extent to which the various strengths of the athletes are favored by the predefined disciplinary structure of the heptathlon [13]. Although the structure of the heptathlon has been created to implicitly consider a well-balanced athlete type [2], athletes with fast-twitch muscle fibers seem to be at an advantage in some disciplines. For example, high performance in speed, explosive strength, and speed strength is mainly associated with a high performance in jump, throw, put, and sprint disciplines, whereas aerobic or anaerobic, endurance-focused factors with a higher share of slow-twitch muscle fibers take weight only in the 800 m run. In this context, Vindusková [14] noted that the heptathlon is a technical discipline with strength and speed character for which "maximum speed", "explosive power", and "speed endurance" are the key performance factors.

2. Methodology

2.1. *Sampling and Survey Procedures*

Data analysis was based on the data recorded for the individual performances of the 10 winning heptathletes in the World Athletics Championships from 1987 to 2013 and the Olympic Games from 1988 to 2012. Previous results were not included because the current conversion formula has been applied only since 1985 [1]. For each athlete, ranking; name; nationality; date of birth; year of competition; results achieved in seconds, centimeters, and meters; points calculated for each discipline;

and the total number of points were determined. Data sources included heptathlon results published in "Leichtathletik" magazine, on the webpage "Sports Reference—Sports Statistics Quickly, Easily & Accurately", and on the official webpage of the International Association of Athletics Federations (IAAF). Comparing the contents of the various media ensured data consistency. Additional specific Internet research on spelling and change of names, dates of births, *etc.*, resulted in a comprehensive list of athletes comprising 200 consistent data records (consisting of 13 datasets for world championships and 7 datasets for Olympic Games, with 10 athletes in each case).

2.2. Data Analysis

The software program used for data analysis was Stata 12. In addition to descriptive analysis methods (e.g., mean values, standard deviation, and frequencies), correlations, bivariate and multivariate linear regressions, and panel data regressions were applied to investigate the research questions mentioned above. Kihlberg and Karvonen (1957) showed that the distributions of the best performances are formally similar to the Pareto and not to the Normal distribution [15]. However the distributions of achieved points in heptathlon resemble a Normal more than a Pareto distribution (Figure 1). Therefore it is possible to compute usual descriptive and inferential statistics.

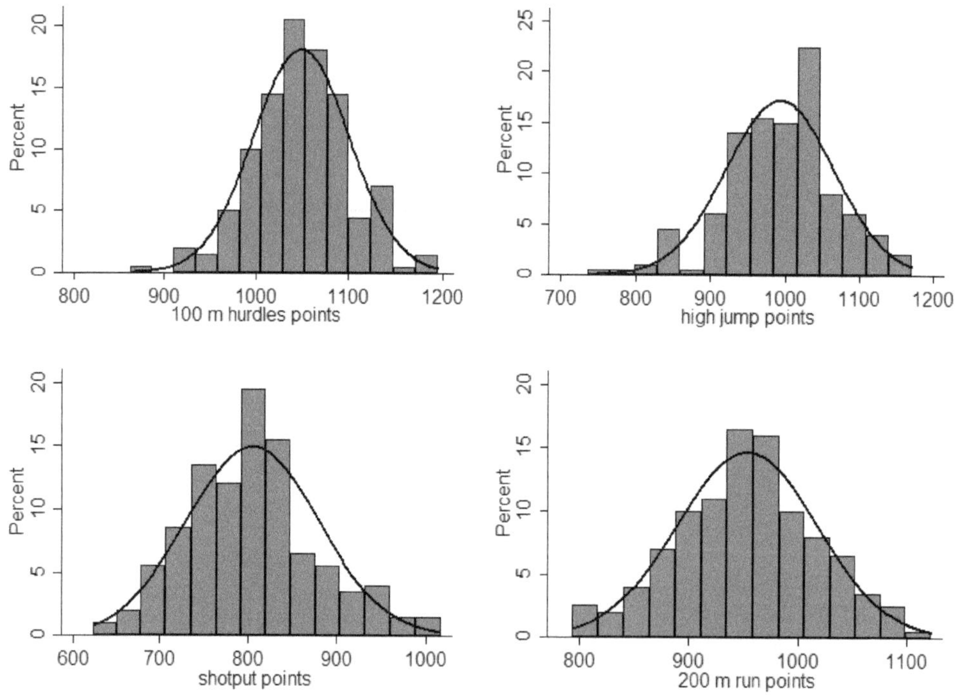

Figure 1. *Cont.*

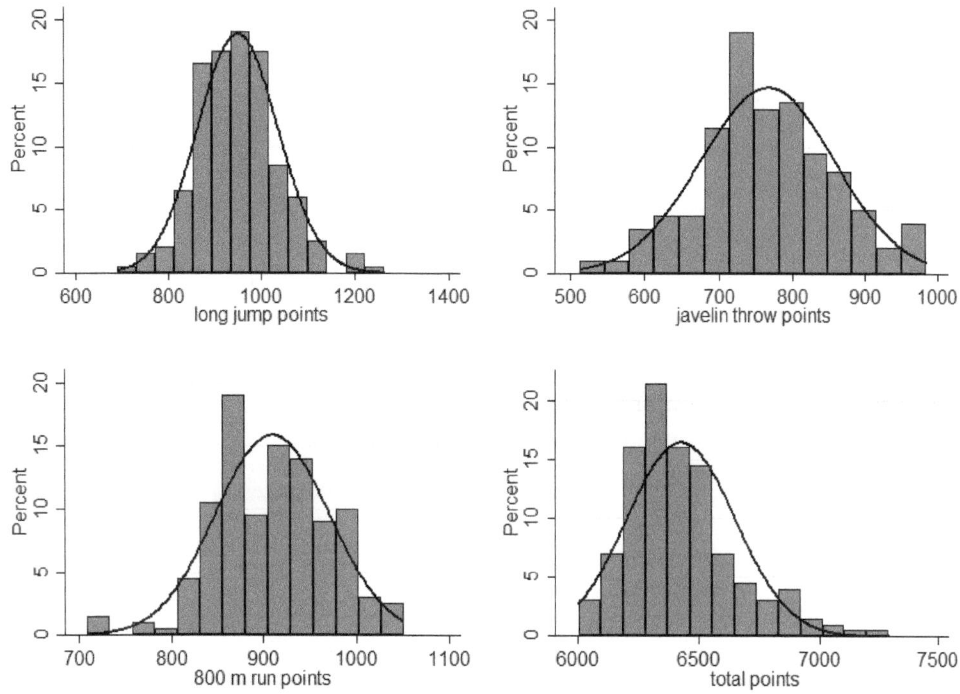

Figure 1. Distribution of the achieved points (n = 200).

To examine the influence of individual performance on the number of points achieved in each discipline, the relevant values needed to be standardized because individual performances are measured in their respective units, and it is naturally impossible to directly compare times, distances, or heights. Therefore, all performances were standardized, or z-transformed.

To analyze the impact of standardized performance on points achieved, seven bivariate linear regressions were estimated and used as a basis for the calculation of marginal effects [16]. Because the curves of the power functions increase positively, sub-disciplines should explain the total amount of variance. For example, to verify that high performance in speed, explosive strength, and speed strength is mainly associated with high performance in jump, throw, put, and sprint disciplines, whereas endurance-focused factors take weight only in the 800 m run, the number of points in the individual disciplines was correlated with the number of total points achieved by means of linear regression, and correlation calculations between the individual disciplines were performed. Owing to potential correlations between performances in the same competitions, we performed seven linear regressions with adjusted standard error for every Olympic Games or world championship.

To obtain additional information on sub-discipline association other than from the correlation matrix, a main component analysis with orthogonalization was performed [17]. "The central idea of principal component analysis is to reduce the dimensionality of a data set in which there are a large number of interrelated variables, while retaining as much as possible of the variation present in the data set" [17]. Through the analysis, a new set of variables is created, including almost all information on the original variables. This factor analysis enables a summary of sub-disciplines. We performed a main component factor analysis with orthogonal varimax rotation. Based on the scree plot of the factor analysis (eigenvalue diagram) and the elbow criterion, the following two implied factors follow: the eigenvalue with two factors is 1.34, compared to 0.98 for a three-factor solution (see Table 1).

Table 1. Results of the exploratory factor analysis via orthogonal rotation, factor loadings (n = 200).

Disziplines	Factor 1	Factor 2
100 m hurdles	0.73	−0.24
High jump	0.50	0.37
200 m run	0.75	−0.39
Long jump	0.83	0.06
Shotput	−0.07	0.54
Javelin throw	−0.07	0.70
800 m run	0.24	−0.73

The disciplines were divided into two factors as follows:

- Factor 1 "Speed": 100 m hurdles, 200 m run, long jump, high jump;
- Factor 2 "Strength": Javelin throw and shotput.

The final 800 m run was not assigned to any factor. Taking the eigenvalue criterion as a basis, a three-factor solution follows with factor 1 comprising 100 m hurdles, 200 m run, and long jump, factor 2 including shotput and javelin throw, and factor 3 consisting of high jump. The 800 m run was again not assigned to any factor (Karlis *et al.*, 2003; Letzelter, 1985).

Because the high jump is primarily determined by speed, explosive strength, and speed strength from a training-scientific point of view and thus correlates much more intensely with the sprint disciplines, we decided to employ the first variant with the high jump being assigned to factor 1.

We performed three multiple linear regressions with each factor, represented through corresponding variables to examine the impact of factors on the total number of points. We used regressions with the cluster option again to indicate that the observations were clustered into the 20 competitions, owing to potential correlations between performances in the same competitions.

In addition, a cluster analysis was performed to examine whether athletes exist with systematic similarities to other athletes in terms of points achieved [18]. "Cluster analysis is an exploratory data analysis tool for organizing observed data into meaningful taxonomies, groups, or clusters, based on combinations of IV's (instrumental variables), which maximizes the similarity of cases within each cluster while maximizing the dissimilarity between groups ... " [19]. We used Ward's method to get an impression of the possible number of clusters, reviewed the dendrogram and performed the K-means cluster analysis [19]). The structure of the heptathlon implicitly applies the athletes' versatility, which is intended to reflect the generalist of athletics (the supreme discipline in women's athletics). Therefore, we aim to verify whether the requirements to live up to this claim are met or athletes specialized in individual disciplines or groups of disciplines have an advantage over generalists.

By means of a cluster analysis using a dendrogram, a two-cluster solution for generalists and specialists has been identified. The level of significance and thus the forecast value were specified to be 5% for all test procedures. The pertinent effect sizes were calculated for the explanatory value.

3. Results

3.1. Performance in Sub-Discipline and Points Achieved in Sub-Disciplines

By means of bivariate regression calculations—based on standardized performances—we could show that athletes attaining javelin throw, long jump, and shotput perform better than one, two, or three standard deviations compared to the average results achieve the highest increase in points (slope coefficient) in relative terms. In contrast, the relative increase in the disciplines of the 200 m and 800 m runs, high jump, and 100 m hurdles is significantly lower. For example, a higher javelin throw result by one standard deviation can lead to a relative performance improvement of 12.5%, whereas an increase by one standard deviation in the 100 m hurdles involves a performance improvement of only approximately 5%. Nevertheless, the analysis in Table 2 shows that a higher javelin throw result by three standard deviations (1047.1 points) corresponds to a merely average performance in 100 m hurdles (1047.3 points).

Table 2. Results of the bivariate linear regressions of the standardized performances on the respective points achieved in the individual disciplines (n = 200).

Individual Discipline	Slope Coefficient	Constant	Marginal Effect		
			(+1 STD)	(+2 STD)	(+3 STD)
100 m hurdles	52.16 ***	1047.3 ***	1099.4	1151.6	1203.8
High jump	71.41 ***	993.7 ***	1065.1	1136.5	1207.9
Shot put	75.73 ***	800.9 ***	876.6	952.4	1028.1
200 m run	63.63 ***	952.0 ***	1015.7	1079.3	1142.9
Long jump	86.66 ***	949.3 ***	1036.0	1122.6	1209.3
Javelin throw	95.23 ***	761.6 ***	856.8	952.0	1047.1
800 m run	60.52 ***	909.8 ***	970.4	1030.9	1091.4

*** $p < 0.001$.

On the basis of the constants, it can also be deduced that the single disciplines on the one hand each contribute differently to the overall result [2], which, for example, becomes strongly evident in positive terms for 100 m hurdles and in negative terms for the javelin throw. However, for the high and long jump, the constants are already quite distinct, an effect that is even more intensified through high slope coefficients.

As shown in Table 2, the slope coefficients of the sub-disciplines of javelin throw, long jump, shotput, and high jump are the highest, whereas lesser coherences are observed in the 200 m run, 800 m run, and 100 hurdles. Therefore, the initial assumption is that athletes with a high performance in these disciplines are rewarded with a high number of points. This is, however, absolutely not the case (with the exception of javelin throw and shotput with their high slope coefficient but low constant) because the average number of points achieved in the disciplines of shotput, javelin throw, and 800 m run is below the number of points achieved in the other disciplines; thus, a performance efficiency that is higher in relative terms takes effect here. At the same time, the athletes achieve a significantly lower number of points owing to the low constant in these sub-disciplines.

3.2. *Points Achieved in Individual Disciplines and Total Number of Points*

Tables 3 and 4 illustrate that all sub-disciplines have a highly significant impact on the final result but with varying explanatory power, which is explained by the different correlation of the points achieved within the sub-disciplines. The strongest influence was evident for the sub-disciplines of long jump, 200 m run, 100 m hurdles, and high jump with a variance clarification of 48% to 21%. The high degree of explanatory power of up to 48% in the case of the long jump is due to the inter-correlation with additional performance factors, such as starting speed (100 m hurdles and 200 m run) and jump impulse (see correlation coefficient of $r = 0.32$ ($p < 0.001$) between the high and long jumps) [5,9,20]. Shotput, javelin throw, and the final 800 m run are also significantly associated with the final result, but they can be deemed marginal in their explanatory power based on the R^2 values (variance clarification 7% to 8%).

Table 3. Results of the bivariate linear regressions of the rounded number of points achieved in the individual disciplines on the total number of points (n = 200).

Individual Discipline	Slope Coefficient	Constant	R^2
100 m hurdles	2.479 ***	3827.1 ***	0.333
High jump	1.533 ***	4903.4 ***	0.208
Shot put	0.705 **	5858.1 ***	0.075
200 m run	2.141 ***	4384.7 ***	0.380
Long jump	1.818 ***	4698.3 ***	0.480
Javelin throw	0.629 ***	5943.1 ***	0.078
800 m run	0.958 **	5553.8 ***	0.069

** $p < 0.01$, *** $p < 0.001$.

Table 4. Correlation matrix of the points achieved in the individual disciplines and the total number of points (significance test in parentheses).

	TP	100	HI	SP	200	LS	JT	800
TP	1							
100	**0.58**	1						
	(0.00)							
HI	**0.49**	0.04	1					
	(0.00)	(0.59)						
SP	0.24	−0.14	−0.06	1				
	(0.00)	(0.04)	(0.44)					
200	**0.61**	**0.61**	0.10	−0.15	1			
	(0.00)	(0.00)	(0.14)	(0.04)				
LS	**0.70)**	**0.45**	**0.32**	−0.03	**0.48**	1		
	(0.00	(0.00)	(0.00)	(0.64)	(0.00)			
JS	0.26	−0.09	0.07	0.19	−0.24	−0.13	1	
	(0.00)	(0.18)	(0.31)	(0.01)	(0.00)	(0.06)		
800	0.26	0.25	−0.01	−0.26	**0.41**	0.12	**−0.35**	1
	(0.00)	(0.00)	(0.89)	(0.00)	(0.00)	(0.09)	(0.00)	

TP = Total points, 100 = 100 m hurdles, HI = high jump, SP = shotput, 200 = 200 m run, LS = long jump, SW = javelin throw, 800 = 800 m run, correlation ⩾ 0.30 are in bold; according to Dancey and Reidy's (2004, p. 171) these are weak correlations.

When looking at the sub-disciplines, significant and moderate correlations can be observed between the 100 m hurdles and 200 m run (0.61), 100 m hurdles and long jump (0.45), high jump and long jump (0.32), 200 m run and long jump (0.48), and 200 m and 800 m runs (0.41) [21]. The javelin throw and 800 m run have a negative correlation (−0.35).

Analyzing the inter-correlation of the disciplines, it becomes evident that a specific type of athlete frequently achieves good performance in these sub-disciplines. Phenotypically, this type shows distinct strengths in the sprint jump area. To develop a better understanding of this information, a factor analysis will examine the extent to which discipline groups can be identified in the heptathlon and which characteristics they carry [5,7,9].

3.3. Factor-Analytic Structure of Heptathlon and Total Number of Points

The following three basic discipline groups are the result of a main component analysis: the "Speed" type included 100 m hurdles, high jump, 200 m run, and long jump. The "Strength" type (maximum strength and speed strength) comprised shotput and javelin throw, and the "Endurance" type consisted of the 800 m run [5].

To examine the impact of factors on the total number of points, we performed three multiple linear regressions with each factor represented by the corresponding variables (Table 5). The "Speed" model with the 100 m hurdles, high jump, 200 m run, and long jump explained 72% of variances (R^2), whereas the "Strength" model explained only 10% and the "Endurance" model 7%. However, given that these regression models consisted of different numbers of variables, we calculated average values by dividing R^2 by the number of independent variables. Again, the "Speed" model explained the largest amount of variance, followed by the "Endurance" and "Strength" models.

Table 5. Results of the multivariate linear regressions of the rounded number of points achieved in the individual disciplines or factors on the total number of points (n = 200).

Disciplines	Model 1 Factor 1 (Speed)	Model 2 Factor 2 (Strength)	Model 3 Factor 3 (Endurance)
100 m hurdles	1.077 *** (4.60)		
High jump	1.064 *** (11.16)		
200 m run	0.872 *** (5.94)		
Long jump	0.925 *** (7.05)		
Shot put		0.578 * (2.54)	
Javelin throw		0.537 *** (4.50)	
800 m run			0.958 ** (3.22)
Constant	2531.1 *** (11.88)	5548.0 *** (30.37)	5553.8 *** (20.64)
N	200	200	200
R^2	0.721	0.102	0.069
Adjusted R^2	0.715	0.093	0.065
Average R^2 (R^2/number of IV)	0.180	0.051	0.069

Regression coefficients and t statistics in parentheses are displayed + $p < 0.10$, * $p < 0.05$, ** $p < 0.01$, *** $p < 0.001$.

3.4. Cluster-Analytic Structure of the Heptathlon Type and Achieved Total Number of Points

The generalists achieved a mean number of points (±SD) of 6349 ± 166 (n = 109), whereas the specialists reached 6518 ± 246 points (n = 85). The generalists' share in the sample was 56% *versus* a 44% share of the specialists (see Figure 2). Six heptathletes could not be assigned to any type in the sample.

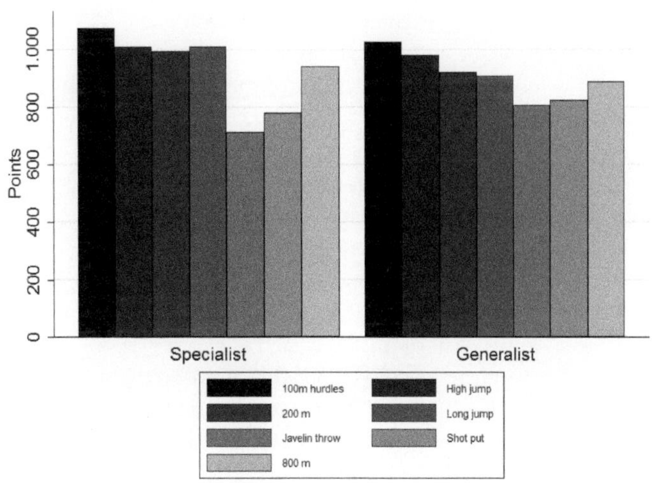

Figure 2. Points achieved by specialists and generalists in the individual disciplines by means of a two-cluster solution.

The sequencing of the analysis of type changes between participations of an athlete in various competitions led to the conclusion that athletes who reached a ranking among the top 10 in Olympic Games or world championships usually abide by their type or do not want to change it. This means that an athlete diagnosed as a specialist was also identified as such in the subsequent competitions. Of the 82 athletes who participated in a total of 194 competitions, only 11 changed their type and 33 stuck by their type during that time.

4. Discussion

The structural analysis of the women's heptathlon yielded empirical evidence that in an allegedly objectively quantifiable form of such sports as the women's heptathlon, the normatively influenced transformation of performance into points using a conversion formula—applied to the ratios between speed disciplines (sprints and jumps), strength requirements (throw and put disciplines) and endurance (800 m)—results in an imbalanced weighting of the performances in the seven disciplines and thus impacts the final result in different ways [4]. This result agrees almost completely with the findings identified for the men's decathlon [6,7,20,22].

Currently, heptathlon performance is disproportionately influenced by a high performance in 100 m hurdles and the performances in the high and long jumps, whereas javelin throw performance is underrepresented in the overall competition performance and thus probably bears the highest training-specific development potential. The long jump in the women's heptathlon is of special importance, as reflected in the high variance clarification of 48% and explainable by the high degree of inter-correlation with the disciplines of 100 m hurdles, high jump, and 200 m run. Physiologically, this can be explained by the high degree of speed, explosive strength, and speed strength in this discipline group, which the cluster analysis with a two-factor solution confirms phenotypically as the sprint-jump type. By comparison, Park and Zatsiorsky [20] found a 43.1% variance clarification in the men's decathlon for the cluster consisting of 100 m run, 400 m run, 110 m hurdles, and long jump, interpreted by the authors as "sprinting performance" [8,10].

The higher shares of maximum strength requirements were attributed to the second factor and were expressed in the disciplines of javelin throw and shotput. The final 800 m as the alleged endurance part in the heptathlon could not be assigned to any factor because, as Letzelter [5] already postulated, it is … "not long enough to check endurance exclusively". (Schomaker & Heumann, 2011; Wimmer *et al.*, 2011) used men's decathlon results to identify a three-factor solution comprising the factors "speed-and-athletic" (100 m, long jump, 400 m, and 110 m hurdles), "strength-and-technique" (shotput, high jump, and discus throw), and "endurance" as a special factor with the final 1500 m run, which largely corresponds to the data presented for the heptathlon.

The following should therefore be considered: (a) the extent to which the dominance of the speed and strength shares could be changed for the benefit of the endurance shares (achieving a balance of the motor capabilities endurance, strength, and speed), and (b) the extent to which the internal respective discipline structures unambiguously represent the basic motor capabilities. To develop these two ideas, further discussion is needed regarding whether the introduction of hammer throw as a more strength-determined discipline to replace javelin throw or the extent to which a final 3000 m or 5000 m run might be more suitable for the representation and weighting of strength with respect to endurance than the 800 m run. These amendments might result in a higher balance within the individual heptathlon disciplines. Implicitly, the specialist in versatility is considered the model athlete in the context of the women's heptathlon, which is expressed, for example, in the German term "Königin der Athletinnen" (queen of female athletes) alluding to the heptathlon as the supreme discipline in women's athletics. Nevertheless, the extent to which historically changed framework conditions, specific selection and support mechanisms, device-based innovations, and the 30-year-old transformation rule influence the chances of even a real specialist reaching a higher performance and thus a higher probability to win is a matter of debate [7,13]. The cluster analysis could show for the present examination sample, pertaining to the participants in world championships and Olympic

Games, that the specialists achieved an average of approximately 170 points more than the generalists and that specialists are found among the world's top athletes approximately 12% more often than generalists, which would explain early selection mechanisms based on good sprint-jump performances. Furthermore, the generalists are relatively more time-stable than the specialists, and the typology applied remained consistent during the competitions.

Analogous to the results identified for the men's decathlon [6], and if equally weighted disciplines are the goal, the present results for the heptathlon show the necessity of a structural reevaluation of the points formula and/or an extension of the disciplines (decathlon or dodecathlon) because the now 30-year-old transformation of performance in the sub-disciplines leads to distortions in the overall result [1]. Thus, in the sense of equality, the women's decathlon instead of heptathlon might be conceivable as an official discipline in women's all-rounder competitions.

Author Contributions: Freya Gassmann, Michael Fröhlich, and Eike Emrich conceived and designed the study; Freya Gassmann, Michael Fröhlich, and Eike Emrich analyzed the data; Freya Gassmann, Michael Fröhlich, and Eike Emrich wrote the paper.

Conflicts of Interest: The authors declare no conflict of interest.

References

1. Trkal, V. The development of combined events scoring tables and implications for the training of decathletes. *New Stud. Athl.* **2003**, *18*, 7–12.
2. Westera, W. Under Attack: The Heptathlon Scoring Method. Available online: http://www.athleticscoaching.ca (accessed on 1 November 2014).
3. Pitsch, W.; Emrich, E.; Fröhlich, M.; Flatau, J. Zur Legitimation von Normen im Sport am Beispiel des Mehrkampfs in der Leichtathletik—Rechtsphilosophische und rechtssoziologische Positionen. *Leipz. Sportwiss. Beitr.* **2006**, *47*, 80–92.
4. Cox, T.F.; Dunn, R.T. An analysis of decathlon data. *J. R. Stat. Soc. Ser. D* **2002**, *51*, 179–187.
5. Letzelter, M. Zur Struktur des Siebenkampfes: Einflusshöhe und interne Verwandtschaft der Einzelübungen. In *Frauenleichtathletik*; Müller, N., Augustin, D., Hunger, B., Eds.; Schors-Verlag: Niederhauen/Taunus, Germany, 1985.
6. Westera, W. Decathlon, towards a balanced and sustainable performance assessment method. *New Stud. Athl. IAAF* **2006**, *21*, 39–51.
7. Kenny, I.C.; Sprevak, D.; Sharp, C.; Boreham, C. Determinants of success in the olympic decathlon: Some statistical evidence. *J. Quant. Anal. Sports* **2005**, *1*. [CrossRef]
8. Schomaker, M.; Heumann, C. Model averaging in factor analysis: An analysis of olympic decathlon data. *J. Quant. Anal. Sports* **2011**, *7*. [CrossRef]
9. Woolf, A.; Ansley, L.; Bidgood, P. Grouping of decathlon disciplines. *J. Quant. Anal. Sports* **2007**, *3*. [CrossRef]
10. Wimmer, V.; Fenske, N.; Pyrka, P.; Fahrmeir, L. Exploring competition performance in decathlon using semi-parametric latent variable models. *J. Quant. Anal. Sports* **2011**, *7*. [CrossRef]
11. Karlis, D.; Saporta, G.; Spinakis, A. A simple rule for the selection of principal components. *Commun. Stat. Theory Methods* **2003**, *32*, 643–666. [CrossRef]
12. Dawkins, B.P.; Andreae, P.M.; O'Conner, P.M. Analysis of olympic heptathlon data. *J. Am. Stat. Assoc.* **1994**, *89*, 1100–1106. [CrossRef]
13. Van Damme, R.; Wilson, R.S.; Vanhooydonck, B.; Aerts, P. Performance constraints in decathletes. *Nature* **2002**, *415*, 755–756. [CrossRef] [PubMed]
14. Vindusková, J. Training women for the heptathlon—A brief outline. *New Stud. Athl.* **2003**, *18*, 27–45.
15. Kihlberga, J.; Karvonena, M.J. Comparison on statistical basis of achievement in track and field events. *Res. Q. Am. Assoc. Health Phys. Educ. Recreat.* **1957**, *28*, 244–256.
16. Greene, W.H. *Econometric Analysis*, 7th ed.; Pearson Education: Upper Saddle River, NJ, USA, 2008.
17. Jolliffe, I.T. *Principal Component Analysis*, 2nd ed.; Springer-Verlag: New York, NY, USA, 2002.
18. Wiedenbeck, M.; Züll, C. Clusterananlyse. In *Handbuch der Sozialwissenschaftlichen Datenanalyse*; Wolf, C., Best, H., Eds.; VS Verlag für Sozialwissenschaften: Wiesbaden, Germany, 2010; pp. 525–552.
19. Burns, R.P.; Burns, R. *Business Research Methods and Statistics Using SPSS*; SAGE: London, UK, 2008.

20. Park, J.; Zatsiorsky, V.M. Multivariate statistical analysis of decathlon performance results in olympic athletes (1988–2008). *World Acad. Sci. Eng. Technol.* **2011**, *5*, 985–988.
21. Fanshawe, T. Seven into two: Principal components analysis and the olympic heptathlon. *Significance* **2012**, *9*, 40–42. [CrossRef]
22. Linden, M. Factor analytical study of olympic decathlon data. *Res. Q. Am. Alliance Health Phys. Educ. Recreat.* **1977**, *48*, 562–568.

15

Radiographic Assessment of Anatomic Risk Factors Associated with Acute, Lateral Patellar Dislocation in the Immature Knee

Thai Trinh [1], Andrew Mundy [2], Matthew Beran [3] and Kevin Klingele [3,*]

1. Mount Carmel Health Systems, Department of Orthopedics 793 West State Street Columbus, Columbus, OH 43222, USA; thai.trinh.12@gmail.com
2. Ohio State University Medical Center, Department of Orthopaedics, 410 W 10th Ave, Columbus, OH 43210, USA; andrew.mundy@osumc.edu
3. Nationwide Children's Hospital, Department of Orthopedics, 700 Children's Drive, Ste. A2630, Columbus, OH 43205-2696, USA; matthew.beran@nationwidechildrens.org

* Correspondence: kevin.klingele@nationwidechildrens.org

Academic Editor: Craig Williams

Abstract: Acute patellar dislocation remains a common injury in both adult and pediatric patients. Non-operative management has been advocated for patients without a history of recurrent instability. Although pathologic thresholds for consideration of operative management have previously been reported in adults, it is largely unknown in children. A retrospective review of all skeletally immature patients diagnosed with acute lateral patellar dislocation who had MRI imaging were included for analysis. An age-based control group was also identified. Six radiographic measurements were compared: lateral trochlear inclination (LTI), trochlear facet asymmetry (TFA), trochlear depth (TD), tibial tuberosity–trochlear groove (TT–TG), sulcus angle (SA) and patellar height ratio. A total of 178 patients were included for analysis (study: $n = 108$, control: $n = 70$). The mean age of patients in the study and control groups was 13.7 and 12.1 years respectively ($p \leqslant 0.001$). Study group patients had significant differences in all radiographic measurements including a decreased LTI ($p < 0.001$), increased TFA ($p < 0.001$) and SA ($p < 0.001$). The mean trochlear depth was 3.4 mm and 5.6 mm for patients in the study and control groups respectively ($p < 0.001$). Study group patients had an increased patellar height ratio ($p < 0.001$) and TT–TG distance ($p < 0.001$). Morphologic abnormalities may predispose skeletally immature patients to an increased risk of acute lateral patellar instability.

Keywords: children; knee; magnetic resonance imaging; morphology; patella; patellofemoral joint

---

1. Introduction

Acute patellar dislocation represents 2%–3% of all knee injuries in adults and children [1–5]. Traditionally, management of patients following primary patellar dislocation has been non-operative, characterized by a short period of immobilization followed by physiotherapy and gradual return to activities [6,7]. Recurrent patellar instability has previously been reported in up to 60% of patients following non-operative management, and has prompted some authors to advocate early surgical intervention aimed at reducing the morbidity associated with recurrent instability, including the time lost from activity and the development of early-onset patellofemoral arthritis [4,8–13].

Radiographic assessment of anatomic risk factors for patellar dislocation has traditionally included the use of plain radiographs and computed tomography (CT) [6,7]. More recently, magnetic resonance imaging (MRI) has become an important diagnostic tool in the evaluation of patients with patellofemoral instability. Although surgical management of recurrent patellar instability continues to evolve, current techniques aim to correct the anatomic risk factors that appear to predispose patients to patellar instability [14,15]. Previous studies have identified morphologic differences between skeletally mature patients with and without patellar instability. Radiographic thresholds that can aid in operative planning have been established based on anatomic differences [9,14,16,17]. It is largely unknown if these thresholds are applicable to skeletally immature patients, as there are only a limited number of studies reporting radiographic norms in pediatric patients with patellar instability [15,18] The purpose of the current study is to report morphological differences between skeletally immature patients with and without acute, lateral patellar instability.

2. Methods

Following the institutional review board (IRB) approval, a retrospective review (August 2009–June 2014) of patients diagnosed with an acute patellar dislocation was performed. Inclusion criteria consisted of skeletally immature patients that had a diagnosis of acute patellar dislocation and had an MRI of the symptomatic knee. The diagnosis of acute patellar dislocation was made clinically with a history and/or physical examination consistent with patellar dislocation. Exclusion criteria included skeletal maturity (defined as closed distal femur physis on plain radiograph and/or MRI), patients with obligatory or habitual patellar instability, and patients who had undergone a previous knee surgery altering their native anatomy (e.g., tibial tubercle transfer, trochleoplasty). A total of 108 patients (108 knees), all between the ages of 9 and 16 years old, were identified. All patients enrolled were skeletally immature with open physes on imaging.

To obtain the control group, a retrospective review of skeletally immature patients presenting between 2002 and 2014, who had undergone MRI imaging to evaluate for knee pathology other than patellar dislocation, was performed. Only MRIs interpreted by a pediatric-trained radiologist as normal or without pathologic features interfering with normal morphology (e.g., popliteal cysts, discoid menisci, and small effusions) were included for analysis. Ten patients were randomly selected at every age within the age range of our acute patellar dislocation study group (9–16 years old) for comparison. This identified a total of 70 patients (70 knees) for analysis (control group).

MRI images were obtained at our institution utilizing MRI scanners possessing a magnetic field strength ranging from 1.5 to 3.0 T. A total of six measurements were recorded utilizing either T2 or proton density (PD) sequences: lateral trochlear inclination (LTI), trochlear facet asymmetry (TFA), trochlear depth (TD), tibial tuberosity–trochlear groove (TT–TG), sulcus angle (SA) and patellar height ratio according to Insall-Salvati [17] (Figures 1–6).

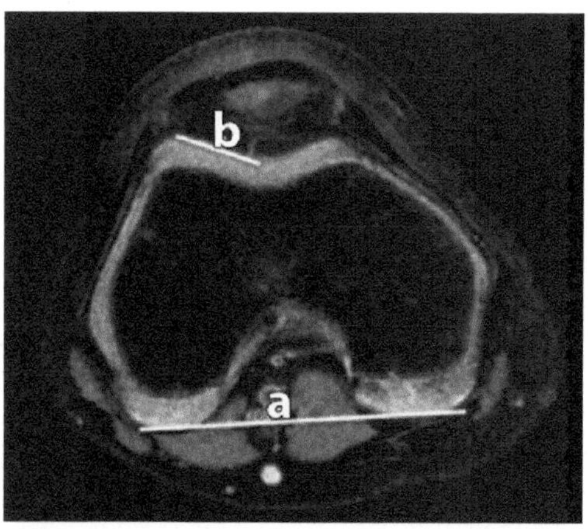

Figure 1. Lateral Trochlear Inclination (LTI). The angle between the lateral trochlear facet (**b**); and the line along the posterior condyles (**a**) is measured.

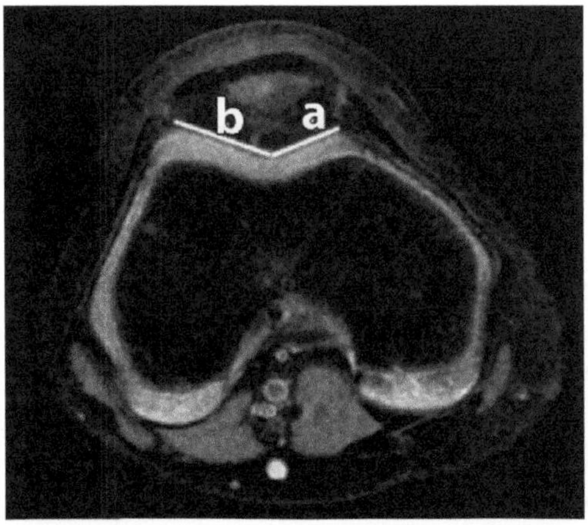

Figure 2. Trochlear Facet Asymmetry (TFA). The distances of the lateral facet (**b**); and medial facet (**a**) are recorded.

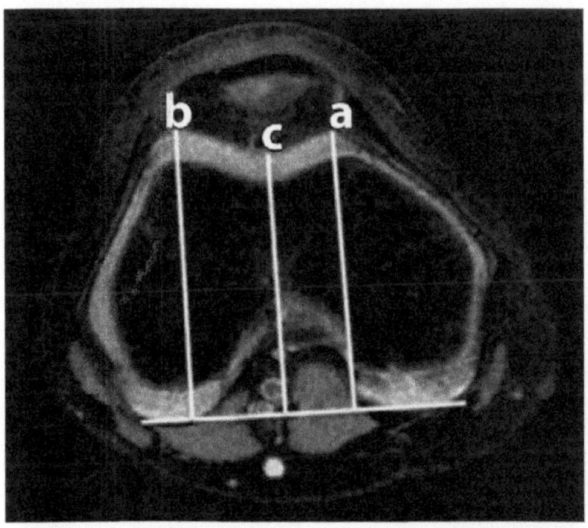

Figure 3. Trochlear Depth (TD). A posterior condylar reference line is created (solid white line). Three lines are drawn from the reference line to the lateral facet apex (**b**); medial facet apex (**a**); and the deepest portion of the sulcus (**c**).

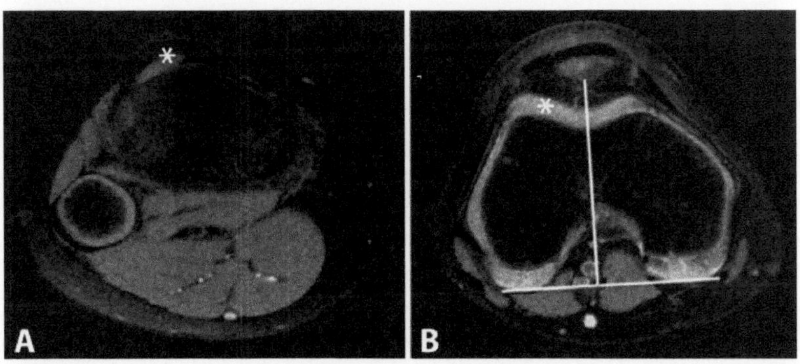

Figure 4. (**A**) and (**B**): Tibial Tuberosity–Trochlear Groove (TT–TG) distance. The superior attachment of the patellar tendon at the tibial tuberosity is marked (**A**); and then transposed on our standard axial sequence (**B**). The distance between the marker (*) and solid white line that is extending through the deep sulcus to the reference line was recorded.

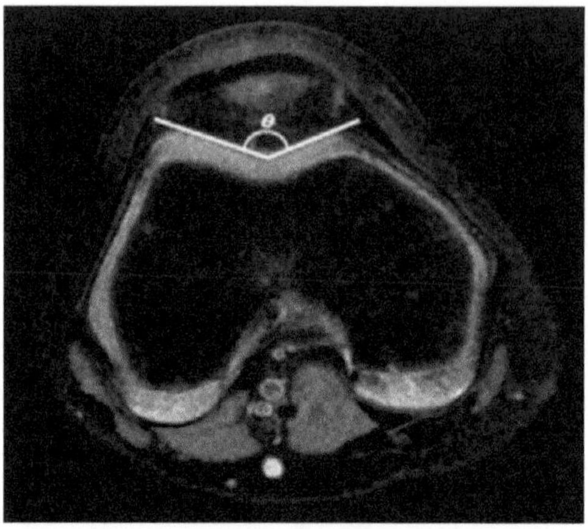

Figure 5. Sulcus Angle (SA). The angle (θ) between the lateral and medial facet is measured.

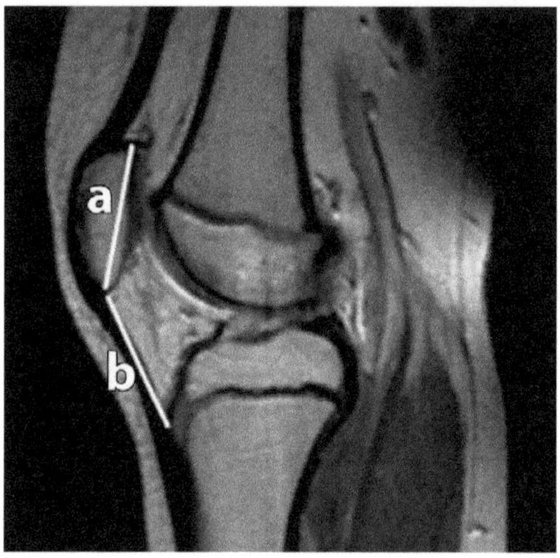

Figure 6. Patellar Height Ratio (PHR) according to Insall-Salvati. Two measurements were recorded, the distance between the superior apex (articular surface) and inferior apex (non-articular surface) (**a**); and the distance of the patellar tendon at its attachments from the inferior patellar apex to the tibial tuberosity (**b**).

These measurements were selected based on their use in previous literature assessing patellofemoral morphology [5,17].

Statistical analysis was performed utilizing the StatPlus LE software (AnalystSoft, Walnut, CA, USA) [19]. All continuous data satisfied the assumption of normality and thus only parametric analysis was performed. Continuous outcome data between study and control groups were analyzed utilizing a two-sample T test. Categorical data between groups were analyzed utilizing a Pearson Chi-square test. Statistical significance was set at $p < 0.05$.

3. Results

A total of 178 patients were included for analysis (study: $n = 108$, control: $n = 70$). The mean age for patients in the study and control groups was 13.7 and 12.1 years, respectively ($p < 0.001$). There was no difference in the distribution of males and females ($p = 0.29$) or laterality ($p = 0.55$) between groups (Table 1).

Table 1. Selected patient demographics.

Variables	All (*n*)	Study (*n*)	Control (*n*)	*p*
Patients	178	108	70	–
Age (Years)	13.1 ± 1.9	13.7 ± 1.42	12.1 ± 2.1	<0.001
Sex				
Male	93	53	40	0.29
Female	85	55	30	
Side				
Left	104	65	39	0.55
Right	74	43	31	

All radiographic measurements of interest were obtained in patients comprising the study and control groups. Summarized data is presented in Figure 7.

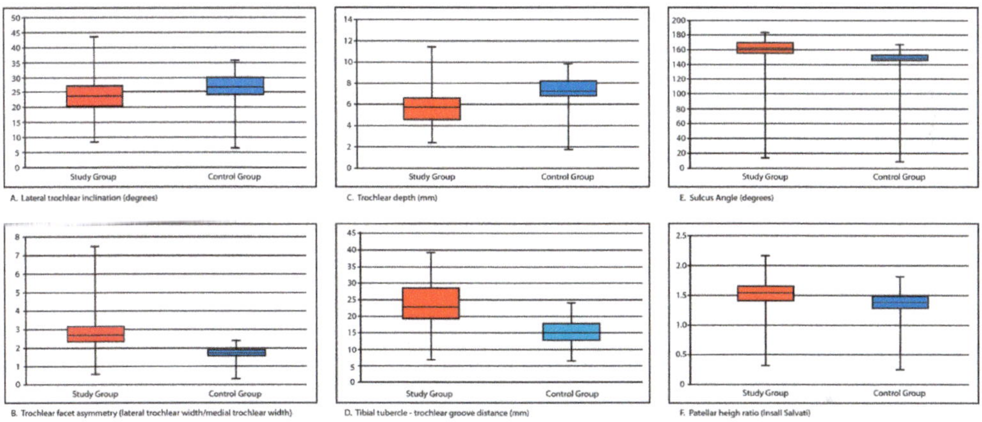

Figure 7. Distribution of lateral trochlear inclination (**A**); trochlear facet asymmetry (**B**); trochlear depth (**C**); tibial tubercle—trochlear groove distance (**D**); sulcus angle (**E**); and patellar height (**F**) between study and control groups.

Measurements characterizing the morphology of the trochlea (LTI, TFA, TD, and SA) were statistically different between patients in the study and control groups (Table 2).

Table 2. Summarized anatomic differences between patients with and without patellar instability utilizing MRI.

Measured Variables	Study Mean ± SD	Control Mean ± SD	*p*
Lateral trochlear inclination (degrees)	15.6 ± 5.5	20.7 ± 3.9	**< 0.001**
Trochlear facet asymmetry (%)	2.3 ± 0.8	1.5 ± 0.3	**< 0.001**
Trochlear depth (mm)	3.4 ± 1.5	5.6 ± 1/1	**< 0.001**
Tibial tubercle trochlear groove distance (mm)	17.0 ± 6.7	8.9 ± 4.1	**< 0.001**
Sulcus angle (degrees)	150.2 ± 10.1	141.6 ± 6.1	**< 0.001**
Patellar height (%)	1.3 ± 0.2	1.1 ± 0.2	**< 0.001**

Patients in the study group were characterized as having a decreased lateral trochlear inclination (15.6° *vs.* 20.7°, $p < 0.001$), increased sulcus angle (150.2° *vs.* 141.6°, $p < 0.001$) and an increased trochlear facet asymmetry (2.3 *vs.* 1.5, $p < 0.001$). The study group also demonstrated a shallower trochlear groove compared to patients in the control group (3.4 mm *vs.* 5.6 mm, $p \leqslant 0.001$). The mean TT–TG distance for patients in the study and control groups were 17.0 mm and 8.9 mm, respectively ($p < 0.001$). A difference in patellar height was also noted between groups with patients in the study group (1.3 ± 0.2 mm) possessing increased patellar height compared to controls (1.1 ± 0.2 mm) ($p < 0.001$).

4. Conclusions

The purpose of the current study was to examine morphological differences between skeletally immature patients with and without acute, lateral patellar instability. Our findings suggest that anatomic differences in trochlear and patellar morphology may result in an increased risk of acute patellofemoral instability in skeletally immature patients. Previous studies examining patellofemoral instability in adults have suggested that surgical correction of aberrant anatomy may decrease the risk of recurrent instability. Although pathologic thresholds for considering surgical treatment in adults have been proposed [7,12,20], it is unclear if these same thresholds are appropriate for the skeletally immature patient, as normal radiographic parameters used to quantify patellofemoral morphology have yet to be established in this population [15]. Mundy *et al.* [18] have shown high inter and intraobserver reliability in the utilization of such measurements in the immature knee. In addition, such measurements develop with maturation, gradually reaching adult norms by age 10 [15,18].

In a retrospective analysis of patients with and without patellar instability, Charles *et al.* [14] reported significant variations in trochlear morphology using MRI. Although the mean age and the status of the distal femoral/proximal tibial physis of patients examined in this study were not disclosed, patients experiencing recurrent patellar instability were shown to have significant differences in trochlear morphology as assessed by the lateral trochlear inclination, trochlear facet asymmetry, trochlear depth, and sulcus angle. The current study reports similar findings in a subset of skeletally immature patients.

Despite the identified differences in trochlear morphology between skeletally mature and immature patients, the clinical implications as it relates to operative management are currently undefined. Previous literature has reported satisfactory outcomes following trochleoplasty in skeletally mature patients experiencing recurrent instability in the setting of trochlear dysplasia [21]. There is likely a limited role for this procedure in the pediatric population due to implications associated with physeal arrest. Furthermore, little is known about the post-operative changes in patellofemoral kinematics and its influence on cartilaginous and bony development following a trochleoplasty procedure. Similarly, tibial tubercle transfers cannot be performed until proximal tibial physeal closure has occurred. Stabilization procedures in the skeletally immature knee thus rely on soft tissue procedures which do not disturb growth.

Limitations of the current study are primarily related to its retrospective design. In order to identify patients for the control group, we retrospectively analyzed all patients who underwent MRI imaging of the knee without a history of patellofemoral instability. In doing so, there is inherent selection bias for patients who presented for evaluation of knee pathology. Differences may exist between this group and those asymptomatic patients who would not have undergone MRI evaluation. Additional limitations include the wide age range of patients in both the study and control groups. For the purposes of the current study, patients were categorized as skeletally immature based on the presence of an open distal femoral physis. There is currently a paucity of literature pertaining to age related changes of the patellofemoral joint. It is possible that different stages of development may alter the anatomy in such a way that what would be considered pathologic at one stage of development, but falls into the spectrum of normal during another. Therefore, considering skeletally immature patients as a group makes the assumption that irregular anatomy contributes to the development of patellofemoral instability equally throughout development. Larger studies are needed to further evaluate the possibility of age related changes to the patellofemoral joint and the implications of these changes as it pertains to management of patients with patellar instability.

Despite these limitations, the current study is the first to compare radiographic differences in patellofemoral morphology between skeletally immature patients with and without acute, lateral patellofemoral instability. Results suggest morphologic abnormalities may predispose skeletally immature patients to an increased risk of such injury. Further research is needed to determine the clinical implications of these differences in order to optimize both surgical and non-surgical management of recurrent instability in skeletally immature patients.

Author Contributions: Thai Trinh and Kevin Klingele conceived and designed the experiments; Thai Trinh performed the experiments; Kevin Klingele and Matthew Beran analyzed the data; Kevin Klingele and Matthew Beran contributed patient data and radiographic images; Andrew Mundy wrote the paper.

Conflicts of Interest: The authors declare no conflict of interest.

References

1. Apostolovic, M.; Vukomanovic, B.; Slavkovic, N.; Vuckovic, V.; Vukcevic, M.; Djuricic, G.; Kocev, N. Acute patellar dislocation in adolescents: Operative *versus* nonoperative treatment. *Int. Orthop.* **2011**, *35*, 1483–1487. [CrossRef] [PubMed]
2. Balcarek, P.; Jung, K.; Ammon, J.; Walde, T.A.; Frosch, S.; Schüttrumpf, J.P.; Stürmer, K.M.; Frosch, K.H. Anatomy of lateral patellar instability: Trochlear dysplasia and tibial tubercle-trochlear groove distance is more pronounced in women who dislocate the patella. *Am. J. Sports Med.* **2010**, *38*, 2320–2327. [CrossRef] [PubMed]
3. Fithian, D.C.; Paxton, E.W.; Stone, M.L.; Silva, P.; Davis, D.K.; Elias, D.A.; White, L.M. Epidemiology and natural history of acute patellar dislocation. *Am. J. Sports Med.* **2004**, *32*, 1114–1121. [CrossRef] [PubMed]
4. Lewallen, L.W.; McIntosh, A.L.; Dahm, D.L. Predictors of recurrent instability after acute patellofemoral dislocation in pediatric and adolescent patients. *Am. J. Sports Med.* **2013**, *41*, 575–581. [CrossRef] [PubMed]
5. Stefancin, J.J.; Parker, R.D. First-time traumatic patellar dislocation: A systematic review. *Clin. Orthop. Relat. Res.* **2007**, *455*, 93–101. [CrossRef] [PubMed]
6. Dejour, H.; Walch, G.; Neyret, P.; Adeleine, P. Dysplasia of the femoral trochlea. *Rev. Chir. Orthop. Reparatr. Appar. Mot.* **1990**, *76*, 45–54.
7. Dejour, H.; Walch, G.; Nove-Josserand, L.; Guier, C. Factors of patellar instability: An anatomic radiographic study. *Knee Surg. Sports Traumatol. Arthrosc.* **1994**, *2*, 19–26. [CrossRef] [PubMed]
8. Camanho, G.L.; Viegas Ade, C.; Bitar, A.C.; Demange, M.K.; Hernandez, A.J. Conservative *versus* surgical treatment for repair of the medial patellofemoral ligament in acute dislocations of the patella. *Arthroscopy* **2009**, *25*, 620–625. [CrossRef] [PubMed]
9. Cofield, R.H.; Bryan, R.S. Acute dislocation of the patella: Results of conservative treatment. *J. Trauma* **1977**, *17*, 526–531. [CrossRef] [PubMed]
10. Hansen, E.B.; Frost, B.; Jensen, E.M. The arthrographic picture following anterior dislocation of the shoulder. A consecutive study of 71 patients. *Ugeskr. Laeger.* **1985**, *147*, 4193–4195. [PubMed]
11. Jacobsen, K.; Metz, P. Occult traumatic dislocation of the patella. *J. Trauma* **1976**, *16*, 829–835. [CrossRef] [PubMed]
12. Koeter, S.; Diks, M.J.; Anderson, P.G.; Wymenga, A.B. A modified tibial tubercle osteotomy for patellar maltracking: Results at two years. *J. Bone Jt. Surg. Br.* **2007**, *89*, 180–185. [CrossRef] [PubMed]
13. Smith, T.O.; Song, F.; Donell, S.T.; Hing, C.B. Operative *versus* non-operative management of patellar dislocation. A meta-analysis. *Knee Surg. Sports Traumatol. Arthrosc.* **2011**, *19*, 988–998. [CrossRef] [PubMed]
14. Charles, M.D.; Haloman, S.; Chen, L.; Ward, S.R.; Fithian, D.; Afra, R. Magnetic resonance imaging-based topographical differences between control and recurrent patellofemoral instability patients. *Am. J. Sports Med.* **2013**, *41*, 374–384. [CrossRef] [PubMed]
15. Dickens, A.J.; Morrell, N.T.; Doering, A.; Tandberg, D.; Treme, G. Tibial tubercle-trochlear groove distance: Defining normal in a pediatric population. *J. Bone Jt. Surg. Am.* **2014**, *96*, 318–324. [CrossRef] [PubMed]
16. Dejour, D.; Byn, P.; Ntagiopoulos, P.G. The Lyon's sulcus-deepening trochleoplasty in previous unsuccessful patellofemoral surgery. *Int. Orthop.* **2013**, *37*, 433–439. [CrossRef] [PubMed]
17. Insall, J.; Goldberg, V.; Salvati, E. Recurrent dislocation and the high-riding patella. *Clin. Orthop. Relat. Res.* **1972**, *88*, 67–69. [CrossRef] [PubMed]
18. Mundy, A.; Ravindra, A.; Yang, J.; Adler, B.H.; Klingele, K.E. Standardization of patellofemoral morphology in the pediatric knee. *Pediatr. Radiol.* **2015**, *46*, 255–262. [CrossRef] [PubMed]

19. AnalystSoft. Available online: http://www.analystsoft.com/en/ (accessed on 14 April 2016).
20. Balcarek, P.; Jung, K.; Frosch, K.H.; Sturmer, K.M. Value of the tibial tuberosity–trochlear groove distance in patellar instability in the young athlete. *Am. J. Sports Med.* **2011**, *39*, 1756–1761. [CrossRef] [PubMed]
21. Von Knoch, F.; Bohm, T.; Burgi, M.L.; von Knoch, M.; Bereiter, H. Trochleaplasty for recurrent patellar dislocation in association with trochlear dysplasia. A 4- to 14-year follow-up study. *J. Bone Jt. Surg. Br.* **2006**, *88*, 1331–1335. [CrossRef] [PubMed]

16

Heart Rate Responses during Small Sided Games and Official Match-Play in Soccer

Alper Aşçı

Haliç University School of Physical Education and Sport, İstanbul 34330, Turkey; alperascii@gmail.com

Academic Editor: Filipe Manuel Clemente

Abstract: Small sided games (SSGs) are a match specific type of training. In addition, there is an insufficient number of studies that compare heart rate (HR) responses of SSGs and official match-play (OM). The purpose of this study was to investigate the heart rate responses during SSGs and OM in young soccer players. Twenty-two male soccer players (mean ± SD; age 17.4 ± 0.9 years, height 174.9 ± 6.6 cm, body weight 67.7 ± 8.1 kg) volunteered to participate in this study. The first session included anthropometric measurements and a maximum running test (RT). Following the RT session, all players participated in five different randomly ordered SSG sessions (3-, 4-, 5-, 7- and 9-a-side with goalkeepers). OMs were also monitored in the fourth week of the study. A one-way multivariate repeated-measures analysis of variance (MANOVA) was then conducted to evaluate the differences between the SSGs and OM. The results showed that 3-a-side elicited significantly higher HR and %HR_{max} than other SSGs and OM, whereas 9-a-side resulted in significantly lower HR and %HR_{max} compared to other SSG formats and OM ($p < 0.05$). In conclusion, 3-a-side, 4-a-side and 5-a-side SSG formats provide players with the opportunity to spend sufficient proportion of time spent in high intensity zones that are specific to match demands.

Keywords: small sided games; soccer; heart rate; time spent

---

1. Introduction

Soccer specific small sided games (SSGs) are often used in soccer training in order to reproduce the physical, technical and tactical requirements of real match-play [1]. SSGs contain many of the elements of soccer match play, such as passing, dribbling skills, and scoring, but typically involve reduced player numbers and/or modified rules [2]. On the technical side, game-specific skill involvements are different during SSGs. Kelly and Drust [3] compared SSG formats according to game-specific skill involvements and found that the number of tackles and shots were higher in SSGs played on smaller pitches than on larger ones. Jones and Drust [4] compared the total number of ball contacts during 4- and 8-a-side games, finding that decreasing player numbers significantly increased the number of individual ball contacts from 13 per game in 8-a-side to 36 in 4-a-side games. Furthermore, game-specific skill involvements are different in SSGs compared to official match play [5]. Capranica *et al.* [5] compared the technical activities of young soccer players in 7-a-side games on a smaller pitch (60 m × 40 m) and in 11-a-side official games on a regular-sized pitch (100 m × 65 m). They found that there were significantly more passes (156 *vs.* 107) in 7-a-side games than in 11-a-side games.

Physiological response during SSGs and match-play has been traditionally determined with the use of heart rate monitors [6,7] because heart rate (HR) measured during soccer exercises effectively reflects the metabolic demands of these intermittent type activities [8]. HR during 5-, 6-, 7- and 8-a-side games has been found to average 169 to 175 bpm [9] corresponding to 85%–90% of maximum heart rate (HR_{max}) [9–11]. For 3-a-side and 4-a-side games, HR averages 173 to 184 bpm, which corresponds to 90%–95% of HR_{max} [4,9,11–14]. While HR responses are between 152 to 184 bpm in SSGs (from 1-a-side to 8-a-side) [15–17], HR during soccer match play averages 150 to 180 bpm [5,18,19], corresponding to 85% of maximum heart rate (HR_{max}) [20].

However, only a few studies have examined the relationship between performance in SSGs and that in competitive matches. Gabbet *et al.* [21] investigated movement patterns in small sided training games (3-a-side and 5-a-side) and compared these movement patterns with those seen in domestic, national, and international standard competitive matches between elite women soccer players. The results of their study suggest that small sided training games simulate the overall movement patterns seen in competitive matches. Dellal *et al.* [22] compared the effects of certain rule changes on the technical and physical demands on elite soccer players in five playing positions in 4-a-side games compared to 11-a-side matches. They found that 4-a-side games played with a rule limiting players to one or two ball touches increased the amount of high-intensity running and the difficulty of performing technical actions, being more specific to match demands. Furthermore, there is no comparative data on physiological responses and proportion of time spent (PTS) in the different heart rate zones to both SSGs and official match-play in male young soccer players. In addition, no study compared physiological responses of 9-a-side and OM. Therefore, this study aims to fill this gap by examining and comparing the heart rate responses and PTS in different heart rate zones during 3-a-side, 4-a-side, 5-a-side, 7-a-side and 9-a-side with similar workout periods and official match play.

2. Materials and Methods

2.1. Subjects

Fifty-one soccer players in the under 18 (U18) and under 16 (U16) soccer teams in Turkey volunteered to participate in this study. However, twenty-two of them who played 90 min in official matches were included in this study (mean $\pm$ SD; age 17.4 $\pm$ 0.9 years, height 174.9 $\pm$ 6.6 cm, body weight 67.7 $\pm$ 8.1 kg, sum of 7-side skinfold thickness 63.1 $\pm$ 19.0 mm, maximum heart rate 196.8 $\pm$ 7.0 bpm and maximum blood lactate 10.0 $\pm$ 2.2 mmol$\cdot$ L^{-1}). All players train for one-and-a-half to two hours a day, five times a week, as well as playing official matches on Saturdays or Sundays. All players and parents were notified of the research procedures, requirements, benefits, and risks before giving informed consent. The study was approved by the Hacettepe University Ethics Committee and was conducted in a manner consistent with the institutional ethical requirements for human experimentation in accordance with the Declaration of Helsinki.

2.2. Procedures

First of all, the four-week training period served as a familiarization period for the subjects to the SSG formats. After the familiarization period, seven sessions were monitored during a six-week in-season period. Small sided games were performed on Tuesdays. In addition, OM played at the end of the fourth week as well as in the SSGs. Anthropometric measurements and a maximum running test (RT) were assessed in the first session. During the RT, each subject's heart rate was continuously recorded using heart rate monitors. Following the RT session, all players participated in five different randomly ordered small sided game formats (3-a-side, 4-a-side, 5-a-side, 7-a-side and 9-a-side games, all including the goalkeeper) over the five weeks including one OM per week. No specific rules were introduced to influence the intensity of the SSGs. Average HR, percent of HR_{max} and time spent in heart rate zones (HRZ) corresponding to $\leqslant$69%, 70%–84%, 85%–89%, 90%–94% and 95%–100% of maximum heart rate were calculated for all bouts and OM for each subject [23]. The time spent in the respective HRZs were reported as a percentage of the total exercise duration of each SSG and OM.

2.3. Field Testing

Each player's individual HR_{max} and maximal blood lactate (La_{max}) was determined using a speed incremental protocol during RT that was performed on an artificial grass soccer pitch. The test included running bouts lasting three minutes and one minute passive rest between bouts. The RT began at a running speed of 8 km$\cdot$h^{-1}, after which the speed was increased to 10 km$\cdot$h^{-1} and then incremental speed increases of 1 km$\cdot$h^{-1} were made for each successive running bout following the rest periods until the subjects were exhausted [24]. The subjects adjusted their running speed to auditory signals at 20 m intervals delineated by visual marks along a 100 m track. Capillary blood samples were drawn from the subjects' earlobes during the one-minute rest periods. Blood lactate was determined using a YSI 1500 Sport Lactate Analyser (Yellow Spring Instruments, Yellow Springs, OH, USA). Subjects' heart rates (recorded at 5 s intervals) were continuously recorded using heart rate monitors (Polar S-610; Polar Electro OY, Kempele, Finland) during the RT. HR data was stored in the heart rate monitors and downloaded to a computer using Polar Interface Plus with the Polar precision performance software (Version 4.01.029, Polar Electro Oy, Kempele, Finland) at the end of each session. The highest value of recorded heart rates in either of the last two bouts was considered the maximum heart rate (HR_{max}).

2.4. Small Sided Games and Official Matches

All subjects played games in the five different formats (3-a-side, 4-a-side, 5-a-side, 7-a-side and 9-a-side games), all of which involved the goalkeeper, official-sized goals and an unlimited number of touches on an artificial grass field. The offside rule was not applied during the SSGs [25]. The SSGs were played at the beginning of each training session, following a standardized 20-min warm-up period. Verbal support was given to all subjects during the SSGs to encourage the maintenance of a high work-rate. Players were allowed to consume available drinking water during all recovery periods of the SSGs. Pitch dimensions used (length-width in meters), pitch size (m^2), pitch size per player (m^2), the number of bouts, bout duration (min), and work time without rest periods (min) are shown in Table 1. In order to record the HR of each subject in one OM, three official matches in total were monitored at the end of the fourth week of this study as the subjects played on different teams. One OM was played between the first and fourth place of U18 league at 13:30 pm on the Saturday while the other OM was between the second and fifth place of the same league at 13:30 pm on the Sunday. The third OM, a U16 league match, was played between the U16 teams of two first division soccer clubs at 11:00 am on the Sunday. All of these OMs were played on artificial grass pitches. In addition, there was no red card and no injury in the OMs.

Table 1. Characteristics of the small sided games including goalkeepers and official match (OM).

Games	Pitch Dimension (m)	Pitch Size (m^2)	Pitch Size per Player (m^2/player)	Number of Bouts	Bout Duration (min)	Total Time Without Rest Periods (min)
3-a-side	25 × 20	500	83	6	2	12
4-a-side	35 × 30	1050	131	4	3	12
5-a-side	45 × 30	1350	135	3	4	12
7-a-side	55 × 40	2200	157	2	6	12
9-a-side	70 × 40	2800	155	2	8	16
OM	105 × 65	6825	341	1	90	90

Heart rates were continuously recorded at 5 s intervals using short-range radio telemetry (Polar Team Sport System, Polar Electro OY, Kempele, Finland) during the SSGs and OM. Recorded HRs were then downloaded on to a computer using the Team system interface unit following each SGG and OM. Average HR and time spent in zones corresponding to ≤69%, 70%–84%, 85%–89%, 90%–94% and 95%–100% of HR_{max} were calculated for all bouts and for each subject. Proportion of time spent (PTS) in the respective HRZs was calculated by dividing the time spent corresponding to HRZ to the total exercise duration for each SGG and OM. Rest periods between exercise bouts were excluded from the analysis.

2.5. Statistical Analysis

Data are expressed as means (M) ± standard deviations (SD). The normality distribution of the data was checked using the Kolmogorov–Smirnov test. A one-way multivariate repeated-measure analysis of variance (MANOVA) was then conducted to evaluate the differences between the SSGs and OM in terms of PTS in each HRZ. HR and $\%HR_{max}$ values were analyzed using a one-way repeated-measures analysis of variance. The Bonferroni procedure was applied to make pairwise comparisons among the different-sided games. The level of statistical significance was set at $p \leqslant 0.05$. Effect sizes (η^2) were also calculated and values of 0.01, 0.05 and above 0.15 were considered small, medium and large, respectively [26]. All statistical analysis was carried out using SPSS statistical software (SPSS Version 15.0 for Windows, Chicago, IL, USA).

3. Results

Figure 1 shows the mean ± standard deviation frequency of HR and $\%HR_{max}$ values during SSGs and OM. The lowest HR and $\%HR_{max}$ responses (156.1 ± 11.4 bpm, 79.4% ± 6.4%, respectively) were found in 9-a-side game, while the 3-a-side game resulted in the highest HR and $\%HR_{max}$ responses (177.1 ± 7.3 bpm, 90.0% ± 3.0%, respectively). One-way repeated ANOVA showed statistical significant differences among SSGs and OM in terms of HR (F = 25.057; $p = 0.001$; $\eta^2 = 0.544$; large effect) and $\%HR_{max}$ (F = 25.594; $p = 0.001$; $\eta^2 = 0.549$; large effect). *Post hoc* pairwise comparisons revealed that 3-a-side elicits significantly higher HR and $\%HR_{max}$ responses than other SSGs and OM, whereas 9-a-side elicits significantly lower HR and $\%HR_{max}$ responses compared to other SSGs and OM.

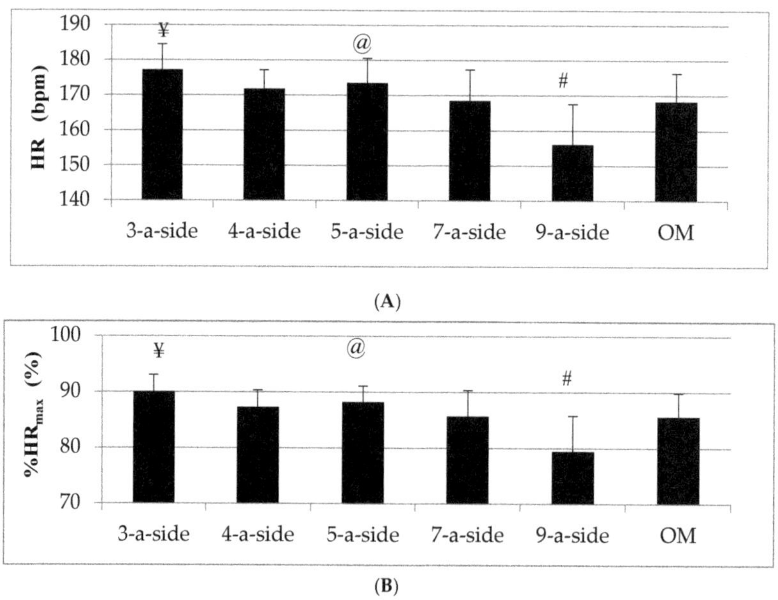

Figure 1. Mean HR (**A**) and $\%HR_{max}$ (**B**) during small sided games (SSGs) and official match (OM). HR: Heart rate; ¥ significantly different from other SSGs formats and OM, $p < 0.05$; @ significantly different from 7-a-side game, $p < 0.05$; # significantly different from all other SSGs formats and OM, $p < 0.05$.

Table 2 shows the mean PTS (± SD) in different HRZs for each SSG format as well as for the OM. One-way repeated ANOVA showed statistical significant differences among SSGs and OM in terms of ≤69% of HRZ (F = 5.242; $p = 0.001$; $\eta^2 = 0.200$; large effect), 70%–84% of HRZ (F = 40.913; $p = 0.001$; $\eta^2 = 0.661$; large effect), 85%–89% (F = 2.644; $p = 0.027$; $\eta^2 = 0.112$; medium effect), 90%–94% (F = 23.805; $p = 0.001$; $\eta^2 = 0.531$; large effect) and 95%–100% of HRZ (F = 6.190; $p = 0.001$; $\eta^2 = 0.228$; large effect). *Post hoc* pairwise comparisons revealed that 3-a-side had a significantly lower PTS in the under

⩽69% of HRZ than other SSG formats. In addition, a 9-a-side game and OM had significantly higher PTS in the 70%–84% of HRZs than all other SSGs. Moreover, 7-a-side had significantly higher PTS in the 85%–89% of HRZ compared to OM. Furthermore, 9-a-side games had significantly lower PTS in the 90%–94% of HRZ than all other SSGs and OM. In addition, OM had significantly lower PTS in the 90%–94% of HRZ than in 3-a-side. Lastly, 9-a-side had significantly lower PTS in the 95%–100% of HRZ than OM and all other SSG formats with the exception of 7-a-side.

Table 2. Mean proportion of time spent (%) in respective heart rate zones during small sided games and official match (± SD).

Zones	Games					
	3-a-Side	4-a-Side	5-a-Side	7-a-Side	9-a-Side	OM
95%–100%	14.2 ± 18.2 §	13.6 ± 16.1 §	16.0 ± 17.9 §	4.9 ± 10.6	1.2 ± 3.0	12.9 ± 11.5 §
90%–94%	48.1 ± 20.8 §	37.3 ± 17.9 §	35.9 ± 17.7 §	35.3 ± 17.3 §	7.9 ± 10.0	24.9 ± 10.0 *,§
85%–89%	21.3 ± 14.7	22.8 ± 14.2	25.2 ± 15.3	32.9 ± 15.3 ¥	20.8 ± 15.7	22.1 ± 5.7
70%–84%	14.6 ± 7.8 §,¥	18.7 ± 11.7 §,¥	17.8 ± 10.5 §,¥	17.8 ± 16.2 §,¥	54.5 ± 18.3 ¥	31.9 ± 12.2 §
⩽69%	1.7 ± 2.5	7.6 ± 6.1 *	5.0 ± 2.9 *	7.3 ± 6.8 *	15.0 ± 17.1 *	8.2 ± 12.2

OM: Official match; * significantly different from 3-a-side game, $p < 0.05$; § significantly different from 9-a-side game, $p < 0.05$; ¥ significantly different from OM, $p < 0.05$.

4. Discussion

The purpose of this study was to investigate the heart rate responses during SSGs and OM in young soccer players. In this study, different formats of SSGs were used when compared the SSGs with a different number of players and OM. The main findings show that 3-a-side, 4-a-side and 5-a-side SSG formats provide players with the opportunity to spend sufficient PTS in high intensity zones, while 7-a-side and 9-a-side SSG formats provide players with the opportunity to spend sufficient PTS in low intensity zones, which are specific to match demands.

Hoff *et al.* [7] found HR and $\%HR_{max}$ to be a reliable way of establishing the exercise intensity carried out in small sided games. Therefore, in the present study, exercise intensity is determined by heart rate and percent of maximum heart rate during 3-a-side, 4-a-side, 5-a-side, 7-a-side, 9-a-side and OM. Mean $\%HR_{max}$ value of SSGs ranged between 79%–90% in the current study. These values are similar to previous studies [9,12,27,28]. In addition, the results of this study show that 3-a-side elicits significantly higher HR and % HR_{max} responses than other SSG formats and OM, whereas 9-a-side elicits significantly lower HR and percent of HR_{max} responses compared to other SSG formats and OM. The present study also shows that 5-a-side elicits significantly higher HR and $\%HR_{max}$ responses than 7-a-side. Little and Williams [9] found that, as the pitch size and the number of players increase in SSGs, HR and $\%HR_{max}$ responses of English professional soccer players decrease. Parallel to findings of Little and Williams [9], the current study shows that when the pitch size per player is increased, the intensity and the involvement into the SSGs might be decreased with the exception of 9-a-side *versus* OM. The reason may be due to different total work duration of these games. OM was played 90 min while total duration of 9-a-side game was played 16 min. Therefore, the increase of game duration may have caused to an increase in heart rate responses in OM compared to 9-a-side game.

This study shows that 9-a-side resulted in significantly lower PTS than 3-a-side, 4-a-side, 5-a-side and 7-a-side games and OM in the high intensity zone, which is 90%–94% of HRZ. In addition, PTS in a very high intensity zone, which is 95%–100% of HRZ, was similar in OM and the SSGs with the exception of 7-a-side and 9-a-side games. Thus, the present study shows that 3-a-side, 4-a-side, 5-a-side games allow match specific high intensity loads. When the pitch size per player is increased, the intensity and the involvement into the SSGs might be decreased. In addition, reductions in the number of players have also been found to increase the number of technical actions such as ball contacts [4,29]. In addition, Jones and Drust [4] reported that backwards and sideways movements increase when the number of the players is decreased. Therefore, backwards and sideways movements may be a possible reason of spending more time in higher HRZ in SSGs when the number of players is decreased. Parallel to the present study results, Owen *et al.* [29] found that 3-a-side games elicited significantly higher exercise intensity in terms of a greater amount of time spent in intense HRZ compared to 9-a-side games. Hill-Haas *et al.* [30] found that the 2-a-side format elicited a greater amount of time spent above 90% HR_{max} than the 4-a-side and 6-a-side formats.

There are some limitations of the present study. One of these limitations, unfortunately, involved not being able to measure the distance covered at various running speeds and technical actions, and, therefore, future studies that investigate time-motion analysis and technical actions during the SSGs and OM are needed. In addition, another limitation of this study was not equal for some variables such as pitch size, pitch size per players, number of bouts, bouts duration and total time in SSGs. For example, players performed 16 min for 9-a-side game, while players performed 12 min for all the other SSGs.

5. Conclusions

Little [2] stated that SSGs that involve more players, such as 5-a-side, 6-a-side, 7-a-side, and 8-a-side games, can be used to develop the anaerobic threshold (85%–90% of HR_{max}), whereas 3-a-side and 4-a-side games might be used with the aim of enhancing maximum oxygen consumption. The results of this study suggest that 3-a-side, 4-a-side and 5-a-side games could be used for high intensity soccer specific aerobic endurance training. However, if coaches want higher %HR_{max} responses and PTS in high intensity zones, they should be organize 3-a-side games. In addition, 7-a-side and 9-a-side games have lower HR responses compared to OM. Therefore, 7-a-side and 9-a-side games seem to not be suitable for high intensity training principles. Finally, 7-a-side and 9-a-side games may be used for low intensity aerobic training by coaches.

Conflicts of Interest: The author declares no conflict of interest.

References

1. Impellizzeri, F.M.; Marcora, S.M.; Castagna, C.; Reilly, T.; Sassi, A.; Iaia, F.M.; Rampinini, E. Physiological and performance effects of generic *versus* specific aerobic training in soccer players. *Int. J. Sports Med.* **2006**, *27*, 483–492. [CrossRef] [PubMed]
2. Little, T. Optimizing the Use of Soccer Drills for Physiological Development. *Strength Cond. J.* **2009**, *31*, 67–74. [CrossRef]
3. Kelly, D.M.; Drust, B. The effect of pitch dimensions on heart rate responses and technical demands of small-sided soccer games in elite players. *J. Sci. Med. Sport* **2009**, *12*, 475–479. [CrossRef] [PubMed]
4. Jones, S.; Drust, B. Physiological and Technical Demands of 4 v 4 and 8 v 8 Games in Elite Youth Soccer Players. *Kinesiology* **2007**, *39*, 150–156.
5. Capranica, L.; Tessitore, A.; Guidetti, L.; Figura, F. Heart rate and match analysis in pre-pubescent soccer players. *J. Sports Sci.* **2001**, *196*, 379–384. [CrossRef] [PubMed]
6. Dellal, A.; Chamari, K.; Pintus, A.; Girard, O.; Cotte, T.; Keller, D. Heart rate responses during small-sided games and short intermittent running training in elite soccer players: A comparative study. *J. Strength Cond. Res.* **2008**, *22*, 1449–1457. [CrossRef] [PubMed]
7. Hoff, J.; Wisløff, U.; Engen, L.C.; Kemi, O.J.; Helgerud, J. Soccer specific aerobic endurance training. *Br. J. Sports Med.* **2002**, *36*, 218–221. [CrossRef] [PubMed]
8. Esposito, F.; Impellizzeri, F.M.; Margonato, V.; Vanni, R.; Pizzini, G.; Veicsteinas, A. Validity of heart rate as an indicator of aerobic demand during soccer activities in amateur soccer players. *Eur. J. Appl. Physiol.* **2004**, *93*, 167–172. [CrossRef] [PubMed]
9. Little, T.; Williams, A.G. Suitability of soccer training drills for endurance training. *J. Strength Cond. Res.* **2006**, *20*, 316–319. [PubMed]
10. Little, T.; Williams, A.G. Measures of exercise intensity during soccer training drills with professional soccer players. *J. Strength Cond. Res.* **2007**, *21*, 367–371. [CrossRef] [PubMed]

11. Rampinini, E.; Impellizzeri, F.M.; Castagna, C.; Abt, G.; Chamari, K.; Sassi, A.; Marcora, S.M. Factors influencing physiological responses to small-sided soccer games. *J. Sports Sci.* **2007**, *25*, 659–666. [CrossRef] [PubMed]
12. Köklü, Y. A comparison of physiological responses to various intermittent and continuous small-sided games in young soccer players. *J. Hum. Kinet.* **2012**, *31*, 89–96. [CrossRef] [PubMed]
13. Koçak, F.U.; Alemdaroğlu, U.; Dündar, U. Comparison of the physiological responses to different small-sided games in elite young soccer players. *J. Strength Cond. Res.* **2011**, *25*, 1522–1528. [CrossRef] [PubMed]
14. Mallo, J.; Navarro, E. Physical load imposed on soccer players during small-sided training games. *J. Sports Med. Phys. Fit.* **2008**, *48*, 166–171.
15. Williams, K.; Owen, A. The impact of player numbers on the physiological responses to small sided games. *J. Sport. Sci. Med.* **2007**, *6*, 100.
16. Köklü, Y.; Albayrak, M.; Keysan, H.; Alemdaroğlu, U.; Dellal, A. Improvement of the physical conditioning of young soccer players by playing small-sided games on different pitch size—Special reference to physiological responses I Unapredenje kondicijske pripremljenosti mladih nogometaša igranjem malog nogometa na igr. *Kinesiology* **2013**, *45*, 41–47.
17. Köklü, Y.; Sert, Ö.; Alemdaroğlu, U.; Arslan, Y. Comparison of the physiological responses and time-motion characteristics of young soccer players in small-sided games: The effect of goalkeeper. *J. Strength Cond. Res.* **2015**, *29*, 964–971. [CrossRef] [PubMed]
18. Bangsbo, J.; Nørregaard, L.; Thorsø, F. Activity profile of competition soccer. *Can. J. Sport Sci.* **1991**, *16*, 110–116. [PubMed]
19. Strøyer, J.; Hansen, L.; Klausen, K. Physiological profile and activity pattern of young soccer players during match play. *Med. Sci. Sports Exerc.* **2004**, *36*, 168–174. [CrossRef] [PubMed]
20. Bangsbo, J.; Mohr, M.; Krustrup, P. Physical and metabolic demands of training and match-play in the elite football player. *J. Sports Sci.* **2006**, *24*, 665–674. [CrossRef] [PubMed]
21. Gabbett, T.J.; Mulvey, M.J. Time-motion analysis of small-sided training games and competition in elite women soccer players. *J. Strength Cond. Res.* **2008**, *22*, 543–552. [CrossRef] [PubMed]
22. Dellal, A.; Owen, A.; Wong, D.P.; Krustrup, P.; van Exsel, M.; Mallo, J. Technical and physical demands of small *vs.* large sided games in relation to playing position in elite soccer. *Hum. Mov. Sci.* **2012**, *31*, 957–969. [CrossRef] [PubMed]
23. Helgerud, J.; Engen, L.; Wisløff, U.; Hoff, J. Aerobic endurance training improves soccer performance. *Med. Sci. Sport. Exerc.* **2001**, *33*, 1925–1931. [CrossRef]
24. Aslan, A. Cardiovascular responses, perceived exertion and technical actions during small-sided recreational soccer: Effects of pitch size and number of players. *J. Hum. Kinet.* **2013**, *38*, 95–105. [CrossRef] [PubMed]
25. Castellano, J.; Casamichana, D.; Dellal, A. Influence of Game Format and Number of Players on Heart Rate Responses and Physical Demands in Small-Sided Soccer Games. *J. Strength Cond. Res.* **2013**, *27*, 1295–1303. [CrossRef] [PubMed]
26. Cohen, J. Statistical power analysis for the behavioral sciences. *Stat. Power Anal. Behav. Sci.* **1988**, *2*, 567.
27. Aroso, J.; Rebelo, A.N.; Gomes-Pereira, J. Physiological impact of selected game-related exercises. *J. Sports Sci.* **2004**, *22*, 522.
28. Fanchini, M.; Azzalin, A.; Castagna, C.; Schena, F.; McCall, A.; Impellizzeri, F.M. Effect of bout duration on exercise intensity and technical performance of small-sided games in soccer. *J. Strength Cond. Res.* **2011**, *25*, 453–458. [CrossRef] [PubMed]
29. Owen, A.L.; Wong, D.P.; Mckenna, M.; Dellal, A. Heart rate responses and technical comparison between small- *vs.* large-sided games in elite professional soccer. *J. Strength Cond. Res.* **2011**, *25*, 2104–2110. [CrossRef] [PubMed]
30. Hill-Haas, S.V.; Dawson, B.T.; Coutts, A.J.; Rowsell, G.J. Physiological responses and time-motion characteristics of various small-sided soccer games in youth players. *J. Sports Sci.* **2009**, *27*, 1–8. [CrossRef] [PubMed]

17

Improvement in 100-m Sprint Performance at an Altitude of 2250 m

Nicholas P. Linthorne

Department of Life Sciences, Brunel University London, Uxbridge, Middlesex, UB8 3PH, UK; nick.linthorne@brunel.ac.uk

Academic Editor: Eling de Bruin

Abstract: A fair system of recognizing records in athletics should consider the influence of environmental conditions on performance. The aim of this study was to determine the effect of an altitude of 2250 m on the time for a 100-m sprint. Competition results from the 13 Olympic Games between 1964 and 2012 were corrected for the effects of wind and de-trended for the historical improvement in performance. The time advantage due to competing at an altitude of 2250 m was calculated from the difference between the mean race time at the 1968 Olympic Games in Mexico City and the mean race times at the low-altitude competition venues. The observed time advantage of Mexico City was 0.19 ($\pm$0.02) s for men and 0.21 ($\pm$0.05) s for women ($\pm$90% confidence interval). These results indicate that 100-m sprinters derive a substantial performance advantage when competing at a high-altitude venue and that an altitude of 1000 m provides an advantage equivalent to a 2 m/s assisting wind (0.10 s). Therefore, the altitude of the competition venue as well as the wind speed during the race should be considered when recognizing record performances.

Keywords: altitude; athletics; Olympic Games; sprinting

---

1. Introduction

Although head-to-head competition is the primary purpose of an organized athletics meeting, the setting of record performances is also of considerable interest to athletes and spectators. Performance in a 100-m sprint can be substantially aided by a strong following wind and so the International Association of Athletic Federations (IAAF) has a limit of 2 m/s for the allowable assisting wind when recognizing 100-m records [1]. However, there is currently no restriction on the altitude of the competition venue, even though there is strong empirical evidence that sprint performances are substantially aided by a high-altitude venue [2–5]. A high-altitude competition venue is believed to improve sprint performance through a reduction in air density, which reduces the aerodynamic drag force acting on the athlete and hence allows the athlete to reach a greater top speed [6]. This benefit is expected to be partly offset by the lower partial pressure of oxygen in the atmosphere, which reduces the aerobic power that can be generated by the athlete's muscles and, hence, increases the time taken to cover the race distance [7].

To date, there is no firmly accepted value for the effect of altitude on a 100-m sprint performance. Several modelling studies have calculated the time advantage of a performance at an altitude of 2250 m (the altitude of Mexico City, site of the 1968 Olympic Games). However, the results range considerably, from as low as 0.05 s to as high as 0.18 s [7–12]. The results from these modelling studies are strongly dependent on the values of aerodynamic and power generation parameters, but some of these parameter values are not particularly well known (e.g., the drag area of the athlete).

Several studies have shown that results from sports competitions can be an extensive source of carefully measured data for use in biomechanical and physiological studies [2,12–14]. By selecting appropriate competition data, an investigator can study the influence of a chosen variable on athletic performance. Therefore, one way of quantifying the effect of altitude on 100-m sprint times is to compare competition performances achieved at high-altitude venues to those achieved at venues near to sea-level. Ward-Smith [6] and Behncke [9] conducted this type of study using competition results from the Olympic Games. Ward-Smith found that the men's 100-m sprint performances at the Mexico City 1968 Olympic Games (altitude 2250 m) were improved by 0.17 (±0.13) s (±90% confidence interval) relative to performances at other Olympic Games, and Behncke calculated that performances were improved by 0.17 (±0.10) s for men and 0.18 (±0.13) s for women. Unfortunately, these studies had large confidence intervals associated with their results because they compared only a few competitions (five and three, respectively) and used performances by only a few athletes in each competition (three and six, respectively). Also, the accuracy of the results is questionable because the studies did not correct the race times for the effect of wind, used a mix of hand times and electronic times, and Behnke did not account for the historical trend in performance.

The aim of the present study was to obtain a more accurate estimate of the effect of altitude on 100-m sprint times by conducting a more substantive analysis of competition results from the Olympic Games. The present study analyzed race times by every 100-m competitor in the 13 Olympic Games competitions between 1964 and 2012. This study had a more thorough account of the confounding factors in the competition data (including the effect of wind and the historical trend in performance), and so was expected to give a more accurate estimate of the time advantage of altitude at the Mexico City 1968 Olympic Games (and with a smaller confidence interval) than those obtained in previous studies.

2. Methods

The electronic times and wind readings for all rounds of the 100-m competitions at the Olympic Games between 1964 and 2012 (about 3250 performances) were obtained from the archives of the Association of Track and Field Statisticians (ATFS). For the Olympic Games prior to 1964 the record of electronic times and wind readings is not complete and so these competitions were not included in the study. The possibility of a gender difference in the effect of altitude on 100-m sprint performance was considered by analyzing the men's and women's competitions separately.

The time advantage of competing at an altitude of 2250 m was obtained by calculating an average performance at each Olympic Games, plotting the results as a function of the year of competition, and then comparing the result from the Mexico City 1968 competition to the data from the other competitions. To obtain an accurate value for the time advantage of an altitude of 2250 m, the confounding factors in the Olympic Games competition data (both between the competitions and within each competition) needed to be considered. In this study the velocity of the wind during the race, the historical trend in 100-m performances, and the sub-maximal performances in the early rounds of the competition were expected to be the largest confounding factors. Other lesser factors were expected to be the non-zero altitude of some of the competition venues, variations in the standard of the athletes at the competitions, and different types of track surface.

2.1. Corrections for Wind and Historical Trend

The competition performances from the Olympic Games were adjusted to a zero wind performance, T_o, using

$$T_o = T + \alpha (V_W - \beta V_W{}^2), \quad (1)$$

where T is the athlete's official race time; V_W is the wind reading; and α and β are constants [14]. For international standard sprinters α = 0.050 s/m, and β = 0.0556 s^2/m for men and β = 0.0667 s^2/m for women. The time advantage of a 2 m/s tailwind is therefore about 0.10 s for men and about 0.12 s for women.

The mathematical form of the historical trend in 100-m performances was determined by examining the world ranking lists for the period between 1950 and 2015. Performances prior to

1975 are hand times and so a correction of 0.24 s was applied to these times [15]. The mean of the twenty highest-ranked athletes in each year was calculated, the mean values were plotted as a function of year, and a selection of mathematical equations was fitted to the data. The fitted curves included a second-order polynomial, a third-order polynomial, a rectangular hyperbola, an exponential curve, a four-parameter symmetric logistic curve, a five-parameter logistic curve, and a six-parameter generalized logistic curve. The decision about the most appropriate curve was guided by a locally weighted regression (loess) fit to the data and by examining the distribution of the residuals [16]. If two or more fitted curves seemed appropriate for the data, a calculation of Akaike's Information Criterion was used to determine which of the curves gave the best fit [17].

2.2. *Calculation of Mean Race Time for an Olympic Games Competition*

Athletes do not always produce a maximum-effort performance in every round of a 100-m competition [14]. Therefore, for each of the 13 Olympic Games competitions, the athletes' best wind-corrected performance in the competition was identified and the athletes were ranked according to this performance (*i.e.*, A_1, A_2, A_3, … A_n, for the athletes ranked 1 to n, where n is the number of athletes in the competition). The mean race time for each Olympic Games competition was then calculated from the ranking list of athletes. However, the uncertainty in a mean race time depends on the number of athletes used in the calculation [18]. In addition, including the highest-ranked athletes (*i.e.*, 1st, 2nd, 3rd, …) in the calculation of the mean race time might not produce the lowest possible uncertainty in the mean race time. To identify the optimum selection of athletes to include in the calculation of the mean race time, the mean race time (and its associated uncertainty) was calculated using (n_{mean} =) 5, 10, 15, 20, 25, 30, 35, or 40 athletes, and for each choice of n_{mean} the middle-ranked athlete in the group (A_{mid}) was systematically varied over a wide range. As an illustration of this process, if the calculation of the mean race time used five athletes and the middle-ranked athlete in the group of five was the 27th-ranked athlete (*i.e.*, $n_{mean} = 5$ and $A_{mid} = 27$), then the calculation used athletes A_{25}, A_{26}, A_{27}, A_{28}, and A_{29}. For each Olympic Games competition the uncertainty in the mean race time was plotted against A_{mid} and n_{mean}. These plots were examined to identify the optimum n_{mean} and A_{mid} that minimized the uncertainty in the mean race time. These optimum values were then used to calculate the mean race time for each of the Olympic Games competitions.

2.3. *Time Advantage of Mexico City*

To calculate the time advantage of competing at Mexico City, the historical improvement in performance was removed by de-trending the Olympic Games competition data with a curve of the same shape as the best fit to the world rankings data. The difference of the Mexico City Olympic Games data from the mean time of the other Olympic Games competitions was then taken as the time advantage of competing at an altitude of 2250 m.

2.4. *Other Confounding Factors*

In this study it was initially assumed that all the Olympic Games competitions between 1964 and 2012 (except Mexico City 1968) were held at venues close to sea-level. However, the Munich 1972 and Atlanta 1996 Olympic Games were held at venues that are at a moderately high altitude (Munich, 520 m; Atlanta, 305 m). The time advantages of competing at Munich and Atlanta were expected to be about 30% and 18% of the time advantage of competing at Mexico City [8]. Therefore, corrections of 30% and 18% were applied to the Munich 1972 and Atlanta 1996 data, and the Olympic Games data were re-analyzed. The effects of the altitude of the Munich and Atlanta competition venues were also tested by removing the Munich 1972 and Atlanta 1996 data from the analysis.

The Olympic Games is the world's premier athletics competition and many of the best 100-m sprinters attended the competitions. However, the 1976 Olympic Games in Montreal was boycotted by 18 nations (mostly African), the 1980 Olympic Games in Moscow was boycotted by many Western nations (most notably USA, Canada, and West Germany), and the 1984 Olympic Games in Los Angeles was boycotted by 17 Eastern Bloc nations (most notably USSR, East Germany, Bulgaria, Poland, and Cuba). The effects of these boycotts were tested by removing the affected competitions and re-analyzing the Olympic Games data.

The Tokyo 1964 Olympic Games was held on a cinders track, but all subsequent Olympic Games competitions were conducted on synthetic tracks. To test for the effects of different types of track surface in the Olympic Games data, the Tokyo 1964 competition was removed and the Olympic Games data were re-analyzed.

3. Results

Figure 1 shows the mean of the twenty highest-ranked athletes in each year between 1950 and 2015. The best fit curve for both the men and women was a four-parameter logistic curve [19],

$$T_{\text{rank}} = \frac{T_{\text{max}} - T_{\text{min}}}{1 + e^{-a(Y - Y_{\text{inf}})}} + T_{\text{min}}, \quad (2)$$

where T_{rank} is the mean time of the top 20 athletes in the world rankings; Y is the year; T_{max} is the asymptotic maximum time; T_{min} is the asymptotic minimum time; Y_{inf} is the year at the inflection point of the curve; and a is a measure of the growth rate. The values of the regression coefficients were T_{max} = 11.37 s, T_{min} = 9.87 s, Y_{inf} = 1955 years, and a = –0.054 per year for the men; and T_{max} = 12.58 s, T_{min} = 10.96 s, Y_{inf} = 1962 years, and a = –0.098 per year for the women.

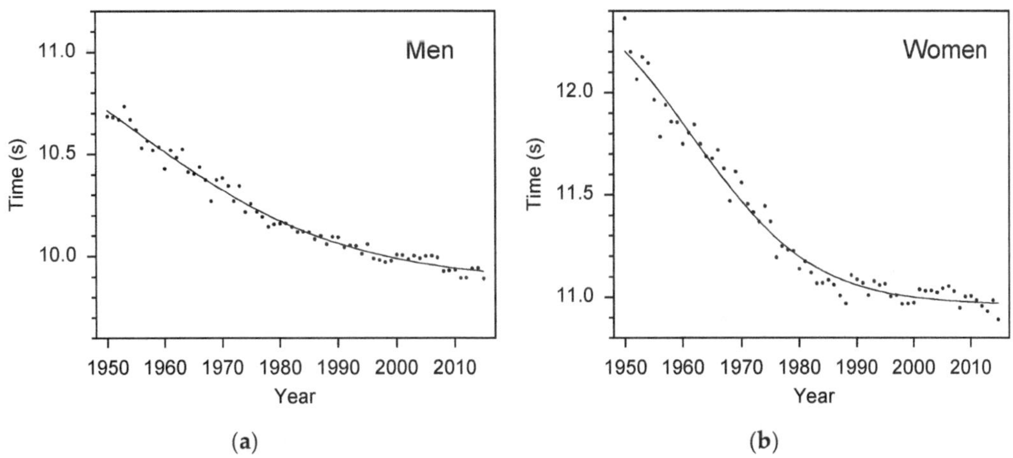

Figure 1. These plots show the historical trend in world 100-m standards; (**a**) men, (**b**) women. Data points are the mean of the top 20 athletes in each year. The fitted curve is a 4-parameter logistic curve (Equation (2)). Coefficient of determination: men r^2 = 0.98; women r^2 = 0.97.

There was an optimum choice of athletes to include in the calculation of the mean race time for an Olympic Games competition. For the men, the uncertainty (90% confidence limits) in the mean race time was lowest when the middle-ranked athlete in the calculation (A_{mid}) was ranked about 20–45, and a reliable value of the uncertainty (with only small random fluctuations) was attained when using greater than about 20 athletes in the calculation (Figure 2). Therefore, the mean race time for the Olympic Games competitions was taken as that calculated with n_{mean} = 20 and A_{mid} = 30. In a similar fashion, for the women the mean race time was taken as that calculated with n_{mean} = 20 and A_{mid} = 20. Figure 2 highlights that the uncertainty in the mean race time is substantially reduced when the top-ranked athletes in the competition are not included in the calculation.

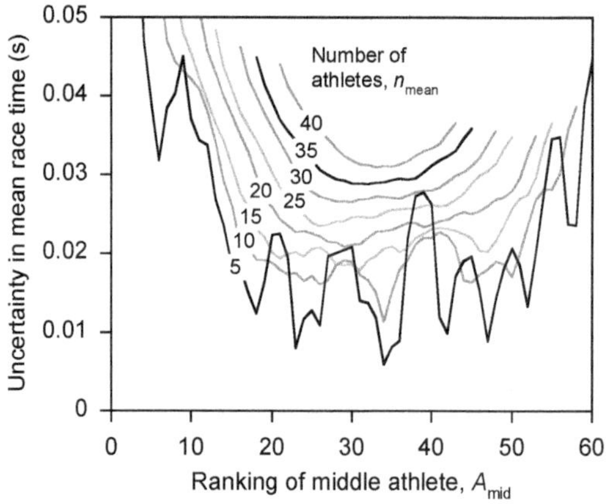

Figure 2. This plot shows there is an optimum choice of athletes to include in the calculation of the mean race time at an Olympic Games competition. The uncertainty (90% confidence interval) in the mean race time is lowest when the ranking of the middle athlete in the group of athletes used in the calculation is about A_{mid} = 20–45. When the number of athletes used in the calculation of the mean race time is less than about n_{mean} = 20, the uncertainty in the mean value is not reliable (*i.e.*, subject to excessive random fluctuations). The optimum values were taken to be A_{mid} = 30 and n_{mean} = 20. Data for the men at the Mexico City 1968 Olympic Games.

A plot of the mean race time for each Olympic Games competition showed a clear historical trend of improving performances, and this trend was similar to that of the world rankings data. The curve that was fitted to the Olympic Games data was constrained to be the same shape as the historical trend in 100-m performances by setting the values of T_{max}, T_{min}, Y_{inf}, and a to be equal to those obtained from the fit to the world rankings data. When calculating the fitted curve, the mean race time at each Olympic Games competition was weighted by the 90% confidence interval in the mean race time. For both the men and women, the deviations of the mean race times at each Olympic Games competition from the fitted curve showed a clear perturbation for the Mexico City 1968 Olympic Games (Figure 3). The time advantage of Mexico City was 0.19 (±0.02) s for the men and 0.22 (±0.05) s for the women.

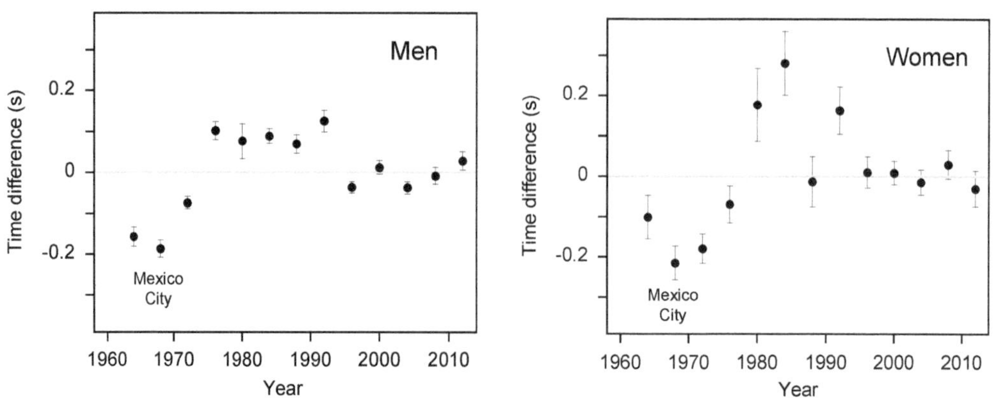

(**a**) (**b**)

Figure 3. These plots show the mean race times at Olympic Games competitions from 1964 to 2012 after de-trending with a curve of the same shape as the historical trend in 100-m performances; (**a**) men, (**b**) women. Vertical error bars indicate the 90% confidence interval in the mean. There is a substantial deviation at the Mexico City 1968 Olympic Games due to the high altitude of this site (2250 m).

The time advantage of Mexico City was insensitive to the number of athletes (n_{mean}) used to calculate the mean race time at the competitions. Using 15 or 25 athletes (rather than 20) changed the calculated time advantage of Mexico City by less than 0.01 s. Similarly, the time advantage of Mexico City was insensitive to the choice of middle-ranked athlete (A_{mid}). For the men, using the 20th or 40th ranked athlete (rather than the 30th) changed the time advantage by less than 0.01 s. For the women, using the 10th or 30th ranked athlete (rather than the 20th) changed the time advantage by less than 0.01 s.

Applying a 30% altitude correction to the Munich 1972 data (0.05–0.07 s) had little effect on the results. The calculated time advantages of Mexico City were increased by less than 0.01 s and there was little change in the uncertainties. Likewise, applying an 18% altitude correction to the Atlanta 1996 data (0.03–0.04 s) had little effect on the results. Removing the data for the boycotted competitions had only a small effect on the results. With the Moscow 1980 and Los Angeles 1984 competitions removed the calculated time advantages of Mexico City were reduced by about 0.01 s, and with the Montreal 1976 competition removed the calculated time advantages of Mexico City were reduced by less than 0.01 s. When the Tokyo 1964 competition (which was held on a cinders track) was removed from the analysis the calculated time advantages of Mexico City were increased by about 0.01 s.

In summary, the calculated time advantage of Mexico City was insensitive to the choices of n_{mean} and A_{mid}, the non-zero altitude of some of the competition venues, boycotts at competitions, and different types of track surface. For the men, the most accurate estimate from this study is probably that with an altitude correction for the Munich 1972 Olympic Games. For this scenario the time advantage of Mexico City is 0.19 ($\pm$0.02) s. For the women, the most accurate estimate from this study is probably that with an altitude correction for Munich 1972 and with the Moscow 1980 and Los Angeles 1984 competitions removed from the data. For this scenario the time advantage of Mexico City is 0.21 ($\pm$0.05) s. The uncertainty in the time advantage of Mexico City was mainly due to the uncertainty in the mean race time at the Mexico City 1968 Olympic Games, rather than due to the uncertainty in the curve fitted to the Olympic Games competition data.

4. Discussion

This study confirmed that athletes derived a substantial performance advantage in the 100-m at the Mexico City 1968 Olympic Games. The estimates of the time advantage were similar to those obtained by Ward-Smith [6] and Behncke [9]. However, the estimates from the present study have a considerably lower uncertainty, which was mostly due to analyzing a more appropriate selection of athletes. Also, the estimates obtained in the present study should be more accurate because the race times were corrected for the effect of wind and for the historical trend in performances.

The results from the present study indicate that there is no substantial difference between men and women in the time advantage of competing at a high-altitude venue. This finding is consistent with results from mathematical modelling studies [7,8], which predict only small gender differences (less than 0.01 s) due to the combined effects of differences in body size, the time to complete the race, and the athlete's velocity profile.

The uncertainty in the calculated time advantage of Mexico City reported for this study is purely statistical and does not include systematic factors. Although considerable care was taken to account for the most likely confounding factors (*i.e.*, wind velocity, the historical trend in performance, submaximal performances in the early rounds, variations in the standard of athletes at the competition, and track surface), Figure 3 shows there is still substantial unexplained variance in the mean race times for the Olympic Games competitions. That is, there might be other confounding factors that were not considered in this study. Potential factors include: the time of year when the competition was held; differences in the time for the sound of the starting gun to travel to the athletes from the starting gun; differences in athlete footwear and track stiffness; inter-athlete differences in frontal area; the effects of differences in air temperature, barometric pressure, and humidity on the aerodynamic drag experienced by an athlete [6,20]; and the effect of temperature on the generation of muscular power.

We cannot exclude the possibility that one or more of these factors (or another unidentified factor) made a substantial contribution to the calculated time advantage of the 1968 Mexico City Olympic Games.

4.1. Other Competition Analyses and Mathematical Models

Hollings and colleagues [2] also used competition data to determine the effect of altitude on 100-m sprint times. However, they did not use data from the Mexico City 1968 Olympic Games. Rather, they used mixed linear modelling to examine performances by elite male athletes in major competitions (6628 performances by 56 athletes) during a ten-year period from 2000 to 2009. They found that performances produced at venues above 1000 m were 0.05 (±0.02) s (±99% confidence interval) faster than those produced at venues below 1000 m. Assuming an average altitude difference of 1000 m between the two groups of performances, and assuming a relation between altitude and time advantage proposed by Arsac [8], the result from Hollings and colleagues indicates that competing at Mexico City (2250 m) should confer a time advantage of about 0.10 (±0.04) s. The accuracy of the altitude result obtained by Hollings and colleagues is strengthened by their result for the effect of a 2 m/s tailwind; 0.08 (±0.02) s, which is similar to the value (0.10 s) obtained by Linthorne [14] in a study of competition results. However, the study by Hollings and colleagues might have obtained more accurate estimates for altitude and wind had it also considered the historical increase in performance (about 0.04 s) over the period of the study. Also, the accuracy of the method used by Hollings and colleagues would be strengthened if an analysis of elite female athletes was conducted and produced a value similar to that obtained for elite male athletes.

Several investigators have used mathematical models to calculate the time advantage of performing a 100-m sprint in Mexico City. For the force models developed by Dapena and Feltner [10], Mureika [11], and Behncke [9], the time advantages were 0.05 s, 0.08 s, and 0.10 s, respectively. For the power models developed by Arsac [8], Ward-Smith [6], and Péronnet and colleagues [7], the time advantages were 0.16 s, 0.17 s, and 0.18 s, respectively. Both types of model produced velocity-time curves that were similar to those for elite sprinters. However, the altitude predictions of the models are sensitive to the athlete's effective drag area, which is only known to an accuracy of about 20% [21]. Also, Ward-Smith [21] suggested that a mathematical model of sprinting should include the effects of changes in aerodynamic drag on the angle of forward lean of the athlete's body, as this is expected to affect the athlete's ability to generate a forward propulsive force. In summary, results from mathematical modelling studies of the effect of altitude on sprint performance should be viewed with caution.

4.2. Implications for IAAF Rules

The breaking of national and world records is an important part of major athletics competitions, and some competitions offer substantial financial rewards to encourage athletes to set a record (e.g., $100,000 for a world record at the IAAF World Championships). For a performance to be recognized as a record, the performance must conform to specific regulations concerning the conduct of the event, the method of measuring the performance, the dimensions and properties of the track, the equipment used by the athlete, and doping control [1]. A fair system of recognizing record performances requires precise quantitative information on the effects of environmental conditions so that limits can be placed on the allowable range of conditions. At present, the only environmental factor that is considered when recognizing a record performance is the strength of the wind in the direction of running. In the 100-m sprint a performance will not be accepted if there is an assisting wind that averages more than 2 m/s.

Two important criteria when selecting the limits on an environmental condition are: (1) the limits should encompass the most commonly experienced conditions at the large majority of competition venues; and (2) the limits should eliminate only those performances that receive a substantial advantage relative to a performance achieved under the most common conditions. For the 100-m races at the Olympic Games between 1964 and 2012, about 94% had wind readings of between –2 and +2 m/s, and only 4% were not eligible for consideration for a record (*i.e.*, an assisting wind greater than +2 m/s). In the 100-m sprint a 2 m/s assisting wind produces a time advantage of about 0.10–0.12 s relative to a performance achieved with a zero wind [14]. If the wind limit were to be set substantially higher than 2 m/s, athletes would be unlikely to set a record under the most common wind conditions.

A similar reasoning can be applied to the selection of the limits on the altitude of a competition venue. About 75% of the Earth's land surface is at an altitude of less than 1000 m [22], as are the vast majority of athletics competition venues [5]. If we assume the shape of the relationship between altitude and time advantage proposed by Arsac [8], the present study indicates that a time advantage of 0.10 s (equivalent to that from a 2 m/s assisting wind) is produced by an altitude of about 1000 m. Therefore, one can argue for an upper limit of about 1000 m when recognizing record performances. This proposed limit is the same as that already used by many athletics statisticians, who recognize the beneficial effect of high altitude by a listing sprinting and jumping performances achieved at venues above 1000 m as 'altitude-assisted' [5].

In addition to the 100-m sprint, the IAAF has a limit on wind assistance for the 200 m, 100 m hurdles, 110 m hurdles, long jump, and triple jump. The wind assistance limit is the same (2 m/s) for all these events, and it would be simplest if any altitude limit was also the same for all affected events. However, the present study of the effect of altitude was restricted to the 100-m sprint because this is the only event in which there is a reliable wind-correction curve [14]. Before studies similar to the present one can be conducted to determine of the effect of altitude on the other events, there needs to be reliable wind-correction equations for these events.

5. Conclusions

The time advantage for 100-m sprinters when competing at the 1968 Mexico City Olympic Games was 0.19 ($\pm$0.02) s for men and 0.21 ($\pm$0.05) s for women. This indicates that 100-m sprinters derive a substantial performance advantage when competing at a high-altitude venue. It is inferred that an altitude of 1000 m provides an advantage that is equivalent to a 2 m/s assisting wind (0.10 s). Therefore, the altitude of the competition venue should be considered when recognizing record performances in the 100-m sprint.

Conflicts of Interest: The author declares no conflict of interest.

References

1. International Association of Athletic Federations (IAAF). *IAAF Competition Rules 2016–2017*; International Association of Athletic Federations: Monaco, Monaco, 2015; pp. 168–169; 269–279.
2. Hollings, S.C.; Hopkins, W.G.; Hume, P.A. Environmental and venue-related factors affecting the performance of elite male track athletes. *Eur. J. Sport Sci.* **2012**, *12*, 201–206. [CrossRef]
3. Hymans, R. The Need for Altitude and Non-Altitude World Records. In *Athletics 1990: The International Track and Field Annual*; Matthews, P., Ed.; Sports World: London, UK, 1990; pp. 145–149.
4. Jokl, E.; Jokl, P. Analysis of winning times of track races for men in Mexico City in 1968 and Munich in 1972. *Olympic Rev.* **1972**, *60–61*, 461–464.
5. Matthews, P. (Ed.) *Athletics 2015: The International Track and Field Annual*; SportsBooks: York, UK, 2015; pp. 255–256.
6. Ward-Smith, A.J. Air resistance and its influence on the biomechanics and energetics of sprinting at sea level and at altitude. *J. Biomech.* **1984**, *17*, 339–347. [CrossRef]
7. Péronnet, F.; Thibault, G.; Cousineau, D.L. A theoretical analysis of the effect of altitude on running performance. *J. Appl. Physiol.* **1991**, *70*, 399–404.
8. Arsac, L.M. Effects of altitude on the energetics of human best performances in 100 m running: A theoretical analysis. *Eur. J. Appl. Physiol.* **2002**, *87*, 78–84. [CrossRef] [PubMed]
9. Behncke, H. Optimization models for the force and energy in competitive running. *J. Math. Biol.* **1997**, *35*, 375–390. [CrossRef] [PubMed]

10. Dapena, J.; Feltner, M.E. Effects of wind and altitude on the times of 100-meter sprint races. *Int. J. Sport Biomech.* **1987**, *3*, 6–39. [CrossRef]
11. Mureika, J.R. A quasi-physical model of the 100 m dash. *Can. J. Phys.* **2001**, *79*, 697–713. [CrossRef]
12. Jánosi, I.M.; Bántay, P. Statistical test of throwing events on the rotating earth: Lack of correlations between range and geographic location. *Eur. Phys. J. B* **2002**, *30*, 411–415. [CrossRef]
13. Lindsey, B.I. Sports records as biological data. *J. Biol. Educ.* **1975**, *9*, 89–91. [CrossRef]
14. Linthorne, N.P. The effect of wind on 100-m sprint times. *J. Appl. Biomech.* **1994**, *10*, 110–131.
15. International Association of Athletic Federations (IAAF). *IAAF Scoring Tables for Combined Events*; International Association of Athletic Federations: Monaco, Monaco, 2001; p. 25.
16. Cleveland, W.S. *The Elements of Graphing Data*; Hobart Press: Summit, NJ, USA, 1994; pp. 126–132; 168–180.
17. Motulsky, H.; Christopoulos, A. *Fitting Models to Biological Data Using Linear and Nonlinear Regression*; Oxford University Press: Oxford, UK, 2004; pp. 147–148.
18. Taylor, J.R. *An Introduction to Error Analysis: The Study of Uncertainties in Physical Measurement*, 2nd ed.; University Science Books: Sausalito, CA, USA, 1997; p. 110.
19. Richards, F.J. A flexible growth function for empirical use. *J. Exp. Bot.* **1959**, *10*, 290–300. [CrossRef]
20. Mureika, J.R. The effects of temperature, humidity, and barometric pressure on short-sprint race times. *Can. J. Phys.* **2006**, *84*, 311–324. [CrossRef]
21. Ward-Smith, A.J. New insights into the effect of wind assistance on sprinting performance. *J. Sports Sci.* **1999**, *17*, 325–334. [CrossRef] [PubMed]
22. Stacey, F.D.; Davis, P.M. *Physics of the Earth*, 4th ed.; Cambridge University Press: Cambridge, UK, 2008; p. 123.

18

Reliability and Validity of the Early Years Physical Activity Questionnaire (EY-PAQ)

Daniel D. Bingham [1,2,*], Paul J. Collings [1], Stacy A. Clemes [2], Silvia Costa [3], Gillian Santorelli [1], Paula Griffiths [2] and Sally E. Barber [1]

1 Bradford Institute for Health Research, Bradford BD9 6RJ, UK; Paul.Collings@bthft.nhs.uk (P.J.C.); Gillian.Santorelli@bthft.nhs.uk (G.S.); sally.barber@bthft.nhs.uk (S.E.B.)
2 School of Sport, Exercise and Health Sciences, Loughborough University, Leicestershire LE11 3TU, UK; S.A.Clemes@lboro.ac.uk (S.A.C.); P.Griffiths@lboro.ac.uk (P.G.)
3 Centre for Diet and Activity Research (CEDAR), MRC Epidemiology Unit, University of Cambridge, School of Clinical Medicine, Cambridge CB2 0QQ, UK; sc808@medschl.cam.ac.uk
* Correspondence: daniel.bingham@bthft.nhs.uk

Academic Editor: Eling Douwe de Bruin

Abstract: Measuring physical activity (PA) and sedentary time (ST) in young children (<5 years) is complex. Objective measures have high validity but require specialist expertise, are expensive, and can be burdensome for participants. A proxy-report instrument for young children that accurately measures PA and ST is needed. The aim of this study was to assess the reliability and validity of the Early Years Physical Activity Questionnaire (EY-PAQ). In a setting where English and Urdu are the predominant languages spoken by parents of young children, a sample of 196 parents and their young children (mean age 3.2 ± 0.8 years) from Bradford, UK took part in the study. A total of 156 (79.6%) questionnaires were completed in English and 40 (20.4%) were completed in transliterated Urdu. A total of 109 parents took part in the reliability aspect of the study, which involved completion of the EY-PAQ on two occasions (7.2 days apart; standard deviation (SD) = 1.1). All 196 participants took part in the validity aspect which involved comparison of EY-PAQ scores against accelerometry. Validty anaylsis used all data and data falling with specific MVPA and ST boundaries. Reliability was assessed using intra-class correlations (ICC) and validity by Bland–Altman plots and rank correlation coefficients. The test re-test reliability of the EY-PAQ was moderate for ST (ICC = 0.47) and fair for moderate-to-vigorous physical activity (MVPA)(ICC = 0.35). The EY-PAQ had poor agreement with accelerometer-determined ST (mean difference = −87.5 min· day^{-1}) and good agreement for MVPA (mean difference = 7.1 min· day^{-1}) limits of agreement were wide for all variables. The rank correlation coefficient was non-significant for ST (rho = 0.19) and significant for MVPA (rho = 0.30). The EY-PAQ has comparable validity and reliability to other PA self-report tools and is a promising population-based measure of young children's habitual MVPA but not ST. In situations when objective methods are not possible for measurement of young children's MVPA, the EY-PAQ may be a suitable alternative but only if boundaries are applied.

Keywords: physical activity; sedentary behaviour; measurement; self-report; preschool; children; accelerometry; ethnicity

---

1. Introduction

The early years (ages 0–5) are vital for establishing healthy lifestyle behaviours including adequate levels of physical activity (PA) and low levels of sedentary time (ST), both of which can have immediate and long-term health impacts [1–3]. In the short term, total PA and moderate to vigorous physical activity (MVPA) both seem to be positively, and ST negatively, associated with multiple health outcomes in children (bone health, motor development, cardiovascular risk factors, cognitive development, psycho-social health and healthy adiposity) [3–5]. In the long term, low PA and high ST are key risk factors for the onset of non-communicable diseases later in life (*i.e.*, cardiovascular disease and type II diabetes) [6–10]. These long-term influences may partly be explained by levels of PA and ST tracking over time [11].

Objective monitoring tools, such as accelerometers, are the first choice for field-based measures of PA and ST in young children [12]. Accelerometers can reliably and accurately measure the frequency, intensity and duration of young children's body movement within everyday settings [13,14]. Hnatiuk and colleagues [15] reviewed the results of studies measuring PA ($n = 40$) and ST ($n = 31$) in young children using accelerometers, and found that the daily proportion of time spent sedentary ranged from 34% to 94%, whereas MVPA ranged from 2% to 41% of awake time. Although accelerometers are becoming common-place in published research [14], like all methods, accelerometers have limitations, including expense, participant burden, and the level of expertise required to process and analyse data [12,16–18]. These factors may preclude large-scale epidemiological studies of young children's (in)activity behaviours, which are particularly required within multi-ethnic and economically diverse populations, as there is a need to better understand health inequalities [19–22].

In 2010, a sub-smaple of the Born in Bradford birth cohort study (BiB-1000) began investigating obesity risk factors for young children living in a multi-ethnic and economically diverse city [23,24]. At the time, there were no available methods deemed appropriate to measure MVPA and ST in this population [24], and an objective measure (such as an accelerometer) was not feasible. For these reasons, a new questionnaire was designed and implemented. A strength of questionnaires over objective measures is the extra contextual information provided about PA and ST (*i.e.*, the activity location and/or type). The new questionnaire generated was the Early Years Physical Activity Questionnaire (EY-PAQ).

The aims of this study were to assess the EY-PAQ's test re-test reliability, and to determine its validity by comparing EY-PAQ data to accelerometry in a sample of young children from a deprived and multi-ethnic population, where English and Urdu are the predominant languages spoken.

2. Materials and Methods

2.1. *Participants and Setting*

The study sample consisted of young children aged 18 months to 4 years and their parents who resided in the City of Bradford, UK. Parents were already recruited as part of a pilot cluster randomized controlled trial [25]. Bradford has an approximate population of 500,000 and is the sixth largest metropolitan area in England [26]. The city is also one of the most ethnically diverse and deprived areas in the UK [26]. Ethical approval for the study was granted by the Bradford Teaching Hospitals Foundation Trust ethics committee, and informed consent was obtained from parents.

2.2. *Procedure*

Parents and children attended two appointments with a trained researcher. The first appointment included completion of the EY-PAQ, measurement of children's height and weight, and positioning of the Actigraph GT3X+ tri-axial accelerometer (ActiGraph, Pensacola, FL, USA). Parents were instructed on how to fit the accelerometer to their child, which was attached around the waist over the right hip. They were also asked that their child wore the accelerometer during all waking hours for seven consecutive days. The second appointment took place approximately seven days later. Accelerometers were collected and the same researcher-parent pair completed the EY-PAQ.

2.3. Measures

2.3.1. The Early Years Physical Activity Questionnaire (EY-PAQ)

The EY-PAQ is a proxy-reported questionnaire that attempts to quantify levels of habitual MVPA and ST in young children. The questionnaire is available in both English and transliterated Urdu (see supplementary material) [26]. Parents were asked to report the frequency and duration of different MVPA and ST activities in which their child engaged during a typical week in the previous month. The activities for MVPA were: (1) playing actively in the house; (2) playing actively in the garden; (3) walking from place to place; (4) engaging in active play causing sweating and increased breathing; (5) playing in the park or playground, and (6) playing at indoor play facilities. The sedentary activities were: (1) colouring, drawing and craft; (2) sitting playing with toys; (3) watching TV/DVDS; (4) playing a non-active computer game; (5) sitting listening or singing to music; (6) reading or being read to; (7) travelling in a buggy/pushchair; (8) being carried while travelling; (9) travelling in the car; and (10) using public transport. A three-stage process was used to calculate daily minutes of MVPA and ST. First, the duration (reporting options were: 1) up to 15 min/day; 2) 16–30 min/day; 3) 31–60 min/day; or 4) free-text for >60 min/day) of each activity was multiplied by the frequency that activity occurred. A pragmatic approach was used with regards to the duration component, as parents tend to over-report PA and under-report ST [27], unless free-text responses exceeding 60 min/day were reported, for the calculation of MVPA, minimum reported durations were used (*i.e.*, 1 min, 16 min, or 31 min), whereas, for ST, the higher values were used (*i.e.*, 15 min, 30 min, and 60 min). Second, the calculated duration of each activity was summed and divided by seven in order to estimate daily minutes of MVPA and ST. Third, daily minutes of MVPA and ST were converted to the proportions of waking time spent in these behaviours, by dividing summed minutes in MVPA and ST, respectively, by 840 min (×100). Fourteen hours (840 min) is typical of a waking day in preschool aged children [28], and is in line with sleep diary data that we have collected from similarly aged children from the source population (data not shown). Proportional values were used as the main outcomes because parents completing the EY-PAQ considered the whole day in which an activity may have taken place, whereas accelerometer measured MVPA and ST was only captured during the time the monitor was worn; this rarely reflected entire waking time. Proportions were therefore used to account for disparities in the reference period [29].

Proxy-reported questionnaires often find large variances in PA and ST due to reporting errors [30]. To non-arbitrarily deal with assumed errors, the validity of the questionnaire was examined using two approaches, firstly by using all EY-PAQ data and secondly only data falling within specific MVPA and ST boundaries. These boundaries reflected the range of published ST and MVPA estimates in young children from objective measures [15]. The boundaries for MVPA were 2% to 41% and for ST 30% to 94% of awake time. The lower boundary for ST was reduced from published value of 34% to account for non-discretionary sedentary behaviours, such as bathroom or meal times, which accelerometry may have captured but the EY-PAQ did not pose questions about.

2.3.2. Accelerometry

The Actigraph GT3X+ (Actigraph Pensacola, FL, USA) is an accurate objective measure that has widely been used to measure young children's PA and ST [17,31–33]. It has been reported to be the favoured device to objectively measure PA in young Bradford children and their mothers [34]. For this study, the accelerometer was set to record data at a sampling rate of 60 Hertz. Raw accelerometer data were downloaded and then transformed into both 5 s and 15 s epoch files. Costa [35] found in a British sample of young children (age 2.9 years (SD 0.60)) that both 10 s and 15 s epochs significantly underestimated ST. From these findings, a new set of accelerometer cut-points were calibrated and validated using 5 s epochs [31]. The Costa cut-points were found to be accurate (criterion measure: direct observation [36]) in estimating young childrens' ST but were inaccurate in measuring MVPA. Therefore, we incorporated an alternative cut-point to assess MVPA in this study. The Pate MVPA cut-points were chosen because they have been reported to be the most accurate and appropriate to estimate MVPA in young children [37,38]. As ST and MVPA were treated as independent behaviours, the choice of epoch length was set in line with with the procedures of the original calibration studies that developed the ST (Costa: $\leqslant$5 counts per 5 s) and MVPA (Pate: 420 counts per 15 s) cut-points [13,31], hence processing data with two epoch lengths. The minimum wear-time for inclusion in the analysis was at least 6 h on any three days, which has been shown to provide reliable activity estimates (ICC = 0.7) in the same population of children used in this study [39]. Non-wear time was defined as $\geqslant$10 min of consecutive zero counts [17]. To calculate the proportion of awake time that each child engaged in behaviours, minutes of accelerometer MVPA and ST were divided by wear time, and multiplied by 100.

2.4. Data Analysis

Descriptive characteristics are presented for all participants and separately for the validity and reliability study participants.

Test/re-test reliability of the EY-PAQ for both MVPA and ST was assessed using a two-way random model intra-class correlation coefficient (ICC(2,1)) with 95% confidence intervals [40]. For the purposes of this study, coefficient values of 0.01 indicated "poor" agreement, 0.01 to 0.20 "slight" agreement, 0.21 to 0.40 "fair" agreement, 0.41 to 0.60 "moderate" agreement, 0.61 to 0.80 "substantial" agreement and 0.81 to 1.00 "almost prefect" agreement [41,42].

For the validity analysis, assessment of whether sex, ethnicity and language modified the relationships between the EY-PAQ and accelerometer MVPA and ST estimates was performed using multiple linear regression analyses. If any demographic variable was found to modify relationships, subsequent analyses were stratified by the influencing variable. All tests were conducted using proportions data, with and without boundaries. Spearman rank correlations (rho) were applied to assess the correlations between the EY-PAQ and accelerometer data. Bland–Altman plots [43] were assembled to assess the agreement between EY-PAQ and accelerometry (before and after applying boundaries). Differences (error) between EY-PAQ and accelerometer estimates of MVPA and ST were calculated (error = EY-PAQ − Actigraph) and plotted against the mean MVPA and ST values of accelerometry and EY-PAQ. The mean difference and direction of systematic error were examined using Pearson error correlations (error = x-axis, Actigraph = y-axis). Heteroscedasticity was examined using Breusch–Pagan/Cook–Weisberg Tests; where heteroscedasticity was present, heteroscedastic ratio limits of agreement (LOA) were calculated on the log scale [44,45].

All tests (reliability and validity) were performed using proportions (*i.e.*, the % of awake time in MVPA or ST), but to ease interpretation of the data and enable comparisons with other published questionnaires, proportions were converted back into minutes based upon a waking day of 840 min [28]. Analyses were conducted using SPSS for windows (version 22) and STATA (version 13), and alpha significance was defined as $p \leqslant 0.05$.

3. Results

The demographic characteristics of children are reported in Table 1. In total, 196 children and their parents took part in the validity analysis and 109 took part in the reliability analysis. A breakdown of the number of participants in each of the components of the study, including details of exclusions, is outlined in Figure 1. The mean age was 3.2 years (SD $\pm$ 0.8), 50.5% were boys and 49% South Asian (Table 1). Most questionnaires were conducted in English (79.6%) and with mothers (98%). There were no significant differences in the sex, ethnicity or age of participants included and those excluded from any aspect of the study. Linear regression models found no significant interactions by sex, ethnicity or language, for the relationships between EY-PAQ and accelerometry; therefore, analyses were not stratified.

Table 1. Demographic characteristics of children in the validity and reliability analyses of the study.

Demographic and Outcome Variables	All *		Validity **				Reliability	
	n = 196		ST (n = 89) ***		MVPA (n = 102) ****		n = 104	
	n (%)	Mean (SD)	n (%)	Mean (SD)	n (%)	Mean (SD)	n (%)	Mean (SD)
Sex								
Boys	99 (50.5)		47 (52.8)		56 (54.9)		52 (48)	
Girls	97 (49.5)		42 (47.2)		46 (45.1)		57 (53)	
Ethnicity								
White British	82 (41.8)		30 (33.7)		37 (36.3)		33 (30)	
South Asian	96 (49)		52 (58.4)		55 (53.9)		67 (62)	
Other	18 (9.2)		7 (7.9)		10 (9.8)		9 (8)	
Age								
Years		3.2 (0.8)		3.2 (0.8)		3.2 (0.8)		3.3 (0.8)
Language								
English	156 (79.6)		69 (77.5)		84 (82.4)		82 (75)	
Urdu	40 (20.4)		20 (22.5)		18 (17.6)		27 (25)	
EY-PAQ								
Proportion estimates (%)				47.0 (13.6)		21.2 (11)		
Actigraph GT3X+								
Wear time (min per day)				594.8 (100.7)		582.1 (127.3)		
Minutes per day				344.1 (88.0)		118.4 (7.5)		
Proportion estimates (%)				57.5 (7.9)		20.3 (7.6)		

* Values presented are for validity analysis before the application of boundaries. ** Values presented are for the remaining sample after the application of boundaries. *** Costa cut-points (⩽5 counts per 5 s). **** Pate cut-points (⩾420 counts per 15 s).

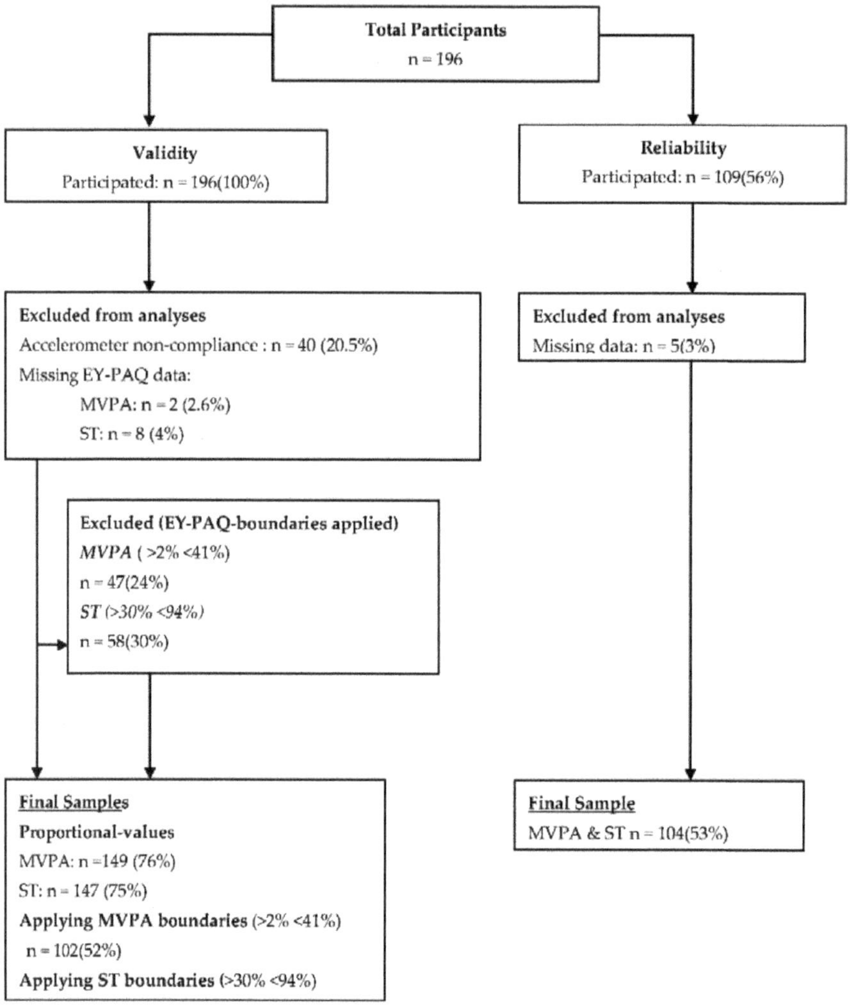

Figure 1. Flow diagram outlining the number of included and excluded participants for the validity and reliability analyses.

3.1. Reliability

The average number of days between the completion of the questionnaire at Test 1 and Test 2 was 7.4 days, ranging from five to 12 days.

Table 2 shows the results of the test/re-test reliability analyses. There was fair agreement for test/re-test reliability of MVPA measured by the EY-PAQ (ICC(2,1) = 0.35, 95% CI: 0.17–0.50)). For ST, reliability was moderate (ICC(2,1) = 0.47, 95% CI: 0.30–0.61)).

Table 2. Intraclass-correlations for moderate to vigorous physical activity (MVPA) and sedentary time (ST) measured by the early years physical activity questionnaire (EY-PAQ).

EY-PAQ Test 1 *vs.* Test 2	Reliability			
	n(%)	Mean Daily Difference in Minutes [95% CI]	ICC (2,1)	95% Confidence Interval
MVPA	104 (93.7)	25.5 [−23.9, 74.8]	0.35 *	0.17–0.50
ST	104 (93.7)	1.7 [−36.5, 39.9]	0.47 *	0.3–0.61

* $p \leqslant 0.05$.

3.2. Validity

Agreement between MVPA and ST estimated by the EY-PAQ and accelerometry are shown in Figure 2. For MVPA, the mean difference was 7.1 min/day (LOA: −185.9 ± 200.1), and, for ST, the mean difference was −87.5 min/day (LOA: −376.6 ± 192.7).

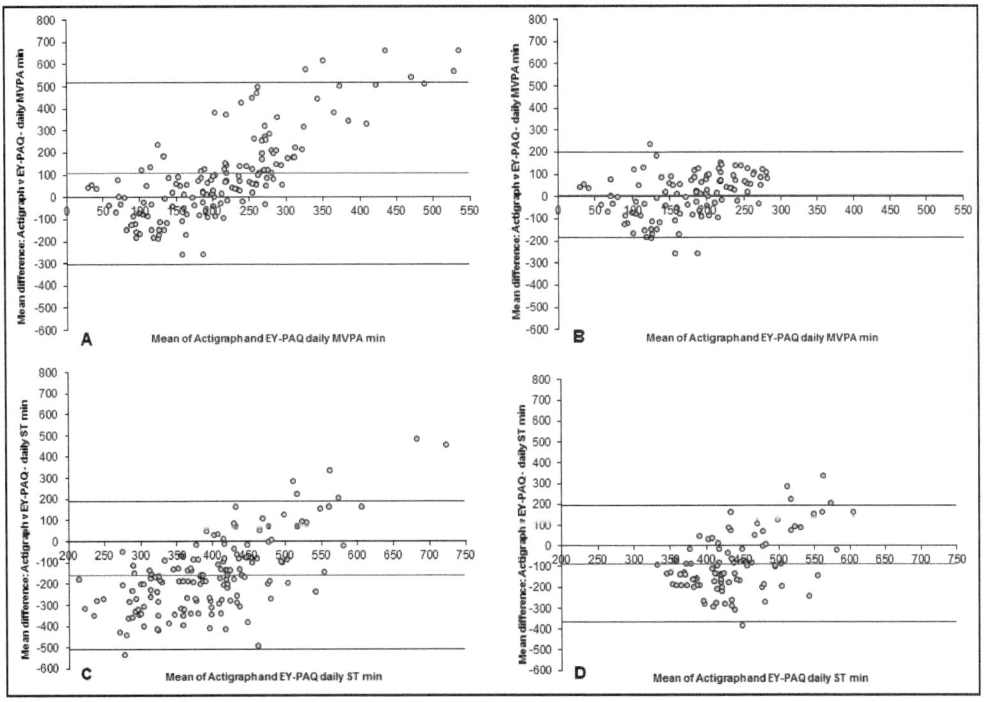

Figure 2. Bland–Altman plots for the difference between time spent in moderate to vigorous physical activity (MVPA) and sedentary time (ST) measured by accelerometry and the Early Years Physical activity questionnaire (EY-PAQ); plotted against the mean average time spent in MVPA and ST measured by the Actigraph and EY-PAQ. (**A**): MVPA plot for EY-PAQ-MVPA no boundaries applied. Mean difference: 106.3 mins/day; 95% limits of agreement (LOA): −303.7, +516.4. (**B**): MVPA plot with EY-PAQ-MVPA boundaries applied. Mean difference: 7.1 mins/day; LOA: −185.9, +200.1. (**C**): ST plot for EY-PAQ-ST no boundaries applied. Mean difference: −160.0 mins/day; LOA: −509.9, +190.0. (**D**): ST plot with EY-PAQ-ST boundaries applied. Mean difference: −87.5 mins/day; LOA: −376.6, +192.7.

The only significant correlation between the EY-PAQ and accelerometer was the proportion of time spent in MVPA after applying boundaries (Table 3). Error correlations for all values were found to be statistically significant (Table 3). The significant correlations highlight that systematic error existed. Breusch–Pagan/Cook–Weisburg tests found heteroscedasticity to be present ($p < 0.05$) in the MVPA values and in the ST values. The MVPA mean bias on the ratio scale found MVPA was overestimated by 20% (1.20) and when the boundary-value was applied this was reduced to an overestimation of 3% (1.03). The ratio mean bias for ST found that it was overestimated by 72% (1.72) which was reduced to an overestimation of 26% (1.26) when the EY-PAQ boundaries were applied. The ratio-limits of agreement were wide for all results (Table 3).

Table 3. Validity of the early years physical activity questionnaire (EY-PAQ) compared to accelerometry.

EY-PAQ *vs.* Accelerometer	Validity						
	N (%)	rho	Mean Daily Difference in Minutes [95% CI]	LOA †	Error Correlations (r)	Heteroskedasicity *p*-Value	Ratio LOA †
MVPA: No boundaries	149 (76.0)	0.03	106.3 [72.5, 140.2]	−303.7 to 516.4	−0.80 *	0.94	1.20 (×/÷ 10.6)
MVPA: Boundary applied >2% (16.8 min)<41% (344.3 min)#	102 (52.0)	0.30 *	7.1 [−12.3, 26.4]	−185.9 to 200.1	−0.37 *	<0.01	1.03 (×/÷ 5.8)
ST: No boundaries	147 (75.0)	0.02	−160.0 [−189.1, −30.9]	−509.9 to 190.0	−0.67 *	<0.01	1.72 (×/÷ 3.6)
ST: Boundary applied >30% (252 min) <94% (789.6 min) #	89 (45.4)	0.19	−87.5 [−117.6, −57.4]	−367.6 to 192.7	−0.50 *	<0.01	1.26 (×/÷ 1.9)

* $p \leqslant 0.05$. # Hnatiuk *et al.* [17] boundaries. † Limits of agreement.

4. Discussion

This study examined the reliability and validity of a new activity questionnaire (EY-PAQ) in a sample of young children from a diverse ethnic background where parents spoke either English or Urdu. Findings of the current study show the EY-PAQ has fair reliability for MVPA and moderate reliability for ST. The validity of the EY-PAQ was assessed against accelerometry. A small mean difference and significant correlation was found for MVPA after applying boundaries, leading to the EY-PAQ being an acceptable population method to measure young children's habitual MVPA. For ST, the mean difference was large and the correlation coefficient non-significant. This was true even after applying boundaries to the data, it therefore appears that the EY-PAQ is not a suitable population measure of ST.

The EY-PAQ is a new tool which measures the habitual levels of young children's MVPA and ST. Other similar tools which have been compared to accelerometry are the Preschool-Age Physical Activity Questionnaire (Pre-PAQ) which was developed in Sydney, Australia and measures MVPA, light activity and ST [27], and the Children's Physical Activity Questionnaire (C-PAQ) which was developed in Cambridge, UK and measures MVPA and total PA [44]. The test/re-test reliability of the MVPA component of the EY-PAQ was found to be fair and acceptable [41,42]. Sedentary time had a greater ICC value than MVPA (0.47 and 0.35). In comparison to other published questionnaires, the EY-PAQ's ST ICC was similar to that of the Pre-PAQ's [27] (0.44). The EY-PAQ's MVPA reliability coefficient was lower than the Pre-PAQ's (0.54) and C-PAQ's [44] (0.39). It is perhaps unsurprising that reliability of all questionnaires were low compared to the 'almost perfect' criteria of ICC = 0.8. Children's PA tends to be highly variable [12], which means levels of MVPA and ST could be very different from one week to the next, thus affecting test/re-test results.

With regards to validity, like the other questionnaires, differences in MVPA and ST were seen between the EY-PAQ and accelerometer. For MVPA, initial results of the EY-PAQ validity assessment revealed larger error values in comparison to the Pre-PAQ and C-PAQ. The EY-PAQ overestimated MVPA by 106.3 min/day, compared to the Pre-PAQ which overestimated MVPA by 50.1 min/day, while the CPAQ underestimated MVPA by −76.5 min. With regards to ST, the EY-PAQ underestimated daily sitting by 160 min/day, which was a smaller difference to the Pre-PAQ's mean difference of −208.6 min/day. However, when the EY-PAQ boundaries were applied differences with accelerometry were reduced to 7.1 min for MVPA and −87.5 min for ST. Like the present study, Corder, van Sluijs [42] also assessed the heteroscedasticity of the C-PAQ and reported the anti-logged ratio limits of agreement. Results showed the C-PAQ at best (depending upon accelerometer cut-points) underestimated MVPA by 32%, which is a greater level of error than the 3% overestimation witnessed with the EY-PAQ after applying boundaries to the data. Limits of agreement for the EY-PAQ, like the Pre-PAQ and CPAQ, were wide but improved with application of boundaries. Applying the EY-PAQ boundaries also improved the correlation coefficient between the two measures for both MVPA and ST. Before the application of boundaries the EY-PAQ had low, non-significant coefficients (MVPA (rho = 0.03, $p \geqslant 0.05$) and ST [rho = 0.02, $p \geqslant 0.05$]) when compared to the accelerometer. After applying boundaries, the EY-PAQ's validity coefficients increased (MVPA: rho = 0.30; ST = 0.19). The MVPA coefficient was statistically significant, thus the EY-PAQ successfully ranked young children's MVPA after applying boundaries. The CPAQ also found that it could rank young children's MVPA (rho = 0.42, $p \leqslant 0.05$). The EY-PAQ's ST coefficient after applying boundaries increased to 0.19, but was still statistically non-significant.

There are numerous reasons that could explain the differences in the reliability and validity coefficients seen between the EY-PAQ, CPAQ and Pre-PAQ. One reason is that the instruments vary in design and question structure. Another possible reason could be the differences in socio-demographic characteristics of the samples used in the three studies. The Pre-PAQ sample consisted of mainly high socio-economic status, white, English-speaking parents and children from Australia. The samples from both the EY-PAQ and C-PAQ validity studies were located in the UK, but the children in the current study were from communities of high deprivation [23], with a high ethnic mix and two different primary languages. Little is known about the sample of the C-PAQ study, other than the sample was from an affluent part of the UK (Cambridgeshire). Future studies should seek to validate multiple questionnaires in the same sample in order to test which of the questionnaires is the most reliable, valid and also feasible. The current study explored interaction by demographic variables such as sex, ethnicity and language on the relationship between the two measures. These variables were not found to impact the association between the EY-PAQ and accelerometry within the present sample.

The error for both MVPA and ST were lowest when mean accelerometer MVPA and ST were highest. This meant that parents were more likely to over or under report MVPA and ST using the EY-PAQ when children's accelerometer-determined levels of MVPA and ST were low. This finding could be explained by the different measurement properties of a proxy-report questionnaire and accelerometer. Dependent upon the placement of the monitor, accelerometry constantly measures movements of the child when worn. However, proxy-report questionnaires are reliant upon what parents observe and remember when completing the questionnaire. Parents will not remember every 15 s of movement or sedentary time that their young child has engaged in throughout the day, but the accelerometer (in the current study) recorded the child's movement (or lack thereof) every 15 s (one of the epoch lengths used). Therefore, a difference between the two measurements was foreseeable. Despite the differences between the two types of methods, accelerometers are the most widely used comparison measure in which new self-report tools are validated against [30] Because of the differences, strong coefficients are seldom reported, with most self-reported validity coefficients with accelerometry ranging between 0.25 and 0.41 [30].

In the current study, the inclusion of boundaries informed by data from a recent systematic review [15] narrowed the limits of agreement and greater accuracy was observed. However, it has to be noted this could lead to a possible exclusion of participants, and reduced sample sizes if the EY-PAQ was applied to future population-level studies. In this study, the percentage of participant loss due to the application of boundaries was 23% (n = 47) for MVPA and 30% (n = 58) for ST. Nonetheless, large scale studies using accelerometry also need to factor in participant loss due to the processing of data (e.g., not enough valid wear time). In comparison to large scale studies using accelerometry, the EY-PAQ's participant loss was similar to that of the Healthy Active Preschool Years study (30%) [46], and less than half of the Millennium Cohort Study (children aged 7–8 years) (53%) [47]. The use of the EY-PAQ and accelerometry share the limitation of possible sample size reduction, but the implementation of accelerometry and other objective measures are limited by the burden to participants (e.g., seven days wearing of monitor), level of expertise required to process data and financial costs, all which do not apply to the EY-PAQ. The results of the current study indicate that the EY-PAQ has the smallest limits of agreement after the application of boundaries when measuring MVPA compared to other similar questionnaires [27,44].

It seems that the EY-PAQ is not suitable for measuring young children's ST. The Pre-PAQ also measures ST in young children, and like the EY-PAQ, it was also found to be a weak measure. Reasons for inaccuracy could include that accelerometry would have likely detected most sedentary behaviours including those not measured by the EY-PAQ (e.g., bathroom and meal times). However, the two techniques are also measuring two different behaviours. The EY-PAQ measures the time and frequency that parents report their child sitting down and doing different activities. Accelerometry measures ST by quantifying the absence of movement. Another reason for inaccuracy could be the design of the EY-PAQ's questions. For example, parents rarely used free-text responses to report engagement in sedentary behaviours ⩾60 min, but it is known that, even in this young age group, TV-viewing is prevalent and possibly prolonged. By having a response category with a maximum of 60 min daily, and free-text responses thereafter, we may have unintentionally given parents the impression that we would not have expect higher values, thereby dissuading truthful responses. Future research should bear this in mind and investigate validity and reliability parameters when using different and more suitable comparison measures (e.g., inclinometers [48]) and adding more domains of ST within the EY-PAQ (e.g., time spent sitting while eating).

A strength of the current study was the relatively large sample of children under the age of five years compared to previous validation studies in young children [27,44]. Furthermore, the EY-PAQ sample were from a low socio-economical, ethnically diverse and bi-lingual population; thereby, this studies' novelty adds to the current measurement literature of young children's PA and ST, which is heavily skewed by white English speaking samples [27]. However, results from the current study may not be generalisable to other populations; therefore, additional validity and reliability studies using this new measure in different populations are required. Although a widely used objective field measure, the use of accelerometers as a comparison measure for ST was a limitation; they do not detect posture and only estimate ST through a lack of movement counts. Accelerometry therefore could be argued to be an unsuitable convergent measure for ST [48]. However, there is currently no other objective measure of habitual ST that has been used with children of this age [49]. Finally, (in)activity levels show variation throughout the day in young children [50], meaning that missing data from particular segments of the day (morning, afternoon, or evening) may have influenced our objective data. In this respect, imparting a time-distribution caveat to the accelerometry data may have been worthwhile [51]. Nonetheless, $\geqslant$360 min of data has commonly been used to define a valid day of accelerometry in young children [14,32,39,52,53], without specifying the pattern of observed data, and our work has shown only small differences in estimated activity levels in the source population with and without specifying that all parts of days must be observed [54].

5. Conclusions

The EY-PAQ has acceptable reliability and validity for measuring habitual MVPA of young children from a bi-lingual (English, Urdu), bi-ethnic (White British, South Asian) low socio-economic community. In situations when objective methods are not possible for measurement of MVPA in young children, the EY-PAQ may be a suitable alternative, but only if boundaries are applied. Having such a questionnaire means researchers can explore the early life determinants of MVPA in an ethnically diverse and low socio economic status population at a low cost. Such evidence will be useful for the development of tailored interventions, with better chances to decrease health inequalities in PA and related health outcomes in young children.

Acknowledgments: The involvement of D.D.B., P.J.C., and S.E.B in this publication was through their affiliation with the Healthy Children Healthy Families theme of the National Institute for Health Research (NIHR). Collaboration for Leadership in Applied Health Research and Care (CLAHRC) Yorkshire and Humber. The views expressed in this publication are those of the authors and not necessarily those of the National Health Service, NIHR or Department of Health. The involvement of S.C. in this publication was under the auspices of the Centre for Diet and Activity Research (CEDAR), a UKCRC Public Health Research Centre of Excellence which is funded by the British Heart Foundation, Cancer Research UK, Economic and Social Research Council, Medical Research Council, the National Institute for Health Research, and the Wellcome Trust. The authors would firstly like to thank all of the children and parents who took part in the study. Secondly, the Bradford children's centres and Born in Bradford community staff who were vital during the data collection. Thirdly, we would like to thank Shaheen Akhtar who aided transliteration of the questionnaire.

Author Contributions: D.D.B., S.A.C., and S.E.B. conceived and designed the study. S.E.B. and D.D.B. led the data collection. S.A.C., S.E.B., P.G., and S.C. designed and created the questions which made up the questionnaire (EY-PAQ). G.S. and P.J.C. developed the coding of questionnaire variables. P.J.C. and D.D.B. analyzed the data. All authors read and contributed to the final manuscript, which was written by D.D.B.

Conflicts of Interest: The authors declare no conflict of interest.

Abbreviations

The following abbreviations are used in this manuscript:

EY-PAQ	Early Years Physical Activity Questionnaire
TPA	Total Physical Activity
MVPA	Moderate to Vigorous Physical Activity
ST	Sedentary Time
BiB	Born in Bradford

References

1. Australian Government Department of Health and Ageing. *Physical Activity Recommendations for Children 0–5*; Australian Government Department of Health and Ageing: Canberra, Australia, 2009.
2. Reilly, J.; Okely, A.; Almond, L.; Cardon, G.; Prosser, L. *Making the Case for UK Physical Activity Guidelines for Early Years: Recommendations and Draft Summary Statements Based on the current Evidence*; UK government: London, UK, 2011.
3. Timmons, B.W.; LeBlanc, A.G.; Carson, V.; Gorber, S.C.; Dillman, C.; Janssen, I.; Kho, M.E.; Spence, J.C.; Stearns, J.A.; Tremblay, M.S. Systematic review of physical activity and health in the early years (aged 0–4 years). *Appl. Physiol. Nutr. Metab.* **2012**, *37*, 773–792. [CrossRef] [PubMed]
4. Tremblay, M.S.; LeBlanc, A.G.; Kho, M.E.; Saunders, T.J.; Larouche, R.; Colley, R.C.; Goldfield, G.; Gorber, S.C. Systematic review of sedentary behaviour and health indicators in school-aged children and youth. *Int. J. Behav. Nutr. Phys. Act.* **2011**, *8*, 1–22. [CrossRef] [PubMed]
5. Ekelund, U.; Hildebrand, M.; Collings, P.J. Physical activity, sedentary time and adiposity during the first two decades of life. *Proc. Nutr. Soc.* **2014**, *73*, 319–329. [CrossRef] [PubMed]
6. Lee, I.M.; Shiroma, E.J.; Lobelo, F.; Puska, P.; Blair, S.N.; Katzmarzyk, P.T.; Lancet, W. Effect of physical inactivity on major non-communicable diseases worldwide: An analysis of burden of disease and life expectancy. *Lancet* **2012**, *380*, 219–229. [CrossRef]
7. Telama, R.; Yang, X.; Leskinen, E.; Kankaanpaa, A.; Hirvensalo, M.; Tammelin, T.; Viikari, J.S.; Raitakari, O.T. Tracking of physical activity from early childhood through youth into adulthood. *Med. Sci. Sports Exerc.* **2014**, *46*, 955–962. [CrossRef] [PubMed]
8. Telama, R.; Yang, X.; Viikari, J.; Valimaki, I.; Wanne, O.; Raitakari, O. Physical activity from childhood to adulthood: A 21-year tracking study. *Am. J. Prev. Med.* **2005**, *28*, 267–273. [CrossRef] [PubMed]
9. Wilmot, E.G.; Edwardson, C.L.; Achana, F.A.; Davies, M.J.; Gorely, T.; Gray, L.J.; Khunti, K.; Yates, T.; Biddle, S.J. Sedentary time in adults and the association with diabetes, cardiovascular disease and death: Systematic review and meta-analysis. *Diabetologia* **2012**, *55*, 2895–2905. [CrossRef] [PubMed]
10. Biswas, A.; Oh, P.I.; Faulkner, G.E.; Bajaj, R.R.; Silver, M.A.; Mitchell, M.S.; Alter, D.A. Sedentary time and its association with risk for disease incidence, mortality, and hospitalization in adults: A systematic review and meta-analysis. *Ann. Intern. Med.* **2015**, *162*, 123–132. [CrossRef] [PubMed]
11. Jones, R.A.; Hinkley, T.; Okely, A.D.; Salmon, J. Tracking Physical Activity and Sedentary Behavior in Childhood A Systematic Review. *Am. J. Prev. Med.* **2013**, *44*, 651–658. [CrossRef] [PubMed]
12. Cliff, D.P.; Reilly, J.J.; Okely, A.D. Methodological considerations in using accelerometers to assess habitual physical activity in children aged 0–5 years. *J. Sci. Med. Sport* **2009**, *12*, 557–567. [CrossRef] [PubMed]
13. Pate, R.R.; Almeida, M.J.; McIver, K.L.; Pfeiffer, K.A.; Dowda, M. Validation and calibration of an accelerometer in preschool children. *Obesity* **2006**, *14*, 2000–2006. [CrossRef] [PubMed]
14. Cain, K.L.; Sallis, J.F.; Conway, T.L.; van Dyck, D.; Calhoon, L. Using accelerometers in youth physical activity studies: A review of methods. *J. Phys. Act. Health* **2013**, *10*, 437–450. [PubMed]
15. Hnatiuk, J.A.; Salmon, J.; Hinkley, T.; Okely, A.D.; Trost, S. A review of preschool children's physical activity and sedentary time using objective measures. *Am. J. Prev. Med.* **2014**, *47*, 487–497. [CrossRef] [PubMed]
16. Lee, I.-M.; Shiroma, E.J. Using accelerometers to measure physical activity in large-scale epidemiological studies: Issues and challenges. *Br. J. Sports Med.* **2014**, *48*, 197–201. [CrossRef] [PubMed]
17. Oliver, M.; Schofield, G.M.; Kolt, G.S. Physical activity in preschoolers: Understanding prevalence and measurement issues. *Sports Med.* **2007**, *37*, 1045–1070. [CrossRef] [PubMed]

18. Fulton, J.E.; Burgeson, C.R.; Perry, G.R.; Sherry, B.; Galuska, D.A.; Alexander, M.P.; Wechsler, H.; Caspersen, C.J. Assessment of Physical Activity and Sedentary Behavior in Preschool-Age Children: Priorities for Research. *Pediatr. Exerc. Sci.* **2001**, *13*, 113–126.
19. Taveras, E.M.; Gillman, M.W.; Kleinman, K.; Rich-Edwards, J.W.; Rifas-Shiman, S.L. Racial/ethnic differences in early life risk factors for childhood obesity. *Pediatrics* **2010**, *125*. [CrossRef] [PubMed]
20. Misra, A.; Khurana, L.; Vikram, N.K.; Goel, A.; Wasir, J.S. Metabolic syndrome in children: Current issues and South Asian perspective. *Nutrition* **2007**, *23*, 895–910. [CrossRef] [PubMed]
21. Bhopal, R. Epidemic of cardiovascular disease in South Asians: Prevention must start in childhood. *Br. Med. J.* **2002**, *324*, 625–626. [CrossRef]
22. Bhopal, R. What is the risk of coronary heart disease in South Asians? A review of UK research. *J. Public Health Med.* **2000**, *22*, 375–385. [CrossRef] [PubMed]
23. Wright, J.; Small, N.; Raynor, P.; Tuffnell, D.; Bhopal, R.; Cameron, N.; Fairley, L.; Lawlor, D.A.; Parslow, R.; Petherick, E.S.; Pickett, K.E.; Waiblinger, D.; West, J.; Born, G. Cohort profile: The Born in Bradford multi-ethnic family cohort study. *Int. J. Epidemiol.* **2013**, *42*, 978–991. [CrossRef] [PubMed]
24. Bryant, M.; Santorelli, G.; Fairley, L.; West, J.; Lawlor, D.A.; Bhopal, R.; Petherick, E.; Sahota, P.; Hill, A.; Cameron, N.; *et al.* Design and characteristics of a new birth cohort, to study the early origins and ethnic variation of childhood obesity: The BiB1000 study. *Longitud. Life Course Stud.* **2013**, *4*, 119–135.
25. Barber, S.E.; Jackson, C.; Akhtar, S.; Bingham, D.D.; Ainsworth, H.; Hewitt, C.; Richardson, G.; Summerbell, C.D.; Pickett, K.E.; Moore, H.J.; *et al.* "Pre-schoolers in the playground" an outdoor physical activity intervention for children aged 18 months to 4 years old: Study protocol for a pilot cluster randomised controlled trial. *Trials* **2013**, *14*, 1–13. [CrossRef] [PubMed]
26. Raynor, P. Born in Bradford, a cohort study of babies born in Bradford, and their parents: Protocol for the recruitment phase. *BMC Public Health* **2008**, *8*, 327–339. [PubMed]
27. Dwyer, G.M.; Hardy, L.L.; Peat, J.K.; Baur, L.A. The validity and reliability of a home environment preschool-age physical activity questionnaire (Pre-PAQ). *Int. J. Behav. Nutr. Phys. Act.* **2011**, *8*, 86. [CrossRef] [PubMed]
28. Collings, P.J.; Brage, S.; Ridgway, C.L.; Harvey, N.C.; Godfrey, K.M.; Inskip, H.M.; Cooper, C.; Wareham, N.J.; Ekelund, U. Physical activity intensity, sedentary time, and body composition in preschoolers. *Am. J. Clin. Nutr.* **2013**, *97*, 1020–1028. [CrossRef] [PubMed]
29. Saint-Maurice, P.F.; Welk, G.J.; Beyler, N.K.; Bartee, R.T.; Heelan, K.A. Calibration of self-report tools for physical activity research: The Physical Activity Questionnaire (PAQ). *BMC Public Health* **2014**, *14*, 1–9. [CrossRef] [PubMed]
30. Helmerhorst, H.J.F.; Brage, S.; Warren, J.; Besson, H.; Ekelund, U. A systematic review of reliability and objective criterion-related validity of physical activity questionnaires. *Int. J. Behav. Nutr. Phys. Act.* **2012**, *9*. [CrossRef] [PubMed]
31. Costa, S.; Barber, S.E.; Cameron, N.; Clemes, S.A. Calibration and validation of the ActiGraph GT3X+ in 2–3 year olds. *J. Sci. Med. Sport* **2014**, *17*, 617–622. [CrossRef] [PubMed]
32. Addy, C.L.; Trilk, J.L.; Dowda, M.; Byun, W.; Pate, R.R. Assessing Preschool Children's Physical Activity: How Many Days of Accelerometry Measurement. *Pediatr. Exerc. Sci.* **2014**, *26*, 103–109. [CrossRef] [PubMed]
33. Hnatiuk, J.; Ridgers, N.D.; Salmon, J.; Campbell, K.; McCallum, Z.; Hesketh, K. Physical Activity Levels and Patterns of 19-Month-Old Children. *Med. Sci. Sports Exerc.* **2012**, *44*, 1715–1720. [CrossRef] [PubMed]
34. Costa, S.; Barber, S.E.; Griffiths, P.L.; Cameron, N.; Clemes, S.A. Qualitative feasibility of using three accelerometers with 2–3-year-old children and both parents. *Res. Q. Exerc. Sport* **2013**, *84*, 295–304. [CrossRef] [PubMed]
35. Costa, S. *The Measurement of Physical Activity and Sedentary Behaviour in a Sample of 2 to 3 Year Old South Asian and White British Children*; Loughborough Univeristy: Leicestershire, UK, 2014.
36. Metcalf, B.S.; Jeffery, A.N.; Hosking, J.; Voss, L.D.; Sattar, N.; Wilkin, T.J. Objectively Measured Physical Activity and Its Association With Adiponectin and Other Novel Metabolic Markers A Longitudinal study in children (EarlyBird 38). *Diabetes Care* **2009**, *32*, 468–473. [CrossRef] [PubMed]
37. Trost, S.G.; Fees, B.S.; Haar, S.J.; Murray, A.D.; Crowe, L.K. Identification and validity of accelerometer cut-points for toddlers. *Obesity* **2012**, *20*, 2317–2319. [CrossRef] [PubMed]

38. Gladstone, M.; Lancaster, G.A.; Umar, E.; Nyirenda, M.; Kayira, E.; van den Broek, N.R.; Smyth, R.L. The Malawi Developmental Assessment Tool (MDAT): The Creation, Validation, and Reliability of a Tool to Assess Child Development in Rural African Settings. *PLoS Med.* **2010**, *7*, e1000273. [CrossRef] [PubMed]
39. Bingham, D.D.; Costa, S.; Clemes, S.A.; Routen, A.C.; Moore, H.J.; Barber, S.E. Accelerometer data requirements for reliable estimation of habitual physical activity and sedentary time of children during the early years—A worked example following a stepped approach. *J. Sports Sci.* **2016**, *2016*, 1–6. [CrossRef] [PubMed]
40. Streiner, D.L.; Norman, G.R. *Health Measurement Scales: A Practical Guide to Their Development and Use*; OUP Oxford: Oxford, UK, 2008.
41. Landis, J.R.; Koch, G.G. The measurement of observer agreement for categorical data. *Biometrics* **1977**, *33*, 159–174. [CrossRef] [PubMed]
42. London, K.C. Q9.10 What Size of Index Indicates "Good Reliability"? Available online: http://www.kcl.ac.uk/ioppn/depts/biostatistics/SAS/faqs9.aspx#a9_2 (accessed on 2 Februray 2016).
43. Bland, J.M.; Altman, D.G. Statistical methods for assessing agreement between two methods of clinical measurement. *Lancet* **1986**, *1*, 307–310. [CrossRef]
44. Corder, K.; van Sluijs, E.M.F.; Wright, A.; Whincup, P.; Wareham, N.J.; Ekelund, U. Is it possible to assess free-living physical activity and energy expenditure in young people by self-report? *Am. J. Clin. Nutr.* **2009**, *89*, 862–870. [CrossRef] [PubMed]
45. Atkinson, G.; Nevill, A.M. Statistical methods for assessing measurement error (reliability) in variables relevant to sports medicine. *Sports Med.* **1998**, *26*, 217–238. [CrossRef] [PubMed]
46. Hinkley, T.; Salmon, J.; Okely, A.D.; Crawford, D.; Hesketh, K. Preschoolers' physical activity, screen time, and compliance with recommendations. *Med. Sci. Sports Exerc.* **2012**, *44*, 458–465. [CrossRef] [PubMed]
47. Lobo, Y.B.; Winsler, A. The effects of a creative dance and movement program on the social competence of head start preschoolers. *Soc. Dev.* **2006**, *15*, 501–519. [CrossRef]
48. Hart, T.L.; Ainsworth, B.E.; Tudor-Locke, C. Objective and subjective measures of sedentary behavior and physical activity. *Med. Sci. Sports Exerc.* **2011**, *43*, 449–456. [CrossRef] [PubMed]
49. Atkin, A.J.; Gorely, T.; Clemes, S.A.; Yates, T.; Edwardson, C.; Brage, S.; Salmon, J.; Marshall, S.J.; Biddle, S.J. Methods of Measurement in epidemiology: Sedentary Behaviour. *Int. J. Epidemiol.* **2012**, *41*, 1460–1471. [CrossRef] [PubMed]
50. Hesketh, K.; McMinn, A.; Ekelund, U.; Sharp, S.; Collings, P.; Harvey, N.; Godfrey, K.; Inskip, H.; Cooper, C.; van Sluijs, E. Objectively measured physical activity in four-year-old British children: A cross-sectional analysis of activity patterns segmented across the day. *Int. J. Behav. Nutr. Phys. Act.* **2014**, *11*. [CrossRef] [PubMed]
51. Collings, P.J.; Wijndaele, K.; Corder, K.; Westgate, K.; Ridgway, C.L.; Dunn, V.; Goodyer, I.; Ekelund, U.; Brage, S. Levels and patterns of objectively-measured physical activity volume and intensity distribution in UK adolescents: The ROOTS study. *Int. J. Behav. Nutr. Phys. Act.* **2014**, *11*, 23–23. [CrossRef] [PubMed]
52. Hinkley, T.; O'Connell, E.; Okely, A.D.; Crawford, D.; Hesketh, K.; Salmon, J. Assessing volume of accelerometry data for reliability in preschool children. *Med. Sci. Sports Exerc.* **2012**, *44*, 2436–2441. [CrossRef] [PubMed]
53. Hislop, J.; Law, J.; Rush, R.; Grainger, A.; Bulley, C.; Reilly, J.J.; Mercer, T. An investigation into the minimum accelerometry wear time for reliable estimates of habitual physical activity and definition of a standard measurement day in pre-school children. *Physiol. Meas.* **2014**, *35*, 2213–2228. [CrossRef] [PubMed]
54. Collings, P.J.; Brage, S.; Bingham, D.D.; Costa, S.; West, J.; McEachan, R.R.C.; Wright, J.; Barber, S.E. Bradford Institute for Health Research, Bradford, UK. Unpublished work. 2016.

PERMISSIONS

All chapters in this book were first published in Sports, by MDPI; hereby published with permission under the Creative Commons Attribution License or equivalent. Every chapter published in this book has been scrutinized by our experts. Their significance has been extensively debated. The topics covered herein carry significant findings which will fuel the growth of the discipline. They may even be implemented as practical applications or may be referred to as a beginning point for another development.

The contributors of this book come from diverse backgrounds, making this book a truly international effort. This book will bring forth new frontiers with its revolutionizing research information and detailed analysis of the nascent developments around the world.

We would like to thank all the contributing authors for lending their expertise to make the book truly unique. They have played a crucial role in the development of this book. Without their invaluable contributions this book wouldn't have been possible. They have made vital efforts to compile up to date information on the varied aspects of this subject to make this book a valuable addition to the collection of many professionals and students.

This book was conceptualized with the vision of imparting up-to-date information and advanced data in this field. To ensure the same, a matchless editorial board was set up. Every individual on the board went through rigorous rounds of assessment to prove their worth. After which they invested a large part of their time researching and compiling the most relevant data for our readers.

The editorial board has been involved in producing this book since its inception. They have spent rigorous hours researching and exploring the diverse topics which have resulted in the successful publishing of this book. They have passed on their knowledge of decades through this book. To expedite this challenging task, the publisher supported the team at every step. A small team of assistant editors was also appointed to further simplify the editing procedure and attain best results for the readers.

Apart from the editorial board, the designing team has also invested a significant amount of their time in understanding the subject and creating the most relevant covers. They scrutinized every image to scout for the most suitable representation of the subject and create an appropriate cover for the book.

The publishing team has been an ardent support to the editorial, designing and production team. Their endless efforts to recruit the best for this project, has resulted in the accomplishment of this book. They are a veteran in the field of academics and their pool of knowledge is as vast as their experience in printing. Their expertise and guidance has proved useful at every step. Their uncompromising quality standards have made this book an exceptional effort. Their encouragement from time to time has been an inspiration for everyone.

The publisher and the editorial board hope that this book will prove to be a valuable piece of knowledge for researchers, students, practitioners and scholars across the globe.

LIST OF CONTRIBUTORS

Amanda M. George, Linda E. Rohr and Jeannette Byrne
School of Human Kinetics and Recreation, Memorial University, St. John's, NL A1C 5S7, Canada

Simon N. Pearson
Sports Performance Research Institute New Zealand (SPRINZ), School of Sport and Recreation, Faculty of Health and Environmental Science, Auckland University of Technology, Private Bag 92006, Auckland 1020, New Zealand
Queensland Academy of Sport, QLD Sport and Athletics Centre, Kessels Rd, Nathan QLD 4111, Australia

Patria A. Hume, John Cronin
Sports Performance Research Institute New Zealand (SPRINZ), School of Sport and Recreation, Faculty of Health and Environmental Science, Auckland University of Technology, Private Bag 92006, Auckland 1020, New Zealand

David Slyfield
Sports Performance Research Institute New Zealand (SPRINZ), School of Sport and Recreation, Faculty of Health and Environmental Science, Auckland University of Technology, Private Bag 92006, Auckland 1020, New Zealand
High Performance Sport New Zealand, PO Box 302 563, North Shore 0751, New Zealand

Hidetaka Hamasaki
Department of Internal Medicine, National Center for Global Health and Medicine Kohnodai Hospital, 1-7-1 Kohnodai, Chiba 272-8516, Japan
Hamasaki Clinic, 2-21-4 Nishida, Kagoshima 890-0046, Japan

Gema Torres-Luque
Faculty of Humanities and Science Education, University of Jaen, Jaen 23071, Spain

Hamid Arazi, Behnam Roozbeh and Alireza Saati Zarei
Department of Exercise Physiology, Faculty of Sport Sciences, University of Guilan, Rasht 1438, Iran

Roger Eston
Alliance for Research in Exercise, Nutrition and Activity; School of Health Sciences, University of South Australia, Adelaide 5000, Australia

Abbas Asadi
Department of Exercise Physiology, Faculty of Sport Sciences, University of Guilan, Rasht 1438, Iran
Roudbar Branch, Islamic Azad University, Roudbar, Iran

Raquel Hernández-García
Faculty of Sport Science, University of Murcia, Murcia 30720, Spain

Raquel Escobar-Molina
Faculty of Sport Science, University of Granada, Granada 18001, Spain

Nuria Garatachea
Faculty of Health and Sport Science, University of Zaragoza, Zaragoza 22002, Spain

Pantelis T. Nikolaidis
Department of Physical and Cultural Education, Hellenic Army Academy, Athens 16673, Greece
Exercise Physiology Laboratory, Nikaia 18450, Greece

Pantelis Theodoros Nikolaidis
Department of Physical and Cultural Education, Hellenic Army Academy, Athens 16673, Greece
Exercise Physiology Laboratory, Nikaia 18450, Greece

Jose Afonso
Faculty of Sport, University of Porto, Porto 4200-450, Portugal

Vicente Javier Clemente-Suarez
Department of Sport Science, European University of Madrid, Madrid 28670, Spain

Jose Rafael Padilla Alvarado
Department of Physical Education, Universidad de Los Llanos Occedentales Ezequiel Zamora, Barinitas 7001, Venezuela

Tarak Driss
UFR STAPS, CeRSM (EA 2931), Université Paris Ouest Nanterre La Défense, Nanterre 92000, France

Beat Knechtle
Instutute of Primary Care, University of Zurich, Zurich CH-8006, Switzerland

Gema Torres-Luque
Area of Corporal Express, Faculty of Humanities and Science Education, University of Jaen, Jaen 3109, Spain

Andrew J. Galpin, Blake Whitcomb, Leonard D. Wiersma, Jakob Rosengarten, JaredW. Coburn and Daniel A. Judelson
Center for Sport Performance, Department of Kinesiology, California State University, Fullerton, CA 92834, USA

James R. Bagley
Department of Kinesiology, San Francisco State University, San Francisco, CA 94132, USA

Jason B. White, and Margaret T. Jones
Health and Human Performance, George Mason University, Manassas, VA 20110, USA

Trevor P. Dorian
Exercise Science and Sport Studies, Springfield College, Springfield, MA 01109, USA

Matthew H. Sharp and Ryan P. Lowery
Applied Science and Performance Institute, Tampa, FL 33607, USA

Kevin A. Shields and Jacob T. Rauch and Eduardo O. De Souza
Department of Health Sciences and Human Performance, The University of Tampa, Tampa, FL 33606, USA

Shane E. Durkee and Gabriel J. Wilson
Maximum Human Performance, West Caldwell, NJ 07006, USA

Juan Ignacio Ortega, Carlos Evangelio and Sixto González-Víllora
Physical Education Department, University of Castilla-La Mancha, Edificio Fray Luis de León,16071 Cuenca, Spain

Filipe Manuel Clemente
Instituto Politécnico de Viana do Castelo, Escola Superior de Desporto e Lazer, Complexo Desportivo e Lazer Comendador Rui Solheiro—Monte de Prado, 4960-320 Melgaço, Portugal
Instituto de Telecomunicações, Delegação da Covilhã, Instituto Superior Técnico—Torre Norte —Piso 10, Av. Rovisco Pais, 1, 1049-001 Lisboa, Portugal

Fernando Manuel Lourenço Martins
Instituto de Telecomunicações, Delegação da Covilhã, Instituto Superior Técnico—Torre Norte —Piso 10, Av. Rovisco Pais, 1, 1049-001 Lisboa, Portugal
Instituto Politécnico de Coimbra, Escola Superior de Educação, Departamento de Educação, IIA, RoboCorp, ASSERT, Rua Dom João III, 3030-329 Coimbra, Portugal

Anja Rossmeissl, Soraya Lenk, Henner Hanssen, Arno Schmidt-Trucksäss
Division of Sports and Exercise Medicine, Department of Sport, Exercise and Health, University of Basel, Birsstrasse 320 B, Basel 4052, Switzerland

Lars Donath
Division of Movement and Exercise Science, Department of Sport, Exercise and Health, University of Basel, Birsstrasse 320 B, Basel 4052, Switzerland

Juliane Schäfer
Division of Sports and Exercise Medicine, Department of Sport, Exercise and Health, University of Basel, Birsstrasse 320 B, Basel 4052, Switzerland
Basel Institute for Clinical Epidemiology and Biostatistics, University Hospital Basel, Spitalstrasse 12, Basel 4031, Switzerland

Robert Ah Sue and Mark DeBeliso
Department of Physical Education and Human Performance, Southern Utah University, Cedar City,UT 84720, USA

Kent J. Adams
Kinesiology Department California State University Monterey Bay, Seaside, CA 93955, USA

Rahel Bürgi and Eling D. de Bruin
Department of Health Sciences and Technology, Institute of Human Movement Sciences and Sport, ETH Zürich, Leopold-Ruzicka-Weg 4, Zurich 8093, Switzerland

Freya Gassmann and Eike Emrich
Department of Economics and Sociology of Sport, Institute for Sport Science, Saarland University, Campus Gebäude B8 1, Saarbrücken 66123, Germany

Michael Fröhlich
Department of Sports Science, University of Kaiserslautern, Erwin-Schrödinger-Street, Kaiserslautern 67663, Germany

Thai Trinh
Mount Carmel Health Systems, Department of Orthopedics 793 West State Street Columbus, Columbus, OH 43222, USA

Andrew Mundy
Ohio State University Medical Center, Department of Orthopaedics, 410 W 10th Ave, Columbus, OH 43210, USA

Matthew Beran and Kevin Klingele
Nationwide Children's Hospital, Department of Orthopedics, 700 Children's Drive, Ste. A2630, Columbus, OH 43205-2696, USA

Alper Aşçı
Haliç University School of Physical Education and Sport, Istanbul 34330, Turkey

Nicholas P. Linthorne
Department of Life Sciences, Brunel University London, Uxbridge, Middlesex,UB8 3PH, UK

Daniel D. Bingham
Bradford Institute for Health Research, Bradford BD9 6RJ, UK
School of Sport, Exercise and Health Sciences, Loughborough University, Leicestershire LE11 3TU, UK

Paul J. Collings, Gillian Santorelli and Sally E. Barber
Bradford Institute for Health Research, Bradford BD9 6RJ, UK

Stacy A. Clemes and Paula Griffiths
School of Sport, Exercise and Health Sciences, Loughborough University, Leicestershire LE11 3TU, UK

Silvia Costa
Centre for Diet and Activity Research (CEDAR), MRC Epidemiology Unit, University of Cambridge, School of Clinical Medicine, Cambridge CB2 0QQ, UK

Index